S0-AJG-257

Women's Health Today

2000

The Latest Breakthroughs for the Female Body

Maximum Weight Loss, Minimum Effort
Feel-Good Plan to Lose 10, 20, or 30 lbs.

Food, Herbs, and Nutrients
How to Add <u>Years</u> to Your Life

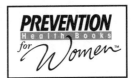

Medicine's Gender Gap
Guide to the Best Care for Women

Disease Defense
• Outsmart Your Genes • Whip Allergies
• Build Bones • Protect Your Breasts

PLUS: Stress Kickers, Intimacy Builders, Beauty Tactics, and More

RODALE

Notice

This book is intended as a reference volume only, not as a medical manual. The information given here is designed to help you make informed decisions about your health. It is
not intended as a substitute for any treatment that may have been prescribed by your doctor. If you suspect that you have a medical problem, we urge you to seek competent medical
help.

Copyright © 2000 by Rodale Inc.
Illustrations copyright © 2000 by Narda Lebo

All rights reserved. No part of this publication may be reproduced or transmitted in any
form or by any means, electronic or mechanical, including photocopying, recording, or any
other information storage and retrieval system, without the written permission of the publisher.

Prevention Health Books for Women is a trademark of Rodale Inc.

Printed in the United States of America on acid-free ∞, recycled paper ♻

The credits for this book begin on page 311.

ISBN 1–57954–240–9 hardcover

2 4 6 8 10 9 7 5 3 1 hardcover

Visit us on the Web at www.rodalebooks.com, or call us toll-free at (800) 848-4735.

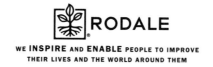

WE **INSPIRE** AND **ENABLE** PEOPLE TO IMPROVE
THEIR LIVES AND THE WORLD AROUND THEM

Women's Health Today 2000 Staff

EDITOR: Jean Rogers

MANAGING EDITOR: Sharon Faelten

CONTRIBUTING WRITERS: Sara Altshul O'Donnell; Marion Asnes; Elizabeth Austin; C. K. Binswanger; Jennifer Cadoff; Rick Chillot; Karen Cicero; Stacey Colino; Deborah Duenes; M. P. Dunleavy; Brooke Eastburn; Julie A. Evans; Allison Fabian; Laura Goldstein; Brian Good; Ginny Graves; Rachel Grumman; Toby Hanlon, Ed.D.; Sarí Harrar; Dalma Heyn; Paula Hunt; Evan Imber-Black, Ph.D.; Donna Jackson; Joely Johnson; Alice Lesch Kelly; Carol Keough; Sherry Weiss Kiser; Sue Landry; Evelyn Leigh; Hallie Levine; Robert Lipsyte; Barbara Loecher; Jenny Lynch; Matt Marion; Linda Marsa; Holly McCord, R.D.; Jeff Meade; Rosie Mestel; Ellen Michaud; Mary Jane Minkin, M.D.; Linda Mooney; Arden Moore; Deborah Moss; Danielle Pergament; Cathy Perlmutter; Maureen Sangiorgio; Jan Sheehan; Dana Silbiger; Stephanie Slon; Nancy F. Smith; Amy Spencer; Michele Stanten; Alice Trevor; Margo Trott; Varro E. Tyler, Sc.D., Ph.D.; Julia VanTine; Zachary Veilleux; Teri Walsh; Densie Webb, R.D., Ph.D.; Lolly Winston; Leslie Yazel; Selene Yeager; Teresa Yeykal

ART DIRECTOR: Darlene Schneck

INTERIOR DESIGNERS: Christopher R. Neyen, Lynn N. Gano

COVER DESIGNERS: Lynn N. Gano, Darlene Schneck

PHOTO EDITOR: James A. Gallucci

ILLUSTRATOR: Narda Lebo

ASSISTANT RESEARCH MANAGER: Shea Zukowski

BOOK PROJECT RESEARCHER AND PERMISSIONS COORDINATOR: Christine Dreisbach

SENIOR COPY EDITOR: Amy K. Kovalski

LAYOUT DESIGNER: Daniel MacBride

ASSOCIATE STUDIO MANAGER: Thomas P. Aczel

MANUFACTURING COORDINATORS: Brenda Miller, Jodi Schaffer, Patrick Smith

Rodale Healthy Living Books

VICE PRESIDENT AND PUBLISHER: Brian Carnahan

VICE PRESIDENT AND EDITORIAL DIRECTOR: Debora T. Yost

EDITORIAL DIRECTOR: Michael Ward

VICE PRESIDENT AND MARKETING DIRECTOR: Karen Arbegast

PRODUCT MARKETING MANAGER: Guy Maake

BOOK MANUFACTURING DIRECTOR: Helen Clogston

MANUFACTURING MANAGERS: Eileen Bauder, Mark Krahforst

RESEARCH MANAGER: Ann Gossy Yermish

COPY MANAGER: Lisa D. Andruscavage

PRODUCTION MANAGER: Robert V. Anderson Jr.

OFFICE MANAGER: Jacqueline Dornblaser

OFFICE STAFF: Suzanne Lynch Holderman, Julie Kehs, Mary Lou Stephen, Catherine E. Strouse

Board of Advisors for *Prevention* Health Books for Women

DIANE L. ADAMS, M.D.
Associate clinical professor and coordinator of the cultural diversity and women's health program at the University of Maryland Eastern Shore in Princess Anne, Maryland

ROSEMARY AGOSTINI, M.D.
Clinical associate professor of orthopedics at the University of Washington and staff physician at the Virginia Mason Sports Medicine Center, both in Seattle

BARBARA D. BARTLIK, M.D.
Clinical assistant professor in the department of psychiatry at Cornell University Medical College in New York City

MARY RUTH BUCHNESS, M.D.
Associate professor of dermatology and medicine at the New York Medical College in Valhalla and chief of dermatology at St. Vincent's Hospital and Medical Center in New York City

TRUDY L. BUSH, PH.D.
Professor of epidemiology and preventive medicine at the University of Maryland School of Medicine at Baltimore and principal investigator for the Heart and Estrogen/Progestin Replacement Study (HERS) and the Postmenopausal Estrogen/Progestin Intervention (PEPI) Safety Follow-Up Study at the Johns Hopkins Women's Research Core in Lutherville, Maryland

LEAH J. DICKSTEIN, M.D.
Professor and associate chairman for academic affairs in the department of psychiatry and behavioral sciences and associate dean for faculty and student advocacy at the University of Louisville School of Medicine in Kentucky and past president of the American Medical Women's Association (AMWA)

JEAN L. FOURCROY, M.D., PH.D.
Past president of the American Medical Women's Association (AMWA) and past president of the National Council on Women's Health in New York City

CLARITA E. HERRERA, M.D.
Clinical instructor in primary care at the New York Medical College in Valhalla and associate attending physician at Lenox Hill Hospital in New York City

JoAnn E. Manson, M.D., Dr.P.H.

Associate professor of medicine at Harvard Medical School and co-director of women's health at Brigham and Women's Hospital in Boston

Mary Lake Polan, M.D., Ph.D.

Professor and chairman of the department of gynecology and obstetrics at Stanford University School of Medicine

Elizabeth Lee Vliet, M.D.

Clinical associate professor in the department of family and community medicine at the University of Arizona College of Medicine and founder and medical director of HER Place: Health Enhancement and Renewal for Women, both in Tucson

Lila Amdurska Wallis, M.D., M.A.C.P.

Clinical professor of medicine at Cornell University Medical College in New York City, past president of the American Medical Women's Association (AMWA), founding president of the National Council on Women's Health, director of continuing medical education programs for physicians, and master and laureate of the American College of Physicians

Carla Wolper, R.D.

Nutritionist and clinical coordinator at the Obesity Research Center at St. Luke's/Roosevelt Hospital Center in New York City and nutritionist at the Center for Women's Health at Columbia-Presbyterian Eastside in New York City

Contents

part one

Medicine's Gender Gap

part two

Health News You Can Use

part three

Disease Defense

Healing with Food, Herbs, and Nutrition

Maximum Weight Loss with Minimum Effort

Introduction

As this book goes to print, I have just returned from a conference on women's health and gender-based medicine—an annual event. Research in gender-based medicine took off in 1992, with the funding of the Women's Health Initiative. Until then, women had been largely excluded from medical research, and when they were included, data often were not analyzed to look for gender differences.

Gender-based medicine is picking up steam and will continue into the next century, not only to "catch up" with male-biased research but also to address the changing needs of women as they continue to outlive men.

Some of the most dramatic male-female differences involve heart disease. For example, women who've had a heart attack are less likely to be given aspirin, even though taking aspirin improves the odds of survival. But doctors are now looking at gender differences across the board—diabetes, cancer, sleep disorders, overweight, pain tolerance, and so forth. My notebook is filled with examples of medical conditions that manifest themselves differently in women and require different treatments. So now more than ever, physicians realize they need to focus on gender differences when diagnosing and treating disease.

"'One-size-fits-all' health care is no longer appropriate," says Wanda Jones, Dr.P.H., deputy assistant secretary for health at the U.S. Department of Health and Human Services. "Aside from the biological difference, there is a culture around being a woman that's different from being a man. So the more we learn, and the more we factor this into our decisions, the better the outcome."

In order to be sure you're getting the best medical care possible, you, too, need to know about "his and hers" health differences. To help you in your efforts, this book functions as a snapshot of current reports on gender-based medicine—news you can use to make smart decisions. And as you'll see, both men and women benefit from gender-based research. For example, doctors now realize that both men and women benefit from taking alendronate sodium (Fosamax), approved for the treatment of osteoporosis in women.

You wouldn't think of buying shoes designed for men if they didn't fit. This book will help you choose health care treatments that best fit you as a woman.

Sharon Faelten

Sharon Faelten
Managing Editor
Prevention Health Books for Women

part one

Medicine's Gender Gap

1

His and Her Health

Is There a Women's Health Center in Your Future?

If there isn't a women's health center in your future, there should be! "A primary-care women's health center is able to offer a comprehensive set of services specifically tailored to women," says Carol Weisman, Ph.D., professor of health management and policy at the University of Michigan School of Public Health in Ann Arbor. "A woman can attend a women's health center and receive all of her basic health-care services in one place—and in a coordinated fashion," says Dr. Weisman, who is also on the board of directors at the Jacobs Institute of Women's Health in Washington, D.C. "If she's seeing an individual physician, who can offer certain services but not others, nobody's going to be coordinating her overall care over time."

According to Dr. Weisman, who published a survey of women's health centers, these centers offer the following services, all under one roof.

❖ Basic preventive services that target the entire body, such as annual physicals and blood pressure tests
❖ Flu shots
❖ Smoking cessation
❖ Alternative treatments
❖ Menopausal counseling
❖ Mental health services
❖ Cancer screenings, such as colorectal exams
❖ Cholesterol tests
❖ Diagnosis and treatment of menstrual problems
❖ Pelvic exams and Pap tests
❖ Family planning services
❖ Prenatal care
❖ Mammography

"These centers pull together physicians from different specialties, including non-physician providers, and coordinate that care for the total woman," says Dr. Weisman. "For example, there are a wide variety of options out there for women dealing with the symptoms of menopause. There is also a great deal of uncertainty about what the most effective options are. A lot of it depends on the individual woman's situation and risk factors. A women-centered approach to care is going to take those into account."

Regarding heart disease, the top killer of women, women's health centers focus on preventing the disease and educating women about their risk. "These centers are going to be tuned into the fact that women may not know their risk for heart disease. Women may not understand what they can do to prevent it. And unlike other physicians who may not understand that heart disease is a major problem for women, those at a center are going to pay attention to it," says Dr. Weisman.

How can you locate a primary-care women's health center near you? Contact local hospitals, or call (800) 994-WOMAN (994-9662). It's the phone number for the National Women's Health Information Center, which is sponsored by the U.S. Public Health Service's Office on Women's Health. The operator can refer you to one of the 18 federally designated National Centers of Excellence in Women's Health located across the country. You can also check out their Web site at www.4woman.gov.

When you locate a center, ask if they are a comprehensive primary-care women's health center. That means they offer a wide variety of services targeting the entire body, not just reproductive services. It's also a good idea to ask if their physicians are board-certified.

1

Why We Need Gender-Specific Medicine

Oh, how it can hurt to have a wisdom tooth pulled, but that prescription the dentist gave you will help ease the throbbing. Right?

It depends.

If you're a woman, the medication could do wonders. If you're a man, you might have to live with the pain.

Then again, if you're a man, it might not hurt as much in the first place.

Researchers are uncovering surprising differences between men and women that could change the ways doctors think about treating patients. Male-female variations occur in metabolism, in responses to medication, in the way organs such as the brain and liver operate, and in the way certain diseases progress.

The growing list is calling into question medicine's practice of treating diseases in men and women the same way. The future, some experts say, involves gender-specific medicine—basing patients' treatment not only on their medical conditions but also on their sex.

"The landscape is so sparse in terms of what we know about the differences between men and women that our first effort is going to be to fill in the gaps," says Marianne Legato, M.D., professor of clinical medicine at Columbia University College of Physicians and Surgeons in New York City. In 1997, she formed the Partnership for Women's Health at Columbia to encourage more research in the expanding world of gender variations.

Aside from obvious reproductive differences, physicians have tended to treat men and women as if they were biologically the same. That's partly because past research studies have concentrated on men.

So Many Unrecognized Differences

Only in recent years, as studies increasingly included women and minorities, have previously unrecognized differences begun to emerge.

"We would extrapolate from the 180-pound man to everyone else, and I mean everyone else," says Judith H. LaRosa, R.N., Ph.D., chair and professor in the department of community health sciences at Tulane University's School of Public Health and Tropical Medicine in New Orleans.

Don't Treat Her like a Man!

For years, doctors have treated diseases the same way in male and female patients. Yet physiological differences exist between the two sexes that make gender-specific medicine a compelling new idea. Here are just a few of the medically significant ways in which men and women differ.

❖ Female brains have more neurons (nerve cells) than male brains.

❖ Women have a higher heart rate than men, even during sleep.

❖ Women wake up significantly faster from anesthesia than men.

❖ Men and women use their brains differently for the same tasks, including language, math, and logic tasks. One example: Men doing rhyming exercises mainly use the left brain; women use both sides of the brain.

❖ Cluster headaches are at least four times more common in men.

❖ Aspirin reduces the risk of stroke in men—but not in women—with high blood pressure.

❖ Men are less susceptible to certain carcinogens, such as those in tobacco smoke.

❖ High blood pressure is two to three times more common in men than women.

❖ Men have a better survival rate after a first heart attack than women: 39 percent of women versus 31 percent of men die in the first year following a heart attack.

HEALTH FLASH

"As research has emerged, all of a sudden people are slapping their heads and the lights are going on and people are saying, 'Wait a minute. There *are* differences,'" says Dr. LaRosa, former deputy director of the federal Office of Research in Women's Health.

In one study, women were found to wake up almost twice as fast from anesthesia as men. In another, an experimental heart drug worked significantly better for women.

Women get heart disease at later ages and less often than men. But when they do, they survive at lower rates in the year following a first heart attack.

Men experience clinical depression at far lower rates than women, but when they do, they respond better to antidepressant medications.

Researchers also have cataloged some basic biological differences. Women have more glucose in their saliva, women's heart rates are higher—even during sleep—and men have fewer nerve cells in their brains.

Dr. Legato spent 6 months combing medical literature to compile what scientists already knew about differences between the sexes.

"I was amazed at the differences," she says. "Everybody assumes that men and women are alike enough that the differences are unimportant or it's not necessary to take them into account."

Dr. Legato doesn't know—and neither does anyone else—just how important these gender variations are. Researchers have only begun to explore their implications for the treatment and prevention of disease. Experts suspect, however, that investigating the variations they have been finding could lead to a host of new medical therapies.

Estrogen for Men?

Heart researchers investigating why men are susceptible to heart disease at earlier ages than women discovered that the female hormone estrogen helps protect against heart disease. Armed with that knowledge, researchers are studying the possibility of giving men small doses of estrogen.

"The new data are so compelling that several of my male colleagues are monitoring their own estrogen levels," Dr. Legato says. Thirty years ago, researchers abandoned attempts to give men estrogen because a few men died from excessive doses.

"Now, because of studying women, we understand more about how to supply the hormone," Dr. Legato says.

Dr. Legato and a handful of others around the country who are calling attention to this issue hope to spur researchers to study other diseases the same way.

"If we begin to understand why men are less susceptible than women to osteoporosis, we may begin to understand important new therapeutic approaches to women," says John Bilezikian, M.D., professor of medicine, pharmacology, and endocrinology at Columbia.

It was Florence Haseltine, founder and president of the Society for the Advancement of Women's Health Research, who coined the term *gender-based biology*. Dr. Legato followed her lead in founding the Columbia partnership and coining the term *gender-based medicine*.

Some in the field of women's health have been puzzled by their efforts, claiming gender-based medicine is just new packaging for old ideas. For example, Vivian Pinn, M.D., who heads the Office of Research in Women's Health under the National Institutes of Health, says her office has been studying differences between women's health and men's health since it was formed in 1990.

But Haseltine and Dr. Legato say gender-based medicine reaches beyond the idea of women's health, to which so much attention has been paid in the past decade. They say too much of women's health has focused on issues unique to women, such as reproduction and breast cancer, or on diseases much more common in women, such as osteoporosis.

"We are trying to capture the concept that if there is a difference between the genders, you can learn something from it," Haseltine says.

"One of the difficulties we had with women's health was that it was 'only women's health,'" Haseltine says. "Actually, women's health should not be isolated. This is a basic attempt to get back to the cellular differences."

The Goal: Improving Health in Both Sexes

Rather than focusing on women, the study of gender differences extends to all aspects of human biology and holds the promise of improving the health of both sexes, says Dr. LaRosa, who worked with Dr. Pinn at the Office of Research in Women's Health.

"This is not just a feminist diatribe," Dr. LaRosa says. "These scientists are saying, 'Look at these differences. Just sheer intellectual curiosity would drive you to want the answers.'"

Because women tended to be left out of clinical trials and research in the past, they may end up benefiting the most from the study of gender differences. But both sexes stand to gain from a deeper understanding of the way male bodies and female bodies function.

"Gender-specific information works both ways," Dr. Legato notes. "If we understand the reasons why women live longer, we can use the information to close the gap and prolong the life span for both sexes.

"For the first time," Dr. Legato says, "we can justify that the study of women is not just a matter of political correctness and social justice. In fact, it makes practical sense."

2

Four Important Ways Women's Health Differs from Men's

When it comes to health, gender does make a difference. In the past, medical researchers conducted studies mostly on men, then simply applied their findings to women. Now, finally, they've begun to study women separately, and an avalanche of intriguing new findings, analyzed by the Society for the Advancement of Women's Health Research, illuminates some marked dissimilarities. Based on these facts, these are the steps you should take to safeguard your health.

Women Are More Vulnerable to Sexual Disease

It's unfair but true: Unprotected sex is much more hazardous to women than men. Women are twice as likely to contract a sexually transmitted disease (STD), such as chlamydia, hepatitis, or gonorrhea, and 10 to 20 times more likely to contract HIV from an infected partner.

"Women have cells on their cervices and vaginal walls that are especially susceptible to invasion by sexually transmitted organisms," explains Kata Chillag, Ph.D., a researcher with the Centers for Disease Control and Prevention's National Center for STD Prevention. "Plus, intercourse can sometimes cause tears and other abrasions in the vagina that make women even more vulnerable."

Women Don't Handle Alcohol as Well

On average, men really *can* tolerate more alcohol than women. Women produce much less of the gastric enzyme that breaks down ethanol in the stomach. Consequently, they absorb almost twice as much alcohol into their bloodstreams as men. And since women's bodies are composed of less water than men's, the alcohol circulation in their blood is less diluted. As a result, women may suffer from alcohol-related heart damage and liver diseases, such as cirrhosis, at lower levels of alcohol consumption than men. Limit your intake accordingly.

Medications Take a Bigger Toll on Women

According to a report from the Society, recent research reveals enormous gender variations in the way women's bodies metabolize certain drugs. In some instances, women may need less medication than men do to achieve the desired effect. Users of oral contraceptives, for instance, are particularly susceptible to the effects of the anti-anxiety drug Xanax. Moreover, "for some drugs, there are far greater risks of serious side effects for women than there are for men," says Raymond Woosley, M.D., Ph.D., chair of the department of pharmacology at Georgetown University Medical School in Washington, D.C.

Several medications can trigger a certain kind of arrhythmia, or irregular heartbeat, in some women, an effect not found in men. These include the antibiotic erythromycin (commonly used to treat chlamydia and upper respiratory ills), the antidepressants Elavil and Ludiomil, and antihistamines such as Seldane and Hismanal. While rarely fatal, irregular heartbeat can sometimes lead to a sudden loss of consciousness. "Women need to watch their responses to medicine carefully," says Dr. Woosley. "At the slightest sign of a bad reaction—heart palpitations, tremors, or dizziness—discontinue the medication until you talk to your doctor."

Smoking Has Worse Consequences for Women

Some women are particularly attracted to smoking because they hope it will help with weight control, but tobacco is a deadly diet aid. That's because women smokers are 20 to 70 percent more likely to develop lung cancer than men smokers, according to a study published in the *Journal of the National Cancer Institute*.

At this point, experts don't know why women appear to be more susceptible to tobacco carcinogens, says Marc Manley, M.D., chief of the tobacco control research branch of the National Cancer Institute. "But the bottom line is that women simply should not smoke."

3 Don't Take Your Medicine like a Man

The gender gap in medicine works both ways. The sexes aren't just treated differently by the medical profession; they also react differently to disease—even the same illness. New York Times *columnist Robert Lipsyte found out this painful truth when both he and his wife were diagnosed with cancer. "As patients, men are impatient, or uneasy, or both," he says. "They need to get a grip, like women." Here's his story.*

Doctors once loved me, or would have if I had gone to them more often. Fix me quick, sawbones, I would say, there's a big land out there to tame and my horse is double-parked. I was heroic and stoic, the stereotypical male health-care consumer. I paid on the way out.

It took 20 years of being a cancer patient and a caregiver, but I think I am on my way to becoming the stereotypical female health consumer, assertive and needy. Glenn E. Good, Ph.D., a psychologist at the University of Missouri, thinks my psychic sex change could add years to my life.

"Of course, you'll be terrible for managed care," he says, "demanding information and taking time to learn about treatment options and side effects."

That there is a vast difference between the way men and women approach their health care is not exactly news. There are statistics: Male patients account for only 40 percent of physicians' visits, according to Dr. Good, and during the last 33 years there have been 4,393 entries in Medline (an Internet database of health information) for "women's health" compared with 94 for "men's health." In addition, a recent nationwide telephone poll conducted by CNN and *Men's Health* magazine found that while 76 percent of American women have had a health exam in the last 12 months, only 60 percent of men have had the same.

Women Are Savvier Medical Consumers

In addition to the statistics, there are theories. For example, there's the theory that men are afraid of appearing dependent and vulnerable, while women, traditionally caregivers for children and the elderly, are savvier medical consumers.

"A woman finds out she has breast cancer because she self-examined or had a mammogram," says Paul Russo, M.D., a urological surgeon at the Memorial Sloan-Kettering Cancer Center in New York City. "She was proactive from the start. Women have an early conditioning toward health; they went to gynecologists, women's doctors. There is no comparable men's doctor."

My medical education began in 1978, when a suburban urologist told me that I probably had testicular cancer. Catatonic, I missed his excitement at dealing with the kind of case he usually only reads about. Thankfully, my wife had pushed her way into the room. She was used to asking questions for the kids.

"How many of these do you do a year?" she asked.

"Two or three," he said.

That was still fine with me. Passively, I signed up for an operation in his hospital. I told Marjorie that it was probably nothing, that I wanted to be close to home, that I didn't want to make a big deal of all this. Back home, I sat numbly until Marjorie nagged me into making an appointment at Sloan-Kettering. Still, I was ready to follow the next alpha male who told me what to do. When the jock surgeon cheerily pronounced my lump "suspicious," I felt a certain thrill at being included in this top doc's excellent adventure.

For 3 weeks, I lived in a company of men as bonded as my old Army basic training squad. We were as intimate and tender with each other as I think girlfriends are, and we mocked the doctors and nurses behind their backs.

But even then, we did not ask the questions about prognosis, treatment, side effects, and sexuality that we needed answered to make informed decisions. We might wear sports gear over our open-ended hospital gowns, but any flash of independence evaporated when the arrogant parade of white coats appeared to poke and pontificate over our heads.

Men Often Play the "Good Patient"

Susan Alfano, a nurse who has worked both in the breast and urology services at Sloan-Kettering, said that men "often shortchange themselves by being our version of the 'good patient'—quiet, more willing to give up control." This makes them easier to take care of, she says, but does not necessarily serve them well.

Through 2 years of chemotherapy, I feigned control by imagining that this was some kind of advanced-placement test. If I survived, I would be tougher than tumors. Week after week, I sat passively in the waiting rooms of Sloan-Kettering, surrounded by other men who had obviously concocted their own fantasies. Men glanced at their watches, annoyed that their trains had been late. Men riffled importantly through spreadsheets, briefs, stock tables, racetrack results, and auto ads in this extension of their offices. Others stared down highways that stretched for years. We rarely acknowledged one another because none of us were quite there.

By contrast, women patients and caregivers buzzed around reception desks and nurses' stations to be sure appointments had not been forgotten. They buttonholed doctors scurrying from room to room. They never stopped talking among themselves, picking up strangers and making them confidantes. Marjorie gathered and shared information about doctors, treatments, nearby restaurants, and parking garages.

She was also asking questions that sometimes made the doctors uncomfortable because they didn't know the answers. By chemo's end, I had grown enough not to respond man-to-man when the doctors rolled their eyes at me after one of Marjorie's sharp queries.

Then she developed cancer and it was a new ball game.

Caregiver: Not Just "Women's Work"

I became a caregiver. While that may still be seen as a stereotypical female role (especially for "the Daughter"), I began to see it as a stereotypical role for a grown-up. Also, it was easier asking questions for my wife than for myself because I could imagine myself in the role of protector instead of scaredy-cat.

"Men and women have similar life processes and needs," says Martin Miner, M.D., a family-practice physician in Swansea, Massachusetts, who has conducted men's-health research for drug companies. "But, typically, as in your case, it took a dramatic event, an illness, a body change, to open up to the process of articulating fears and confronting them."

Men, Dr. Miner points out, are often under pressure to be providers for their families, which includes hiding their anxieties so as not to alarm their wives and children. "Men feel they are not allowed to manifest illness unless it's overt," he says. "One reason men die 7.2 years earlier than women is because of the length of time before they go for treatment. And even if they survive, their quality of life tends to be less than a woman's."

By the 1990s, when Marjorie and I each had second rounds with cancer, the patient had become the health-care consumer, a citizen with rights, a person whose illness was not a punishment, a customer who should be allowed to make informed decisions.

This concept did not come from the powerful white men who managed the system but from those traditionally marginalized by medicine—male homosexuals, Black and Hispanic intravenous drug users, and women. The gallantry and political energy of AIDS and breast cancer groups certainly informed me when I was diagnosed with cancer again.

My old surgeon had retired, and I didn't like his replacement. A few years earlier, I might have left the hospital in a huff or just passively grumbled and taken it like a man. Now, I demanded a choice, which was no simple matter but eventually brought me to the open and accessible Dr. Russo.

Finally, Changes in Male Attitudes

"I think we're beginning to see some changes in male attitudes," Dr. Russo says. "When you have a General Schwarzkopf ordering men to get prostate exams and a Michael Milken looking to conquer health problems the way he conquered junk bonds, you have the beginnings of a movement. But can they raise awareness the way women did for breast cancer?"

Nurse Alfano sees any change complicated by basic male-female relationships: Men are used to being cared for by women, who are often economically dependent on a man's good health. "When a male patient starts to have difficulty emotionally after discharge, the phone call I get is usually from his wife or daughter," she says. "She'll ask me to give him a pep talk without letting him know she called. It often works. This is what's interesting to me: I'm not sure if the reason it works is because I am a health-care worker or because I am a woman."

This sort of conspiracy of women is seen by some pragmatists as the best way to get men healthier—appeal to wives and daughters to bring men in for checkups and follow-ups by expressing their concern or by downright nagging.

Conversely, psychologist Dr. Good thinks that men can be brought into the medical tent by language changes. Because the "care" in health care sounds feminine, he writes, phrases like "tune-ups" and "executive coaching" and "a chance to enhance optimal functioning" might help.

Both scenarios seem to have the drawback of playing the gender card without really changing the system or sensibility.

For Men, Good Health = Great Sex

Dr. Miner thinks sex is the hook, since most men seem to equate good health with sexual functioning. That view is supported by the covers of popular health magazines, which usually promote articles on sexual performance (and on tightening the abdominals to impress dates so that one gets a chance to perform). Even the *Harvard Men's Health Watch*, a serious newsletter, seems to publish a prostate story in every issue.

Dr. Miner wants to broaden men's definition of sexual health to include intimacy, feelings, and the mind-body connection; women, he noted, have always used these as aids to wellness and healing. He also thinks that there will be a boom in men's health as soon as the pharmaceutical companies figure out how to exploit the market beyond drugs like Viagra.

Now that gives me anxiety I can't hide. The merchandisers of men's drugs, which include cars and beer sold as sex aids, know our insecurities and our twisted self-images all too well. Will they help us deal with the underpublicized problems of male depression and suicide, or will they keep us running with the cash bulls of natural baldness and relaxed stomach muscles?

Or, with old generals barking orders and old financiers pulling strings, will men enter a vast new frontier where we will confront our physical and psychological fears, get healthier, and live longer? When will we learn to take our medicine like a woman?

"You keep saying that," Dr. Good complains. "Why do you call the results of your revelations becoming more 'female'? Why not that you're finally becoming a good patient?"

part two

Health News You Can Use

His and Her
Health

T.S. Eliot once wrote, "Men live by forgetting—women live on memo-ries." Today, modern science shows that the differences between the sexes don't stop there. According to a recent study by the Society for the Advancement of Women's Health Research, there are a number of major differences in the way men and women are affected by disease or med-ical treatments. At the top of the list are the country's leading killers—heart disease and cancer.

"Heart disease is more lethal in women than it is in men," notes Trudy Bush, D.Ph., Ph.D., professor of epidemiology and preventive medicine at the University of Maryland School of Medicine in Baltimore. "Women are more likely than men to die with their first heart attack. If they do sur-vive it, they are also more likely to have a second heart attack within a year of the first."

During treatment, angioplasty and bypass surgery aren't as successful in women as they are in men. "Doctors suspect this is because women's hearts are smaller than men's, with smaller vessels," says Dr. Bush. "Women's hospital stays are even longer. There are usually more complications.

"Another major problem is that many women associate heart disease with their husbands," Dr. Bush continues. "Women need to start thinking about it in terms of themselves." The first step is to recognize the early warning signs of a heart attack and get to the hospital emergency room immediately. Those signs are:

❖ Sudden pressure, fullness, squeezing, or pain in the center of your chest that lasts more than a few minutes or that goes away and comes back

❖ Pain that radiates from the center of your chest to your shoulders, neck, or arms

❖ Chest discomfort with lightheadedness, fainting, sweating, nausea, or shortness of breath

In addition to heart disease, there are also differences between the sexes regarding cancer. "We currently have an epidemic of lung cancer in women," says Dr. Bush. "We are all concerned about breast cancer, but more women die each year of lung cancer. In men, lung cancer rates have stopped increasing. But in women, the rate is increasing tremendously. Women need to stop smoking, as men have."

According to Dr. Bush, many women don't quit because they fear they will gain weight. We are much more concerned with body image than men—and it's that attitude that's killing us. "The fact is that if they stop smoking, exercise regularly, and eat a low-fat, well-varied diet, these women will not gain weight," she says.

Another misconception women have is in regard to colon cancer. "It's the third leading cancer killer of both men and women," notes Dr. Bush. "But unlike men, women don't seem to think they are at risk for it." The American Cancer Society recommends that at age 50, both men and women should have a fecal occult blood test and either a flexible sigmoidoscopy or a colonoscopy.

4

Dangerous Symptoms Your Doctor May Miss

Women are three times more likely than men to have their physical problems diagnosed as mental ills. Don't let this happen to you. Here's how to get the right diagnosis and treatment.

Medical student Vicki Ratner was rushing to the bathroom dozens of times a day and frequently at night. She could barely work. She couldn't sleep. And she felt constant pressure and pain in her lower abdomen. Her pelvis felt like it was on fire.

But when Ratner went to her doctor, standard urine cultures showed nothing wrong. The problem wasn't in her bladder, said her doctor. It was in her head.

Ratner, today a 48-year-old orthopedic surgeon in San Jose, California, ended up visiting 14 doctors before figuring out through her own research that she had interstitial cystitis (IC). A urologist later confirmed this diagnosis. A little-studied illness, IC is a painful inflammatory condition of the bladder that probably occurs when urine seeps through a weakened section of the bladder's protective lining and settles within the bladder wall.

Although she's not cured, today Dr. Ratner is doing well with treatment. But what happened to her is still far from uncommon. In fact, if you're a woman, no matter where your particular medical problem may be—bladder, thyroid, even your heart—study after study shows that your doctor is often likely to tell you "it's all in your head."

This is a potentially dangerous situation. Along with IC, there are several

other physical conditions that are often misdiagnosed in women as emo█
They include a lazy or overactive thyroid and a frighteningly rapid heartb█
(Heart disease in women is also still being misdiagnosed.) Here's what the e█
perts say you should do if misdiagnosis happens to you.

Interstitial Cystitis: An Irritated Bladder

An estimated 450,000 Americans, 90 percent of them women, have IC, says Dr. Ratner. But because many more remain undiagnosed, closer to 1.5 million are affected. Forty is the average age of onset.

Unfortunately, many people suffer for years without a proper diagnosis, in part because many doctors refuse to believe IC exists. "We still get letters from patients whose doctors tell them there's nothing wrong and send them to psychiatrists," says Dr. Ratner, who started the Interstitial Cystitis Association (ICA) after her own frustrating experience. "In the last two months, we've received three separate letters about young women in their forties who had been in severe pain from interstitial cystitis. The pain wasn't being adequately treated. With no end to their pain in sight, all three killed themselves."

The diagnosis: Part of the problem in diagnosing IC may be that standard urine cultures won't detect the condition. A doctor tests your urine, finds out it's normal, then tells you there's nothing wrong.

If your problem is persistent, your doctor should take a closer look. The only way to do that is to perform an invasive outpatient procedure called a hydrodistention and cystoscopy.

The procedure, which should be performed by a urologist, requires general anesthesia. A thin tube equipped with a miniature camera is inserted through your urethra, the opening that allows urine to flow from your bladder. Your bladder is filled with water and then, with the camera, the doctor looks for tiny blood spots on the bladder wall, explains Dr. Ratner. While the procedure is invasive, it may not only reveal IC but also temporarily relieve the pain by stretching the bladder wall and breaking up scar tissue.

The solution: Though there's no cure, the vast majority of women find that the following strategies—either alone or in combination—bring relief.

Avoid acidic foods and beverages as well as alcoholic, caffeinated, and carbonated beverages. A survey by the ICA found that 50 percent of those with IC report their pain is increased by these types of foods and beverages. Steering clear of them can sometimes provide dramatic relief, says Dr. Ratner.

Consider medication. Talk to your doctor about Elmiron (pentosan polysulfate sodium), a new drug that may help repair a damaged bladder lining. Studies show that 38 percent of patients taking Elmiron for 3 months had improvement in their symptoms. Other medications that may bring relief are anti-inflammatories, antispasmodics, antihistamines (hydroxyzine), and tri-

ssants (amitriptyline), which are known to relax muscles and ...es of pain. If oral medication doesn't work, you may want to ...octor about an office procedure that places a solution of di-...DMSO), a drug that reduces pain and inflammation, directly through a catheter. The over-the-counter oral and topical ...on't work.

...re information, contact ICA at (800) HELP-ICA (435-7422) or visit their Web site at www.ichelp.org.

Thyroid Problems: A System-Wide Screwup

A couple of years ago, Los Angeles screenwriter Susan Shepard felt really run-down. "It was as though I couldn't wake up," says Shepard. "My thinking was fuzzy. My vision was off. I went to the eye doctor for a new eyeglass prescription—and had to go back six times because my eyesight kept fluctuating." Plus, her hair thinned, her skin got dry, and her periods became erratic. She thought it was the start of menopause. It wasn't. But what was it?

Her naturopath couldn't figure it out. Neither could her herbalist, her M.D., or her gynecologist, who "concluded I was just stressed," says Shepard. An earache that sent her to an ear, nose, and throat specialist turned out to be fortuitous. The slight lump he spotted in her neck made him check her thyroid, a bow tie–shaped gland at the base of the throat that regulates metabolism.

The diagnosis: A simple test revealed that Shepard had hypothyroidism (often called underactive thyroid). Low levels of the hormone produced by the thyroid—thyroxin—caused her symptoms. Hypothyroidism affects mainly women, although it's not known why. In fact, 1 in 20 women, mostly in their thirties and beyond, have some kind of thyroid disorder, says Jack Baskin, M.D., past president of the American Association of Clinical Endocrinologists and director of the Florida Thyroid and Endocrine Clinic in Orlando.

One reason hypothyroidism and its opposite disorder, hyperthyroidism (an overactive thyroid), are often misdiagnosed is that they can both cause emotional problems. Mood swings, mild depression, and decreased concentration are characteristic of underactive thyroid. People with an overactive thyroid often suffer with an agitated and nervous form of depression. In fact, Dr. Baskin's research suggests that many people treated for depression, including those taking medication for it, actually have an unrecognized thyroid problem.

Left untreated, an underactive thyroid disorder can raise your cholesterol, increasing your risk of heart disease. An overactive thyroid can lead to heart problems and osteoporosis.

Other symptoms of underactive thyroid can include fatigue, dry hair, bloating, infertility, miscarriage, sore muscles, painful joints, muscle cramps, and ab-

H
E
A
L
T
H

F
L
A
S
H

How to Get the Right Diagnosis

What do you do when troubling symptoms are dismissed by a doctor?

First, trust your instincts, says Vicki Ratner, M.D., an orthopedic surgeon in San Jose, California, who started the Interstitial Cystitis Association after her own long search for diagnosis and treatment of agonizing bladder pain. "If you think something is wrong, there is."

The next step is to get a health professional on your side. Here are some tips offered by the experts.

Give your doctor all the facts. "Don't go to the doctor saying, 'Oh, I feel terrible!'" says internist Marianne Legato, M.D., who directs the Partnership for Women's Health at Columbia University College of Physicians and Surgeons in New York City. Be specific about what's happening to you and when and where you experience symptoms. Describe exactly how they feel and what makes the symptoms appear or go away.

Do your homework. Check out your symptoms in medical dictionaries or encyclopedias at your local library. Or turn to Web sites from top medical centers such as the Mayo Clinic (www.mayohealth.org) or Johns Hopkins (www.intelihealth.com). If you find a condition that seems to match your symptoms, ask your doctor point-blank: "Can this be the problem?" Then ask him to justify the answer: "Yes, but how do you know?"

Show your doctor in print. Copy the information that seems to describe what you have and hand it to your doctor, recommends Dr. Ratner. Holding it in his hand will make a difference.

Be insistent and persistent. "The squeaky wheel does get the grease," says endocrinologist Jack Baskin, M.D., past president of the American Association of Clinical Endocrinologists and director of the Florida Thyroid and Endocrine Clinic in Orlando. "And patients who squawk and holler get the most done."

dominal pain. Those with overactive thyroid may experience restlessness, insomnia, heat intolerance, and irritability.

The solution: If any of these symptoms sound familiar, call your family doctor and ask him to set up a blood test called a TSH, advises Dr. Baskin. Be sure to ask for it by name, because not all doctors have heard of it. (Or in today's cost-cutting medical climate, they may be under pressure to save money by using an older, cheaper, and much less accurate test, called the T4.)

If a TSH test reveals an underactive thyroid, adds Dr. Baskin, treatment is easy: a daily thyroid pill to boost your thyroid level back to normal. If the test shows an overactive thyroid, the most common treatment is a one-time radioiodine pill, which is extremely safe.

PSVT: A Heart Gone Haywire

You're relaxed. You're happy. Maybe you're watching a movie or talking to friends. Suddenly, your heart is pounding like it's about to jump out of your body. In seconds, you feel faint, you can't catch your breath, and your chest hurts. You fear you're having a heart attack. But it's soon over. And by the time you reach a doctor, she can't find a thing wrong.

Paroxysmal supraventricular tachycardia—or PSVT—is the mouthful that describes a particular kind of irregular heartbeat that affects more than half a million Americans. It strikes mostly women: some every day, others every couple of years.

Unfortunately, the problem is frequently misdiagnosed, especially in women. Two years ago, cardiac electrophysiologist Michael H. Lehmann, M.D., and his former colleagues at Wayne State University in Detroit interviewed 107 patients with PSVT and found that only 45 percent had been correctly diagnosed at their first physician visit.

"We were amazed to learn what tortured paths many of these patients had taken," says Dr. Lehmann, who is currently clinical professor of medicine at the University of Michigan in Ann Arbor. The PSVT patients were mislabeled with all kinds of diagnoses, from menopause to caffeine jitters. More than half were told their symptoms were due to panic disorder, anxiety, or stress. Further, women were more than twice as likely as men to be told they had a psychiatric problem.

The diagnosis: A PSVT attack can last a few seconds or a half-hour, says Dr. Lehmann. It's triggered by an abnormality in the electrical impulses that power the heart. Instead of firing in an orderly fashion—upper chamber first, then the lower—cascading electrical impulses chase each other up and down the heart. This speeds up the heart and prevents it from filling and pumping adequately. The cycle may abruptly stop on its own or require intravenous medication to restore the normal rhythm.

It's basically an anatomical problem. "People who have PSVT are born with an extra fiber connection between the upper and lower chambers of their hearts," says Dr. Lehmann. "When conditions are right, such as when what's called a premature or 'trigger' heartbeat occurs, an electrical impulse can go down one pathway and up the other. In a normal heart, that could not occur."

It took roughly 3 years for the men and women in his study to get the right diagnosis, says Dr. Lehmann. Panic disorder may have been the most logical of all the wrong guesses their doctors made. Its symptoms are virtually identical to those of PSVT: palpitations, dizziness, shortness of breath, sweating, chest pain, flushing, numbness, nausea, choking, fear of dying, and fear of going crazy. That doesn't explain, however, why women were more frequently misdiagnosed with the psychiatric disorder, raising the possibility of gender bias among physicians. (Some of these symptoms also mimic those of heart attack.)

The solution: If you experience unexplained attacks of rapid heartbeat, have a complete cardiac exam and then follow it with an electrocardiogram from a loop recorder–type of event monitor.

An event monitor consists of a small pagerlike box worn on the waist, connected by wires to a couple of adhesive pads on the chest. It's worn all the time—except while showering.

When you experience an episode of rapid heartbeat, you press a button and the device then permanently records on a memory "loop" your heart rhythms for the minute or so before and after you press it. The monitor is then hooked up to a telephone, and the information is transmitted to a doctor. With those data in hand, the doctor can clearly see whether PSVT is the problem or not.

The device that usually doesn't detect PSVT, yet continues to be prescribed by many doctors, is something called a Holter monitor. This device records the heart's rhythm over a 24-hour period. "Unless you're having one or more episodes of PVST that day—which most people don't have—the Holter monitor won't find anything," says Dr. Lehmann.

Three PSVT options: If PSVT is diagnosed, says Dr. Lehmann, you have three options: Learn to live with it, which may mean trips to the emergency room as needed; treat it with medication; or have a surgery to correct it.

Since PSVT is almost never life-threatening, you need treatment only if it causes severe symptoms such as fainting or if it significantly affects the quality of your life, says Dr. Lehmann. Or you may need treatment if you're in a profession where safety is an issue, such as an airline pilot or bus driver. Your doctor can prescribe medications such as beta-blockers or calcium channel blockers.

You can have a procedure that destroys the heart fiber causing the problem. Electrophysiologic study and ablation are done under local anesthesia with sedation. In this outpatient procedure, your doctor passes flexible, thin wires through veins in the groin or neck to the heart. They record your heart's electrical activity and permit your doctor to electrically trigger PSVT. The recorded signals reveal where the troublemaking extra fiber is. Then your doctor touches the fiber with a wire and applies an electrical current that destroys the fiber.

The procedure doesn't hurt, says Dr. Lehmann, and it's effective. The overall success rate is better than 90 to 95 percent, and the complication rate is less than 2 percent.

5

Six Medical Tests You Really Need

Health screenings save lives, but advice about who needs them is fuzzy at best. Consider this: Within a 2-month span in 1997, the recommendation about who should receive a mammogram changed three times. Doctors have long debated how often Pap tests are needed, and the battle about which women need bone-density testing is heating up. When the government, medical organizations, HMOs, and your own physicians can't agree about which screening tests you need and when you should have them, how are *you* supposed to know what to do?

Here are straight answers from experts in women's health about the most common tests—as well as pointers about making the results more accurate and how the test will improve in the next decade.

1. Pap Test

A Pap test screens for cervical cancer, precancerous lesions, and some sexually transmitted diseases such as herpes and human papillomavirus. At least one-third of the 13,000 annual cases of cervical cancer in the United States are detected in women who haven't had a Pap test in 5 years.

When to get it: The Preventive Health Services Task Force, established by the government's Department of Health and Human Services, recommends

The Painless Alternative to Uterine Biopsy

An ultrasound device resembling a large plastic tampon works as well as endometrial biopsy for determining the cause of vaginal bleeding in postmenopausal women, according to an analysis of 35 ultrasound studies.

Biopsy, used to check for endometrial cancer, is invasive and uncomfortable. An endovaginal ultrasound is painless and may be more reliable at detecting cancer, says study coauthor Rebecca Smith-Bindman, M.D., assistant adjunct professor of radiology at the University of California in San Francisco. (Some women may still need biopsy if cancer is detected.) Endovaginal ultrasound is already in use by some gynecologists.

that women in a monogamous relationship who've had two consecutive normal Paps get the test every 3 years. The American College of Obstetrics and Gynecology in Washington vehemently disagrees, however, contending that the Pap test should be performed annually, because even in the best labs there can be a 15 percent chance of missing an abnormality.

"If you wait 3 years between Paps, a precancerous condition missed on your last test may have had time to develop into something more serious," says Andrew Good, M.D., chief of medical gynecology at the Mayo Clinic in Rochester, Minnesota. Still, the task force is unlikely to change its recommendation, because the group weighs the cost of medical testing against how many lives it saves, and there is little evidence that women who get annual Paps have a lower risk for invasive cervical cancer than those who get checked every 3 years. In fact, in a landmark 1986 study published in the *British Medical Journal*, a Pap test every 3 years picked up 91 percent of malignancies, while an annual Pap test detected about 94 percent.

The bottom line: Yearly exams seem slightly more effective, so if you're at the gynecologist's anyway, go ahead and get one done.

What's involved: Your gynecologist inserts a speculum into your vagina, then scrapes a few cells from your cervix for analysis at a lab.

Extra credit: Schedule the test for about 2 weeks after your period starts, when the specimen is least likely to contain blood and other natural secretions that make it difficult to get an accurate result, advises Susan Tannenbaum, M.D., a fellow of the College of American Pathologists in Port Chester, New York.

Grading system: Chances are, you'll pass with flying colors. Less than 5 percent of Pap tests turn up something suspicious, and most of those are "atypical squamous cells of undetermined significance/favor reactive." All that jargon sounds scary, but in a study of more than 10,000 Paps done at Mayo, doctors found that this kind of mild abnormality almost never indicated a problem. "Most physicians recommend that a woman with this type of Pap get rescreened in 6 months," says Dr. Good. If your next test reveals another abnormality, your doctor will help you decide whether to get rescreened or opt for a colposcopy, a procedure in which your gynecologist examines your cervix and vagina with a magnifying tool and takes a sample of problem cells.

Future possibilities: A computer, rather than a lab technician, will likely be judging your Pap tests within the next decade. In May 1998, the FDA approved AutoPap, a computer screening system, to examine Paps that aren't high risk. A 1997 study of 31,500 specimens, published in *Cancer Cytopathology*, showed that the system was as good at picking up problems as technicians were. Previously, AutoPap and a similar system, PapNet, had been approved only to recheck tests that technicians had labeled negative. The probable result of computerization: a test that's at least as accurate as those administered by a technician. But for now, most doctors don't think it's worth the money to get your Pap rescreened by a computer. A 1998 study in the *Journal of the American Medical Association* used PapNet to recheck 5,000 negative Paps. The system identified just six abnormalities that the technicians had missed, and all were conditions extremely unlikely to lead to cancer.

2. Mammogram

A mammogram screens for breast cancer. Combined with a clinical breast exam, it may cut the risk of dying from the disease by at least one-third.

When to get it: After a much-publicized cloud of controversy, the National Cancer Institute finally conceded that most women should be getting their first mammograms when they turn 40 and should have the test every year or two afterward. (If you have a family history of disease, talk to your doctor about starting earlier.) The American Cancer Society stands firm on its recommendation of annual mammograms starting at age 40. Both groups agree that a baseline mammogram at age 35 is a waste of time and money. "Most women at that age have such dense breasts that a mammogram is difficult to read," says Paul Fisher, M.D., chief of breast imaging at Allegheny University Women's Hospital in Philadelphia.

What's involved: A radiology technician compresses your breasts between plastic plates while x-rays are taken.

Extra credit: Schedule the test for 2 weeks after your period starts, when your breasts should be least tender. "Accuracy depends on proper compression," says Dr. Fisher. If your breasts are sensitive, he suggests you take a pain reliever 1 to 2 hours beforehand.

Grading system: Radiologists study your mammogram for finely stippled white dots about the size of a pencil point. If these suspicious spots are detected, your doctor will probably schedule a biopsy. The good news: At least

80 percent of all biopsies are now done as outpatient procedures and use a needle, not a scalpel.

Future possibilities: Digital mammography, which uses computer technology (rather than film) to produce a picture of the breast, has the potential to provide sharper images in half the time with less radiation than conventional mammograms, says Dr. Fisher. A digital mammography system from Lorad of Danbury, Connecticut, is awaiting FDA approval. The digital images are at

Get That Mammogram Now!

HEALTH FLASH

Many experts have long advocated annual mammograms for women in their forties. But others have argued against the practice, saying that because it's so difficult for mammography to penetrate younger women's dense breast tissue, it's not as useful at saving lives as it is in older women.

Now, the latest research shows that getting yearly mammograms in your forties may indeed save your life. When researchers at the University of Chicago looked at the medical histories of more than 800 women with breast cancer, they found that women under age 50 whose cancer was found through mammography had a 90 percent chance of survival, compared with 77 percent for women who first identified a lump through clinical breast palpation.

The reason? While mammography may be more difficult in women under 50, "palpation is also difficult in younger women," says lead study author Ruth Heimann, M.D., Ph.D., assistant professor of radiation oncology at the university. By the time a tumor can be felt in a breast check, it's twice as big—and correspondingly more dangerous—in a 40-year-old than in someone over 50.

Take these steps now.

❖ Follow up. Check with your doctor to verify your results after each mammogram.
❖ Follow through. Don't be lulled into a false sense of security if your mammogram is normal. You still need to check your breasts monthly and inform your doctor if you feel anything unusual.

If you need help finding an accredited radiologist, call the American Cancer Society at (800) ACS-2345 for a list of qualified doctors near you. It could save your life.

least as good as those of a traditional mammogram, Dr. Fisher says, but the amount of radiation isn't yet reduced. "This is just the beginning," he notes.

3. Bone-Density Scan

A bone-density scan measures bone thickness to give an indication of a woman's risk for osteoporosis, a disease that affects more than 28 million Americans, most of them women.

When to get it: "If cost weren't an issue, I think every woman at menopause should have the test," says Felicia Cosman, M.D., clinical director of the National Osteoporosis Foundation (NOF). But money does count, at least when making recommendations, so NOF suggests the test for women who are struggling to make the decision to take birth control pills during perimenopause or hormone-replacement therapy (HRT) after menopause. The test is also advised for postmenopausal women taking medication to maintain bone density as well as for those who are at significant risk for osteoporosis because they are longtime smokers or have a family history of the condition, a thin frame, or other risk factors.

The bottom line: If your insurance company doesn't cover the test (only about half do), you should appeal its decision. If that doesn't work and you can afford to pay the $50 to $200 fee (depending on the equipment used), spring for it: It's worth the money.

What's involved: It depends on what test is available to you. The Cadillac of the industry is a central dual energy x-ray absorptiometry (DEXA) machine.

How Fast Should You Expect Test Results?

When it comes to getting test results, many doctors have a "don't call us, we'll call you" policy, says Michael Donio, director of projects at the People's Medical Society in Allentown, Pennsylvania. That's not good enough, he says, because a study in the *Archives of Internal Medicine* showed that one-third of physicians don't have a reliable system to make sure your test results come back in the first place. So be sure to ask your doctor when you can follow up. Below is how long you should wait before you dial your doctor for the results of these common checks.

❖ Pap test: 10 to 14 days
❖ Mammogram: 1 to 2 days
❖ Bone density: 7 to 10 days
❖ Fasting plasma glucose: 1 to 2 days
❖ Cholesterol: 1 to 2 days

You lie on a padded table with your feet slightly raised on a soft block while the machine takes images of your hip and spine, the two most serious fracture sites. If there's not a central DEXA near you (there are only 5,000 nationwide), you may have to settle for its cousin, the peripheral DEXA, which looks at bone mass in the forearm, finger, or heel. About 15 percent of women with low bone density in their hips or spines will have normal peripheral DEXA readings.

Extra credit: When having a central DEXA, don't wear clothes with a zipper near your spine or pelvis. The metal will interfere with the reading—and the technician will insist you change into one of those horrid hospital gowns.

Grading system: Both machines calculate your bone mass and compare it with an average for women of your age and body size. If you're at the norm or above, great; if not, and you have a peripheral DEXA, your doctor may want to confirm the findings with a central DEXA. If the measurements still look low, she'll probably suggest taking HRT or bone-maintaining drugs.

Future possibilities: While current tests simply measure how much bone you have, equipment is being developed to determine how structurally sound the bone is, says Dr. Cosman.

4. Fasting Plasma Glucose Test

The fasting plasma glucose test checks for type 2 diabetes, a condition that plagues about 15 million Americans, about 8 million of them women.

When to get it: The American Diabetes Association recommends a test every year, beginning at age 45. Start at 35 if you have risk factors such as obesity, gestational diabetes, or a family history of the disease.

What's involved: After avoiding food and beverages except water for 8 to 12 hours, you'll have blood drawn.

Extra credit: Reschedule the test if you're not feeling well; even something as minor as a cold could interfere with results, says John Hare, M.D., director of the affiliated centers program at Joslin Diabetes Center in Boston. Alert your doctor if you're on a low-carbohydrate eating plan such as the Zone diet; it may throw off your results, too.

Grading system: If your result is below 110 milligrams per deciliter, you're as good as gold. If it's over 125, your doctor will likely recommend a repeat test. If the result is over 125 again, you have diabetes. If your first test result is between 110 and 125, your doctor will suggest having a glucose tolerance test, in which you fast overnight and then drink a super-sweet solution. Blood will be drawn 1 hour and 2 hours after the drink. If the 2-hour glucose tolerance test measurement is 200 or more, you have diabetes.

Future possibilities: Researchers at the University of Toronto have developed a sweetened wafer that won't cause the nausea produced by the sugary drink given as part of the glucose tolerance test. Another alternative: Doctors at St.

John Hospital and Medical Center in Detroit perform the test using jelly beans. Look for these patient-friendly options to become more widely available.

5. Blood Pressure Check

A blood pressure check helps assess your risk for heart attack, stroke, and liver and kidney damage. More than one-fifth of American women have high blood pressure. Cutting it back just a little can reduce the risk of heart attack by about 15 percent and stroke about 40 percent.

When to get it: Women who are 21 or older with no family history of hypertension should have their blood pressures checked a minimum of once every 2 years. Those with a family history should be tested at least annually.

What's involved: An inflatable cuff is wrapped around your upper arm to help your doctor measure the pressure of your blood against your artery walls as your heart contracts and relaxes.

Extra credit: This is one test you really shouldn't be nervous about, since anxiety can make it appear as if you have high blood pressure when you don't— a phenomenon known as white-coat hypertension. Also, if the circumference of the middle of your upper arm is less than 12½ inches, ask your physician to use a small blood pressure cuff. Most offices have at least two sizes. Loose cuffs can artificially lower your reading, while ones that are too tight can elevate it.

Grading system: If your pressure is below 140/85, you pass. If the bottom number is 86 to 90, your doctor will probably ask you to return soon for another reading. Have a reading greater than 140/90? Your doctor will take it a few more times to confirm that you have high blood pressure.

6. Cholesterol Screening

Cholesterol screening is a key component in determining your risk for heart disease. About 20 percent of women have cholesterol levels that put them at an elevated risk.

When to get it: The National Heart, Lung, and Blood Institute (NHLBI) and the American Heart Association recommend that adults 20 and older have their cholesterol checked once every 5 years if they don't have a history of high cholesterol. The Preventive Health Services Task Force is a bit less stringent, however, suggesting periodic (it doesn't define exactly how often) screening only for women 45 and over (and men 35 and over). But the task force will soon be reviewing its cholesterol recommendations. For now, it's probably better to follow the NHLBI's.

What's involved: You fast for 12 hours (water and black, unsweetened coffee or tea are permitted) and head to your doctor's office or lab to get blood drawn.

Persuade Your Guy to Get a Checkup

Medical research has finally acknowledged what women have known for centuries: Men don't like to go to the doctor.

When focus groups of family physicians were interviewed about how men handle their health care needs, researchers got an earful. Men, it seems, tend to worry about being perceived as vulnerable or weak. They may also have difficulty relinquishing control to doctors for a variety of social and personal reasons. And unlike women, guys generally don't like discussing their health with each other—unless it is about something superficial, such as a sports-related injury.

On the other hand, female partners emerged from the focus-group discussions as the most popular confidantes. "Women were the most prepared to listen to men's health concerns and to encourage them to seek medical help," says Fred Tudiver, M.D., director of the Center for Evidence-Based Practice and professor in the department of family medicine at the State University of New York Health Sciences Center in Syracuse. Mothers are influential in the case of adolescent boys, he adds. Sisters and daughters may also be a source of support for men.

If you want to help a special guy in your life, first and foremost be a good listener, says Dr. Tudiver. Next, be a good initiator. Encourage him to talk about his health. Ask him about his family history of disease and if he knows what screening tests he should have at his age. Ask if he is aware of his risks for various diseases and if he is comfortable with his current doctor. If all else fails, make the doctor appointment for him. Offer to go with him, if he'd like.

In the case of really stubborn guys, try subtle persuasion. "This is a classic in family medicine: A wife calls up before her husband's appointment, asking the doctor to bring up this symptom or that, just to make sure the guy talks about it," says Dr. Tudiver.

"Sometimes it takes a reminder of his important role in the family to get him to the doctor's office," notes Robin DiMatteo, Ph.D., professor of psychology at the University of California at Riverside.

If you are truly concerned about a serious or chronic condition, it might be worth applying a bit of gentle pressure. Say, "I'm worried about you" or "What would happen to the kids and me if something bad happened to you?" Your concern may make a big difference in your guy's willingness to take care of himself, says Dr. DiMatteo.

Extra credit: Avoid exercise for up to 4 hours before the test, because it could falsely elevate your level, says Margo Denke, M.D., professor of internal medicine at the University of Texas Southwestern Medical Center in Dallas. If you're tracking your test results, she recommends scheduling every appointment approximately the same number of days after your period begins, because your cholesterol level naturally rises and falls over the course of your cycle.

Grading system: Since your cholesterol can naturally vary 20 to 40 points daily, doctors should consider the results of several tests before making a diagnosis. You're shooting for a low-density lipoprotein (LDL) level under 130, a high-density lipoprotein (HDL) level of above 45, and triglycerides under 200. An LDL between 130 and 160 and triglycerides between 200 and 400 are considered borderline high; your doctor will probably retest you in a few weeks and recommend changes in your diet and activity level. If you have an LDL level above 160, an HDL level below 45, or triglycerides over 400, your doctor will suggest a second test right away. If your levels are still out of line, you'll most likely be given cholesterol-lowering drugs to take in addition to making lifestyle changes.

Future possibilities: In the next few years, your cholesterol checks will likely become much more detailed. A test developed by LipoMed of Raleigh, North Carolina, sorts the particles of HDL and LDL present in your blood by size and gives measurements for each of the four sizes of HDL and five sizes of LDL. You also get readings for six sizes of very low density lipoprotein (VLDL), another substance that has been linked to heart disease. A 1998 study in the *Journal of the American Heart Association* links small HDL or large VLDL with a three to four times greater than normal risk of heart disease.

6

What Your Ob/Gyn Isn't Telling You

Like most smart women, you probably come to your annual gynecological exam armed with a list of health concerns. But you may never ask your obstetrician/gynecologist the critical question: "What aren't you telling me?"

Your doctor can't inform you of things that she herself doesn't know—for example, important new research findings that she hasn't read up on yet. And she certainly won't mention things she'd rather keep hidden, such as any blots on her professional record or gaps in her training. To make sure you're getting the whole story, here's a list of things your doctor may not be telling you, plus advice on how to get the knowledge you need for the good health care you deserve.

That Vaginal Infection Could Spell Trouble

Bacterial vaginosis (BV) is the most common vaginal infection—so common, in fact, that many physicians don't take it seriously. Even when a routine pelvic exam turns up BV, some doctors don't bother to inform their patients, because they may have been taught in medical school that it isn't harmful to a woman's health. Now, however, a growing number of researchers are campaigning to raise awareness of BV, citing recent studies that link it to a greater risk for preterm birth and pelvic inflammatory disease (the latter can ultimately lead to infertility and ectopic pregnancy). Because BV disrupts the normal levels of infection-fighting acids in the vagina, it also can increase your risk of contracting gonorrhea or HIV from an infected partner.

In women with bacterial vaginosis, the "good" bacteria that normally populate the vagina are overwhelmed by another strain that can produce a grayish discharge and release a fishy-smelling odor—one that's particularly noticeable after intercourse or at the end of your period. Many women try to mask the odor with douches or feminine deodorant sprays. "We've been taught to be very clean," says Sharon Hillier, Ph.D., associate professor at the University of Pittsburgh School of Medicine. "But it's extremely important not to use products that disguise the symptoms and signs of this infection before seeing a doctor." In fact, douching appears to make matters worse by killing healthy bacteria.

BV is easily treated with antibiotics once it's diagnosed—but patients are often too embarrassed to mention their symptoms. "And doctors don't look for BV if patients don't complain," says Dr. Hillier. "It's a conspiracy of silence." Even if you haven't noticed any symptoms (many women with BV are asymptomatic), if you're concerned, ask your doctor to check a sample of your vaginal fluid, especially if you are pregnant or trying to conceive.

She Doesn't Know Who's Checking Your Pap Test

A Pap test, which screens for signs of cervical cancer, is only as good as the pathologist who reads it—and if your doctor doesn't know who's evaluating your test, you're not getting the quality control you deserve. If your doctor and the lab aren't in regular contact, the pathologist may not have all the information necessary to diagnose a problem. Sometimes, for instance, certain key details of a patient's medical history can help a pathologist interpret murky results.

Don't be afraid to question your doctor about the reputation of the lab she uses and whether she's familiar with the people who work there. If your managed-care plan dictates that she use an out-of-state lab that's unfamiliar to her, consider paying out-of-pocket to have your test results rechecked by a local pathologist your doctor trusts. The cost for the added peace of mind: $15 to $20.

You can also check up on your health plan's lab yourself: All pathology labs must be state-licensed, but those accredited by the College of American Pathologists (CAP) often must meet higher standards. CAP may also know whether a lab has lost its accreditation because of problems. Call CAP at (800) LAB-5678 (522-5678) to find out whether your doctor's lab makes the grade.

Ultimately, though, your best protection against screening oversights is simply to get a Pap test every year. "Sheer repetition will virtually ensure that any abnormalities are picked up," says Robert J. Kurman, M.D., a Richard TeLinde distinguished professor of gynecologic pathology at the Johns Hopkins University School of Medicine in Baltimore. "Most problems don't appear out of nowhere. Since cervical cancer is generally very slow-growing, if

There's an Easier Way to Remove Fibroids

HEALTH FLASH

Removal of fibroids can spell hysterectomy for some women. But a new procedure called hysteroscopic resection is changing that. A telescope-like instrument called a hysteroscope is inserted through the vagina and cervix into the uterus, allowing the doctor to look inside. Attached to the hysteroscope is an electrode through which electric current passes. The current shaves off the fibroid and breaks it into small pieces for easy removal. No incisions are necessary, and the procedure is done on an outpatient basis.

Hysteroscopic resection is best done when fibroids are small (about 6 centimeters) and only if they're the type growing from the uterine wall into the uterine cavity. Often fibroids can be shrunk with medication first to make the procedure easier. Advantages over hysterectomy include enhancement of fertility, return to normal activity within a few days, less blood loss, and minimal risk of surgical adhesions or scar tissue.

you are checked on a regular basis, the risk of not catching a problem until its latter stages is extremely low."

You May Be Using Your Birth Control Incorrectly

You may not realize it, but those reassuring effectiveness statistics cited on the insert that's tucked inside your birth control's packaging refer to "perfect use," which, in the language of contraceptive manufacturers, means using your method with extraordinary attention to detail. Guess what? In real life, most women don't do that. The more meaningful statistic, which is also included inside the package, is the pregnancy rate for "typical" users, which can be anywhere from 5 to 20 percent greater.

The trouble is that most doctors don't review patients' birth control habits or warn them of potential lapses in effectiveness. That's why it's in your interest to learn all you can about your contraceptive. Your best bet: Follow the instructions on the package. It may save you a lot of grief.

For example, a woman on the Pill who suffers a bout of vomiting or diarrhea should use a back-up method (a condom, say) for the rest of her cycle. If you're on a mini-pill (Ovrette, Nor-QD), be sure to take it at the same time every day. Diaphragm users should insert a dose of spermicidal jelly or cream with each act of intercourse and have the device refitted after childbirth. Couples who use condoms should check the package's expiration date and store them in a cool, dry, dark place, as heat can cause latex to break down. After intercourse, take special care in removing the condom: Your partner should withdraw his penis immediately after ejaculation while holding the rim of the condom snugly against the base of his penis to avoid leakage.

If your gynecologist seems reluctant to discuss these details, find another doctor. "Look for someone you're comfortable with who will answer your questions, someone who will help you decide on the contraceptive that will work best for you," advises Tina Hoff, director of media relations for the Kaiser Family Foundation.

Your Doctor Could Be on Probation

When you're choosing a gynecologist from an HMO's seemingly endless list of providers, it's easy to assume that all of them are competent—or else they wouldn't be there, right? Don't count on it. Your doctor is under no legal obligation to inform you that a hospital has put her on probation or that another state has revoked her medical license. So if you're picking out a doctor at random, it pays to check credentials before you sign up.

As a first step, call your state's medical licensing board and check on the status of your doctor's license: Ask specifically about any disciplinary actions. In most states, hospitals advise the state when they put a doctor on probation for 30 days or more, says Alicia Mitchell, assistant director of media relations for the American Hospital Association.

You can also call the doctor's affiliated hospital and talk to a patient representative, consumer advocate, or social worker. "Say, 'I'd like to check on the admitting status of Dr. X,'" advises Michael Donio, director of projects at the People's Medical Society in Allentown, Pennsylvania. If your doctor isn't affiliated with any hospital, that's a red flag that something is wrong.

You can check that your doctor is board-certified by calling the American Board of Medical Specialties at (800) 776-CERT (776-2378) or by checking their Web site at www.certifieddoctor.org. (Board certification means that she has met even more stringent standards than those required by the states.) In 14 states, you can get additional information on your physician's background from the Association of State Medical Board Executive Directors' Web site at www.docboard.org. The site may provide a list of actions taken against your doctor by state licensing boards as well as information on malpractice suits filed.

It's Okay to "Schedule" Your Period

If you've ever planned a romantic vacation around your period, you'll see the appeal of trying to work it the other way around. The idea of using oral

Stop Monthly Breast Pain

Breast pain around the time of your period is common among women in their thirties and forties, but it's often easily treated. Try these approaches.

❖ Go on the Pill. Some doctors report a 60- to 70-percent success rate in treating breast pain with oral contraceptives, which balance the hormones in your system.

❖ Cut out caffeine. Research has shown that the methylxanthines in caffeine sources such as coffee, tea, cola, chocolate, and even over-the-counter painkillers can worsen breast discomfort.

❖ Apply cold compresses. These help by easing the swelling.

❖ Take a nonsteroidal anti-inflammatory pill such as ibuprofen (Motrin) or naproxen sodium (Aleve).

❖ Try a supplement. One study found vitamin E to be effective in 41 percent of breast-pain cases. "The typical recommendation is 400 international units a day," says A. Marilyn Leitch, M.D., a surgical oncologist and professor of surgery at the University of Texas Southwestern Medical Center in Dallas.

Research also suggests that evening primrose oil may be effective for almost half of the women who complain of period-related breast pain. To soothe pain, Jill Stansbury, N.D., a naturopathic physician and director of the Battleground Naturopathic Family Practice in Battleground, Washington, suggests taking one or two capsules (either 500 or 1,000 milligrams) of evening primrose oil three times a day for several months. Dr. Stansbury is also the chairman of the botanical medicine department at the National College of Naturopathic Medicine in Portland, Oregon.

❖ Wear a comfortable, supportive bra. Trade your binding underwire bra for one with a broad band of fabric on the sides and wide straps that lend sufficient support.

❖ Ask your doctor about prescription drugs. Danocrine, which is derived from the male hormone androgen, has been shown to be 70- to 90-percent effective in relieving breast pain. Unfortunately, it has a number of unwelcome side effects, such as increased body hair, weight gain, and acne.

HEALTH FLASH

contraceptives to manipulate your menstrual cycle may make your doctor uneasy, but there's no reason to have an inconveniently timed period, says James A. McGregor, M.D., professor of obstetrics and gynecology at the University of Colorado School of Medicine in Denver.

Yes, most doctors and patients think of a period as a monthly event, and most birth control packs come with 3 weeks of active pills and one week of "dummy," or inert, pills. If you take them as directed, you'll usually have a period during the week you take the placebo, "but it's not really necessary," according to Dr. McGregor.

If you have no health problems that keep you from taking oral contraceptives, you can reschedule your cycle to suit your needs—like if you're going on a scuba diving vacation or your honeymoon. Ask your doctor if you can take two packages of pills back-to-back for a 7-week cycle with no placebo week.

The Food and Drug Administration (FDA) hasn't officially approved using the Pill for making periods more convenient, but researchers point out that continuous pill use is often prescribed for women with endometriosis, with the result that they never menstruate.

You Can Exercise Your "Sex Muscles"

The Kegel exercise, a rhythmic tightening of the pelvic floor muscles, is one of the easiest things a woman can do to improve sexual response and avoid incontinence as she ages. Studies have shown that women who regularly do Kegels—which strengthen the same muscles used to stop the flow of urine midstream—have more frequent, intense orgasms. Yet the vast majority of gynecologists never check a woman's pelvic muscle tone or even discuss it with her. "Gynecologists will rarely broach the topic unless you're pregnant or incontinent," says Lauri J. Romanzi, M.D., clinical assistant professor of gynecology at Weill Medical College of Cornell University in New York City. "But it should be part of every routine exam. These muscles are just like the muscles in the arms and legs; if you work them, they'll get stronger."

During a pelvic exam, your gynecologist should ask you to clench your pelvic muscles as hard as you can. If your doctor checks every patient regularly, she should be able to tell you how your strength compares with other women your age and prescribe a regular regimen of Kegels if necessary.

Researchers don't know exactly how many Kegels are needed for optimal strength, but "I tell my patients to do them when they're on the bus or driving in their cars," Dr. Romanzi says. (To do a Kegel, tighten your pelvic floor muscles as if you were stopping the flow of your urine midstream and hold for several seconds. Work up to 10 contractions at a time. Repeat several times a day.)

Regulate Your Period with Vitex

The herb vitex, also called chasteberry, may help to normalize irregular menstrual cycles. In fact, Germany's herbal authority, Commission E, has approved it for a variety of menstrual disturbances, including painful breasts and menopause symptoms.

Commission E recommends only 20 milligrams daily, but higher doses (even as much as 1 gram, three times a day) seem to be safe. Commercial preparations (alcohol extracts and capsules) vary greatly in strength, so follow label instructions for the product you take. You may have to use this remedy for several months to see significant improvement.

Note: Consult with your physician before using vitex. Pregnant women should never use vitex.

"Women who exercise regularly should do them during their warmup or cooldown."

If your gynecologist doesn't seem interested when you ask about Kegels, it may be a sign that you have the wrong doctor. "I still get referrals from women who say they've been to four, five, six doctors and were told that incontinence is just part of aging and that they should live with it—or go buy pads," Dr. Romanzi says. "That's the same as taking someone who has cataracts and telling them to just get a Seeing Eye dog."

The Pill Can Interfere with Prescription Medications

Any good gynecologist should talk to you about the common side effects of oral contraceptives, such as menstrual changes and breast tenderness. But it is just as important that she make sure you're not taking any other medications that might interact with the Pill, including those prescribed by other doctors.

For instance, several antibiotics can interfere with the Pill's effectiveness. If you're taking penicillin for strep throat, you need to use a back-up method of birth control for the rest of the month. Additionally, several antiseizure medications can make birth control pills ineffective. Alternately, oral contraceptives can heighten the effects of theophylline, a common asthma drug. And the hormones in oral contraceptives may boost the effects of certain tricyclic antidepressants—including Elavil and Tofranil—and tranquilizers, such as Valium or Xanax, leaving you woozy or even dangerously impaired. Finally, birth control pills can heighten the impact of alcohol, so go easy on wine, beer, and liquor.

She Needs More Practice

Your doctor may be delighted with her new medical gadgets, but you don't want to be a guinea pig while she learns how to use them, especially if she's working with no supervision. Although some doctors are conscientious about getting trained when a new medical device or procedure comes out, "there are too many doctors who go to a weekend seminar, watch a video, then operate on Monday morning," says Donio.

John Marlow, M.D., president of the Gynecologic Surgery Society, recommends that you ask: Who trained you in this procedure? How many cases have you done? What kind of complications have occurred?

There are no legal limits on a licensed doctor's ability to use any new FDA-approved device, notes William Parker, M.D., chairman of obstetrics and gynecology at Santa Monica–UCLA Medical Center and author of *A Gynecologist's Second Opinion*. Some hospitals do keep tabs on their doctors' training, requiring them to be closely observed during their first few go-rounds with unfamiliar equipment. But other hospitals have no such requirements. To be safe, call your hospital to check on its policies, and if you're facing an unsupervised procedure in your doctor's office or a private clinic, seek a second opinion.

You Need an Above-the-Belt Checkup, Too

If you're like many women, your gynecologist may be your primary care physician, the one you call about everything from sinus infections to chest pains. But if that's the case she needs to provide more than just a yearly pelvic exam and Pap test.

"The question is, what's a good 30,000-mile checkup?" says Eric Steen, M.D., assistant professor of internal medicine at the University of Texas Southwestern Medical Center at Dallas. The two biggest long-term threats are cancer and heart disease, so your office visit should include a skin cancer screening as well as periodic screenings for major risk factors for heart disease—diabetes, hypertension, high cholesterol—and a record of your family history. "I also make a big deal about smoking and being overweight," he says.

Your primary care doctor should remind you to keep your immunizations up-to-date and have a tetanus shot every 10 years. She should also be discussing substance abuse and mental health issues. "Women have higher rates of depression," Dr. Steen says, "but if a doctor is just asking about vaginal discharge, she won't detect these kinds of problems." A good primary care physician will even nag you about visiting the dentist and eye doctor.

"These are the things that need to get done," Dr. Steen says. "If your doctor doesn't cover them, ask her to do so—or go to someone who does."

Natural Progesterone: Miracle or Hype?

7

Maybe you've heard other women talking about the new "miracle in a jar" that whips menopausal symptoms. Maybe your doctor has mentioned it. Maybe you've seen the raves of "satisfied customers" in the ads of the companies that sell it.

It's natural progesterone, a plant hormone derived from wild yams or soybeans. If you have heard about it, you no doubt have two questions: What is it? And should you be using it?

There are some good reasons to consider taking natural progesterone—it may help reduce your health risks and ease the discomfort of menopause—but not by itself and not in overhyped cream that may not contain any progesterone at all.

Here's the straight scoop on the "other" menopause hormone.

What Is Progesterone—And Why Do I Need It?

Progesterone is the other female hormone your body produces besides estrogen. It helps regulate your cycle, nourishes the lining of your uterus in preparation for pregnancy, and helps maintain it should conception occur. But its job is also to prevent estrogen from causing the lining to thicken too much. So when an egg is not fertilized, progesterone levels drop, causing the lining to be shed in a menstrual period.

The New Herbal Estrogen

Given in supplement form, herbal estrogen decreased hot flashes without unpleasant side effects in 26 women who took it, according to researchers at New York University Medical Center and New England Medical Center. It's available as Promensil, an over-the-counter supplement made from plant estrogens found in red clover.

As you approach menopause, your ovaries slow down and stop producing progesterone since you ovulate less frequently or not at all. By the time you reach menopause, the drop in progesterone is almost 100 percent. Estrogen, on the other hand, drops by about 90 percent, since there are other sources of estrogen in the body.

If you're given estrogen at menopause, a progestin (or synthetic version of progesterone) is added to your hormone therapy to prevent the estrogen from causing a buildup of tissue in your uterus that can lead to endometrial (uterine) cancer.

Though a progestin acts like your body's own progesterone in some ways, it's not its chemical twin—with good reason. When taken by mouth, natural progesterone is quickly digested, broken down by the liver, and excreted. That means it doesn't get to the uterus in sufficient doses to offer any protection. So researchers developed synthetic substitutes: progestins that are easily absorbed. The latest breakthrough, however, is micronized progesterone, which is formulated by breaking the particles into very tiny pieces so they pass untouched through the liver and are absorbed by your body.

Unlike estrogen, which has been shown to protect your heart, prevent osteoporosis, lower your risk of colorectal cancer, and perhaps even prevent Alzheimer's disease, there's no scientific evidence that progesterone does anything more than counteract the effects of estrogen on your uterus. So other than that, why do you need it? And why do you need a natural version when a synthetic will do?

Synthetic Progesterone: HRT "Bad Guy"

The synthetic progestins—which experts often refer to as a necessary evil—in current hormone-replacement therapy (HRT) formulations appear to produce most of the unpleasant side effects associated with HRT: mood changes, depression, irritability, bloating, breast tenderness, and headaches. "None of these is common," says Vanessa M. Barnabei, M.D., Ph.D., associate professor of obstetrics and gynecology at the Medical College of Wisconsin in Milwaukee. "But they can be significant enough to cause problems for some women." And they can be significant enough to encou

as 38 percent—to stop filling their prescriptions for H

more—60 percent—stop taking it after 2 years. Natural

other hand, has far fewer side effects in most women.

There may be other reasons to take a natural progesterone,
it gets controversial. Its advocates claim that natural progest
relieve the symptoms of menopause with none of the risks of
pleasant side effects than progestin. Some, like John R. Lee, M.
stave off osteoporosis, calm premenstrual syndrome and endome   , and
eliminate fibrocystic breasts and ovarian cysts, among other problems. Dr.
Lee, a retired California family physician, has also suggested that menopausal
symptoms aren't caused by lack of estrogen but by lack of progesterone. He
promotes his highly controversial view in a popular book, *What Your Doctor
May Not Tell You about Menopause.*

Critics scoff, calling these claims quackery. And many health experts worry
that women will turn to readily available over-the-counter natural progesterone creams instead of HRT, depriving themselves of the scientifically
proven benefits of estrogen to protect their hearts and bones.

Beware the Yam Scam

The "all natural" wild yam cream you bought promises to banish all
your menopausal ills. Will it? Some women say the progesterone creams
work wonders for them and make them feel better. But there's no reliable
scientific evidence that these creams can provide relief from menopausal
symptoms. It could be the powerful placebo effect: If you think you're
getting a benefit from something, you will.

But if you want to try these creams, experts say it's unlikely they can
hurt you. Just be sure you're getting the best product for your money by
checking what's on the label.

❖ A cream contains natural progesterone if the progesterone is biologically
   identical to what your body makes. It doesn't refer to the source of it.
❖ Unless a cream contains pharmaceutical-grade progesterone—look for
   "progesterone USP" on the label—it's likely to do nothing more than
   make your wallet a little skinnier.
❖ Proponents of natural progesterone creams agree that it takes a minimum of 400 milligrams of progesterone per ounce to alleviate
   menopausal symptoms.
❖ Be especially wary of creams that say they contain diosgenin, "a precursor to progesterone." Though the label might imply that your body
   can turn the yam compound into progesterone, it can't.

sy aside, there is some evidence that natural progesterone can be
neficial—if you're also taking estrogen postmenopausally. For example,
tural progesterone may be better than synthetic at preserving more of estrogen's beneficial effects on the heart. And in at least one set of studies,
women who took natural progesterone along with estrogen said they felt better emotionally.

Get the Facts

Unfortunately, there have been few scientific studies on natural progesterone. In fact, science knows very little about the progesterone you make in
your body, let alone the kind made in a lab. But this much we do know: Natural progesterone—which, despite its name, is also created in a lab—is chemically identical to the hormone secreted during the luteal phase of your
menstrual cycle (the two weeks after you ovulate).

The reason you need a lab to intervene is that wild yams and soybeans don't
contain progesterone but rather another chemical—a plant compound called
diosgenin—that can be turned into a facsimile of your own progesterone, but
only in a lab. You can't get it by eating the vegetables or by smearing them on
your skin. Your own body can't transform a plant hormone into a human one.

In fact, over-the-counter creams that contain natural progesterone actually
have a pharmaceutical grade of progesterone added. And while natural progesterone is readily absorbed through your skin, studies have found that it's very
difficult for a woman to achieve normal levels of circulating hormone by applying it that way.

So what's your best choice right now? Several forms of natural progesterone—suppositories, lozenges, and capsules—have been available by prescription from pharmacies that specialize in compounding (making individual
formulations in the exact dose your doctor orders). But your best bets may be
the two newest products on the market.

The pill form. The chief advantages of this form are that it's as convenient
as, well, popping a pill. Also, scientific evidence says it protects your heart and
uterus.

Called Prometrium, it has been approved by the FDA for use in hormone-
replacement therapy. Because it's micronized, it can be absorbed by your body
before it's destroyed by your liver.

Micronized progesterone has proven itself superior to progestins in a major
study, the Postmenopausal Estrogen/Progestin Intervention (PEPI) Trial.
Progestins can diminish the protective effect estrogen has on the heart—
mainly by blunting the estrogen-triggered rise in HDL, the "good" cholesterol. Natural progesterone taken orally, on the other hand, preserves more of

New Choice in Hormone Replacement

H E A L T H F L A S H

Many women who are eligible for hormone-replacement therapy (HRT) decide against starting it. Of those who do start, one-third stop filling their prescriptions within a year because of concerns about unpleasant side effects. If you fit either description, here's a new option you can discuss with your doctor: estratab, estrogen in pill form extracted from soy and yams.

A two-year study conducted by Morris Notelovitz, M.D., Ph.D., founder and president emeritus of the Women's Medical and Diagnostic Center in Gainesville, Florida, showed that a 0.3-milligram daily dose of Estratab did not increase the incidence of endometrial hyperplasia, a noted side effect of estrogen taken without progesterone or a progestin. In March 1998, the FDA approved the 0.3-milligram dose for the prevention of osteoporosis. This lower dose still provides all the benefits of higher doses of estrogen. It reduces symptoms of menopause and improves cholesterol profiles.

What about breast cancer risk? Dr. Notelovitz speculates that such a low dose of estrogen may not carry the same risk of breast cancer that some women fear when taking standard HRT.

estrogen's beneficial effects on the heart while preventing estrogen from building up tissue in your uterus.

In the PEPI study, the only real side effect noted by study participants was drowsiness. But that is "easily managed by taking the drug at bedtime," says principal investigator Trudy Bush, D.Ph., Ph.D., professor of epidemiology and preventive medicine at the University of Maryland School of Medicine in Baltimore.

Vaginal gel. There are a number of chief advantages to vaginal gel. For example, progesterone is delivered directly to the uterus. Further, study subjects report an emotional boost. Crinone is a natural progesterone-containing gel that's applied to the vagina, where it's readily absorbed and concentrated in the uterus. Unlike vaginal creams and suppositories, the gel doesn't cause a messy discharge. And in a series of studies involving 610 patients, it was effective at protecting women taking estrogen from endometrial cancer.

Those studies were conducted by Michelle P. Warren, M.D., director of the Center for Menopause, Hormonal Disorders, and Women's Health at

Columbia–Presbyterian Medical Center in New York City. "Our clinical trial also showed women felt better on progesterone than on estrogen alone. When we added the progesterone, we got a decrease in reports of headaches, depression, and mood swings that we did not expect," she says.

In fact, the drowsiness reported by the women in the PEPI study may be related to the calming effect the women experienced in the Crinone studies. Progesterone was used as an anesthetic during the 1930s.

Like Prometrium, Crinone has been FDA-approved for uses other than HRT, but physicians can still prescribe it as part of HRT.

If you are now taking or are a possible candidate for HRT, talk to your doctor about using natural progesterone with your estrogen. But hold off on treating yourself with over-the-counter preparations until the scientific proof is in that they're something more than very expensive skin cream.

Amazing Facts about the Pill

Pop quiz! Name the drug that can do all this: Treat your acne. Tame those killer cramps and menstrual migraines. Wipe out perimenopausal symptoms. Prevent several common cancers. Strengthen your bones. Possibly even boost your fertility.

Here's one more clue. This drug has a nifty "side effect": Taken daily, it is 99 percent effective in preventing pregnancy. That's right—it's the Pill (as in oral contraceptives), which just celebrated 38 years as one of the most studied, debated, cursed, and praised drugs ever developed.

An Easier Pill to Swallow

If you're like most women, you've had a complicated relationship with birth control pills. True, they are by far the most popular reversible contraceptive, to the tune of 18 million American users. (Some 80 percent of women have used them at some point, according to a new Gallup survey.) After all, it's hard to quibble with nearly foolproof birth control. But even though we take it in droves for years on end (or start and stop and start again), many women still have complaints about side effects and lingering doubts about its safety.

Now hear this: Those fears are, quite literally, history. When the Pill was

Hidden Benefits of the Pill

The experts are unanimous: Most women (and even some doctors) wildly overestimate the risks of the Pill and vastly underestimate its many health benefits. Did you know it could do all this?

Day-to-Day Pill Pluses

❖ Clockwork-regular periods
❖ Lighter flow
❖ Fewer days of bleeding
❖ Less cramping
❖ Clearer skin

Lower Health Risks

❖ Lower incidence of benign breast disease
❖ Lower risk of endometriosis
❖ Fewer ovarian cysts
❖ Lower risk of pelvic inflammatory disease
❖ Lower risk of tubal pregnancy

Special Benefits

❖ Reduces risk of anemia in women with heavy bleeding
❖ May lessen severity of rheumatoid arthritis
❖ May reduce heavy bleeding and cramping from fibroids
❖ May help preserve fertility in women over 30

Long-Term Health Bonanza

❖ Builds stronger bones
❖ Reduces the risk of endometrial cancer (the most common gynecologic cancer in this country) by half
❖ Decreases by up to 80 percent the risk of ovarian cancer, the most deadly gynecologic cancer

first introduced in the 1960s, it contained much higher doses of hormones than it does now—five times as much estrogen and nine times as much progesterone. It was also given to women who would, today, be advised to steer clear, such as smokers over age 35. In the interim, side effects (both the truly dangerous and the merely annoying) have plummeted.

Not only is the Pill safer than ever, it has turned out to be positively good for women. Thirty-eight years ago, who knew that the Pill would have at least as much to contribute to our health as it does to our sex lives? "Today's Pill is truly a wonder drug," says Carolyn Westhoff, M.D., medical director of family planning at Columbia Presbyterian Medical Center in New York City.

Benefits at Every Age

The proof is in the prescribing. Doctors are so impressed by the power of the Pill that they now give it to women who don't even need it for birth control.

"More and more, I prescribe oral contraceptives specifically for their non-contraceptive benefits, and I also emphasize those benefits to women who are interested in birth control," says Andrew M. Kaunitz, M.D., professor and assistant chairman of obstetrics and gynecology at the University of Florida Health Science Center in Jacksonville.

For women in their teens and twenties, the Pill can alleviate acne, soothe painful cramps, and smooth out erratic cycles. For women in their thirties who have fibroids, the Pill can tame crampy, heavy periods, often eliminating the need for surgery. For women in their late thirties and forties, it can obliterate perimenopause symptoms like hot flashes and irregular or heavy bleeding, easing the transition to menopause (while shoring up bone density).

Another astonishing possibility: Taking the Pill might actually help women stay fertile longer. "Women who get pregnant after age 30 have a higher incidence of abnormal chromosomes in their fetuses," says Lane Mercer, M.D., professor of obstetrics and gynecology at Northwestern University Medical School in Chicago. "Part of the reason for this may be related to the fact that, over time, you're using up your eggs. One very good recent study suggests that women who take birth control pills for more than 9 years before the age of 30 may have a significant decrease in miscarriages caused by chromosome abnormalities."

Why? "The Pill works by suspending ovarian function," Dr. Mercer explains, "basically putting your eggs on hold. In the study, it took 9 years on the Pill to see this effect. And it didn't work to take the pills later in life. The idea that you might be able to get to age 40 and still have, essentially, a 30-year-old's eggs is very compelling."

Pill Basics

Although there's a bewildering array of oral contraceptives on the market, most are actually quite similar. They contain two active ingredients: an estrogen and a progestin (or synthetic progesterone). "All recently introduced pills have the same estrogen: ethinyl estradiol. It's the amount of estrogen and the amount and type of progestin that varies," explains Dr. Kaunitz. There are also mini-pills that contain only progestin, which are used much less commonly.

Oral contraceptives work mainly, as noted above, by stopping ovulation. The low levels of hormones are just enough to "trick" your body into thinking you're pregnant, so the brain doesn't signal the uterus and ovaries to start up a new menstrual cycle. In addition, the progestin thickens the cervical mucus, making

When You Forget a Pill— And Other Disasters

The exceptional effectiveness of birth control pills depends on using them correctly and consistently. But sometimes things go awry. Here's what to do when:

You forget a pill. If you miss one pill (a surprising 47 percent of women do so at least once a month, according to a 1996 study), double up once. If you miss two pills, double up twice. If you miss three or more, toss the pack and start a brand-new one on Sunday, no matter what day of the week it is. Use a back-up method of birth control until you've taken the new pack for 7 days. (Your doctor may want you to handle the situation slightly differently, and you can always call her if you're not sure what to do or if you're on a phasic pill, which is a little more complicated.)

You are sick as a dog. If you're vomiting or have severe diarrhea, use a back-up method until you've taken pills for a week after you're feeling better. Or just forget your pills for the duration and start a new pack the next Sunday, says Carolyn Westhoff, M.D., medical director of family planning at Columbia Presbyterian Medical Center in New York City.

You don't get your period. Most women's first thought is that they're pregnant. But if you've been taking your pills regularly, that's extremely unlikely. It's just that the low dose of estrogen in the pills may not build up the uterine lining enough for it to need to bleed. "Whatever you do, don't stop taking the Pill," says Dr. Westhoff. "Go ahead and get a pregnancy test if you want to. Even if you are pregnant and you decide to continue the pregnancy, the Pill is not dangerous to you or the embryo. I've seen so many women who don't have a period say, 'I guess the Pill failed,' and stop taking it. By the time I finally see them a couple weeks later, they *are* pregnant."

You need last-chance contraception. At your next checkup, ask your doctor for emergency contraception instructions. You may be able to use your current birth control prescription in the specific formula prescribed for unprotected sex. Or you can get a prescription for the newly FDA-approved PREVEN Emergency Contraceptive Kit—which includes the pills you need, a pregnancy test, and detailed instructions. In either case, you have to act fast: The first dose of pills has to be taken within 72 hours (48 hours for the mini-pill).

HEALTH FLASH

it harder for sperm to get through. Progestin also inhibits implantation, although the chances of a fertilized egg getting that far are remote.

Any pill with 35 micrograms or less of estrogen is considered low-dose. With very few exceptions (some detailed below), that's the amount you should be taking, says Elizabeth Connell, M.D., professor emeritus of obstetrics and gynecology at Emory University School of Medicine in Atlanta and an early Pill researcher.

There are a handful of different progestins used in pills. Two of the newest ones, sometimes referred to as third generation progestins, were designed specifically to have less of an androgenic, or male hormone, effect on the body. It's the progestin that's usually blamed for side effects like weight gain, acne, and unwanted hair growth.

The new progestins (norgestimate and desogestrel) were under a cloud a couple of years ago, when reports from Europe blamed them for an increase in blood clots. Upon closer analysis of the data, they have been exonerated. One fact that threw a monkey wrench into the original numbers: In Europe, women were taking the Pill who would not be considered good candidates in this country. It is worth noting, however, that all birth control pills approximately triple the risk of blood clots, although you're tripling a very small number. "Probably an additional 12 per 100,000 users annually would experience a blood clot, usually without major consequences," estimates Dr. Kaunitz. "To put that in perspective, pregnancy increases clot risk six times, or twice as much as the Pill."

With traditional Pill packs, which are designed to last a month apiece, every tablet contains exactly the same dose, and you take one every day for 3 weeks. Then there's a week off, when you take either no pills or placebo pills from your pack. During this "hormone withdrawal," the uterine lining sloughs off and you get a period—though not a true period, since no egg has been released.

Beyond the fact that we're all accustomed to menstrual cycles being about 28 days long, there's nothing magical or medically necessary about this three-week-on, one-week-off cycle. Oral contraceptives were developed to mimic the menstrual cycle because Pill manufacturers believed that women would want to have a period. In theory, you can safely take the pills for several months without a monthly bleeding break. In fact, some doctors prescribe such a regimen for patients with certain conditions, like endometriosis or debilitating menstrual cramps. (Naturally, you should try this only under a physician's guidance.)

In recent years, we've seen some new variations on the old Pill theme: With so-called cyclic or phasic pills, the amount of estrogen and/or progestin varies over the 3 weeks to more closely mimic natural hormone surges. And one new pill, called Mircette, really veers from the norm: Instead of a full week "off," it has just 2 hormone-free days, followed by 5 days of pills containing a half-dose of estrogen.

Who Shouldn't Take the Pill

There are, of course, some women who should not touch the Pill. Heading the list are smokers over the age of 35. Please don't cheat; the cardiovascular risks really do rise with this combo. "The Pill's safe; smoking stinks," is the way one expert put it.

Also, if you've had a stroke or heart attack, the Pill is not for you. Women who have health problems that affect the cardiovascular system—high blood pressure, diabetes, certain types of migraines—are almost always better off using a different method. (Dr. Mercer does believe that some women with high blood pressure can take the Pill if their pressure is well-controlled by a single medication.)

Sometimes progestin-only mini-pills are an alternative, since it's the estrogen in regular combination pills that's thought to be responsible for any effect

The Right Pill for the Right Problem

For most women, experts say, any low-dose oral contraceptive will do an excellent job of preventing pregnancy. If you're already taking a particular pill and you're happy with it, don't mess with success. But there are some symptoms and situations where the subtle differences between pill formulas may make a difference. Here are suggested substitutes and tips from doctors on sidestepping irksome side effects and handling special situations.

Acne. It has long been recognized that many oral contraceptives help soothe troubled skin, but only Ortho has actually gone to the trouble and expense of documenting the proof and getting FDA approval for it. Ortho Tri-Cyclen is the only pill specifically approved for acne.

Spotting. A little light bleeding during the cycle is a start-up symptom that usually stops in 2 to 3 months. If not, a pill with slightly more estrogen—up from 20 micrograms to 30 or 35—or Mircette, with its little bit of estrogen during the off week, might do the trick.

Lax libido. It's not common for the Pill to have a negative impact on libido, but it can happen—probably because of the decrease in androgen levels. Much more often, something else is to blame—relationship problems, job stress, kids, lack of sleep, a drug side effect (antidepressants head that list). But if the Pill seems to be the culprit, you might try one with a different progestin—perhaps an "old" (more androgenic) one, such as Ortho-Novum 7/7/7 or Triphasil.

"Nuisance" symptoms. Symptoms such as breast tenderness, nausea, and headaches are more common during the first several months on any new pill but usually disappear after 2 to 3 months. If not, a pill with just 20 micrograms of estrogen (like Alesse) might work better for you.

on the blood vessels. Recent studies on the new very low dose pills (20 micrograms), though, suggest that they have absolutely no effect on blood vessel linings, according to Dr. Mercer.

Women on certain medications have to be careful about Pill use, too. The birth control authority *Contraceptive Technology* lists more than a dozen drugs—everything from acetaminophen, alcohol, and megadoses of vitamin C to antidepressants, corticosteroids, and asthma drugs—that can potentially interact with oral contraceptives, either intensifying or lessening the effect of the Pill or of the other drug. The experts also say that significant effects are very unusual, except with three specific drugs: Dilantin, for seizures; griseofulvin, for fungal infections; and rifampin, an antibiotic used to treat tuberculosis. Each of these can lessen the Pill's effectiveness enough to warrant a back-up method of birth control or a switch to another method. (Always keep your gynecologist and any other doctors you see apprised of your use of the

Excessive hair growth. This is one sign of a pill with a bit more of an androgenic (male hormone) effect. If that's a problem for you, try one with a new progestin, such as Desogen, Ortho Tri-Cyclen, Ortho-Cyclen, Ortho-Cept, or Mircette.

Weight gain. Studies show that women are just as likely to lose weight as to gain it. The experts advise eating carefully and healthfully, particularly during the first few "adjustment" months on oral contraceptives, to ease your body's adaptation. Both estrogen and progestin have been blamed for weight gain: In theory, estrogen could encourage "female" fat buildup on hips and thighs; progestins might increase appetite, according to the birth control authority *Contraceptive Technology*. A pill with a different estrogen/progestin balance, or one with less of both, may have less effect on weight.

Migraines or cramps. Mircette, the new pill with the short hormone-free interval, as the experts call it, can be a godsend for women who get menstrual migraines, which seem to be largely caused by estrogen withdrawal. (Note, however, that not all women with migraines can take the Pill.) Another approach: Take the Pill you're already on without a break for several months straight. Fewer periods will mean fewer migraines. The same strategy also works for women with incapacitating menstrual cramps. As always, it's important to run your game plan by your doctor.

Nursing moms. Progestin-only mini-pills such as Micronor, Ovrette, and NorQD are safe for nursing moms, who can start them as soon as 2 to 4 weeks after delivery. Since they are slightly less effective in preventing pregnancy and have a higher likelihood of breakthrough bleeding, most women will want to go back to combination pills after the baby is weaned.

Pill and other medications—including over-the-counter drugs, vitamin supplements, and herbal treatments—just in case there could be a problem.)

Here's a surprise: Although women who have had breast cancer should not take the Pill, age alone is no longer an issue. "There's no such thing as being on the Pill too long," says Dr. Kaunitz. "It's perfectly safe to use the Pill straight into menopause, as long as you're healthy and do not smoke."

Cancer Fear Unfounded

That leads to the question: What about the feared link between oral contraceptives and breast cancer? (Almost a third of women associate the Pill with an increased cancer risk, according to the Gallup survey cited above.) There's good news in this department, too, from a mammoth study conducted at Oxford University that reanalyzed more than 90 percent of the research (some 54 studies involving more than 150,000 subjects) published worldwide on the subject of breast cancer risk and oral contraceptive use. The data, says Dr. Kaunitz, "demonstrated convincingly that a decade or more after women stop taking the Pill, which is to say as women get into that time in their lives when breast cancer becomes more prevalent, there was no increased risk of breast cancer." This held true no matter what type of pill women took, how long they used it, or even—perhaps most significantly—if they had a family history of breast cancer.

It's natural that women fear breast cancer, says Dr. Connell, "but they don't have the risk in perspective. The irony of it to me is that women will pass up proven protection against two major killers—endometrial cancer and ovarian cancer—because of the unproven possibility of an increased risk of breast cancer."

When it comes to ovarian cancer, in fact, Dr. Mercer goes so far as to recommend the Pill for women who have a family history of the disease, a strategy bolstered by a recent study. "If you have one first-degree relative with ovarian cancer, it markedly increases your risk. If you have two, your chances are more than quadrupled—from a 1.6 percent to 8 percent lifetime risk. But if you take birth control pills for up to 9 years, you cut that risk in half; if you take them for 10 years or more, you actually reduce it to normal." This is yet more proof that birth control pills have earned a rightful place in your medicine chest.

What Alternative Medicine Can Do for You

Alternative medicine. By the very nature of the words, it sounds odd. Out there. But when you come right down to it, alternative medicine is very simply this: any sort of healing that's not typically found in the office of your M.D. It's not necessarily odd at all. It's just different. Of course, different can be disconcerting. So whether your M.D. has recently begun recommending herbal remedies or you're considering a visit to an alternative practitioner, you deserve to know what works—and what to expect. Here's a consumer-friendly guide to seven of the hottest cures in the alternative medicine arena.

Acupuncture: Restore Your *Qi*

How can becoming a human pincushion possibly make you healthy? The answer is that those hair-thin needles inserted just under your skin are actually stimulating the flow of a life-giving energy called *qi* (pronounced chee). Chinese medical practitioners believe that this *qi* flows through meridians (invisible channels in your body) to nourish your organs and limbs. When these meridians become blocked by unhealthy living or injury, the result is illness and pain. Acupuncturists believe that inserting the needles at specific points along the meridians restores the flow of *qi*—and your overall health.

Mystical as it sounds, this ancient treatment is well-researched and accepted. In 1997, a consensus panel at the National Institutes of Health (NIH) concluded that acupuncture can help treat the nausea of pregnancy, chemotherapy, and surgery as well as postoperative dental pain. And although solid evidence is still lacking for its success in treating other problems, some researchers feel that it may also relieve the pain of arthritis, headaches, menstrual cramps, back injury, and fibromyalgia. It may even lessen the symptoms associated with withdrawal from drug and alcohol addictions.

Although many Western scientists don't attribute its action to qi, they know that acupuncture triggers the release of endorphins—the body's natural pain relievers. Plus, it may release the mood-lifting brain chemical serotonin and the anti-inflammatory hormone cortisol.

The needles used are extremely thin and flexible. So while inserting them might sting a bit, the needles don't really hurt. Treatment lasts from 15 to 60 minutes. The practitioner may twirl the needles for greater effect. Make sure the acupuncturist uses disposable needles to avoid infection.

Qualifications: Look for certification by the National Commission for the Certification of Acupuncture and Oriental Medicine or an M.D. with 200 hours of acupuncture training.

Licensure: Most states provide licensing or certification. States currently without regulations on acupuncture include Idaho, Oklahoma, South Dakota, and Wyoming.

Cost: $35 to $125 per session.

Insurance coverage: Increasingly covered. In 1997, the NIH consensus panel on acupuncture recommended that it be covered by Medicare.

Ayurveda: Live Right for Your Type

Dubbed the "science of life" 5,000 years ago in India, Ayurveda may be the oldest medical system in existence. Its premise is that your body's biological intelligence (or ability to heal itself) acts through three forces called doshas. These are *vata* (space and air), *pitta* (fire and water), and *kapha* (water and earth).

All of us are made of a combination of these doshas, giving us a special metabolic type—or *pakruti*, as it's known in Ayurveda. Most folks have one dosha that dominates and gives them characteristics associated with their primary elements. *Vata* people, for instance, are thin and energetic; *pittas* tend to be hot tempered; and *kaphas* are slow and solid.

So long as your doshas remain balanced, your health is fine, say ayurvedic doctors. But high stress, a diet of fast-food hamburgers, and even changing seasons can throw them off balance, and that, in turn, causes the symptoms of disease. Generally, ayurvedic practitioners use herbs, meditation, exercise, diet, and other treatments to restore your dosha's balance and thus make you well.

Ayurveda is best known for disease prevention, and centuries of anecdotal evidence suggest that it can also treat many chronic diseases. Unfortunately, there are few clinical studies to verify this, though some research has shown that meditation, exercise, and many of the herbs that are used in Ayurveda will help lower blood pressure, cholesterol, and stress.

If you go to an Ayurvedic practitioner, expect to spend 45 to 90 minutes answering all kinds of questions about your interests, emotions, and lifestyle. The practitioner will also take your pulse and may take urine, blood, or stool samples as part of the diagnosis. He or she may even analyze your tongue to assess your health.

Qualifications: A Bachelor of Ayurvedic Medicine and Surgery degree from India, which equals 5½ years of medical school there. U.S. schools don't offer the degree, but some offer courses on Ayurveda as a specialty.

Alternative Medicine Gains Acceptance

HEALTH FLASH

If you're new to alternative medicine, you may be wondering, "What's the major draw?" It's simple: Its practitioners generally take a holistic approach to your health. If you have asthma, for example, an alternative practitioner won't just see constricted airways and give you an inhaler; he'll see a person whose body isn't working as it should. He'll examine your diet, exercise habits, lifestyle, environment, and mental state to find the root of the problem, then suggest noninvasive remedies like herbs or massage to solve it.

Of course, along with draws come drawbacks. And alternative medicine's biggest drawbacks are:

❖ Fewer studies support its claims than do those of mainstream medicine.
❖ Insurance companies rarely cover it.
❖ One treatment can work well for one person but not at all for another.

Combine these drawbacks with the fact that these whole-body remedies usually work more slowly than symptom-specific drugs, and you can see why many people are intrigued but cautious.

The good news is that conventional doctors are starting to see the value of alternative medicine. Workshops, seminars, and lectures on alternative health care are being held across the country—each triggering more discussion and debate. As doctors weigh the pros and cons, many are beginning to accept the notion that alternative medicine can complement their current healing methods.

Licensure: None in the United States.

Cost: $40 to $100 for the initial consultation.

Insurance coverage: Generally limited to M.D.'s or other licensed practitioners who specialize in Ayurveda.

Chiropractic: Manipulating Your Health

If there is strength in numbers, chiropractic is one of the strongest alternative health care professions. With approximately 50,000 practitioners in the United States, chiropractors are second only to medical physicians in providing primary care. While chiropractic theory focuses on enhancing the body's ability to heal itself, today's chiropractors deal largely with spine-related problems of a neuromusculoskeletal nature. They use spinal adjustments to care for problems such as headaches, neck pain, back pain, chronic pain, and pain from injuries.

You probably know how common back pain is. It strikes about 80 percent of us at some point in our lives, which may explain why one in three people has tried chiropractic care. And now the Agency for Health Care Policy and Research agrees that spinal manipulation can indeed help lower-back pain. There are no well-controlled studies, however, to support that manipulation relieves gastrointestinal distress, breathing troubles, and other nonmechanical problems.

Chiropractors—by choice of their profession—don't prescribe drugs, but you can expect them to use x-rays when clinically necessary.

If you go to a chiropractor, you're in for a physical experience. The chiropractor will adjust or manipulate your joints and spine to correct any misalignment. On the average, it takes 5 to 10 treatments before you can expect to see results, depending on your condition.

Qualifications: Look for a licensed Doctor of Chiropractic who is a member of either the American Chiropractic Association or the International Chiropractors Association. All doctors of chiropractic must have a state-issued license.

Licensure: Chiropractors are licensed in every state.

Cost: $50 to $100 for the initial visit and $25 to $65 for follow-ups.

Insurance coverage: Most insurances, including Medicare and many state Medicaid programs, cover chiropractic.

Homeopathy: The Ultimate Paradox

Homeopathy is based on the idea that what causes your illness will cure it. If that sounds strange, keep in mind that doctors use Ritalin—a stimulant—to keep hyperactive children calm.

Who Will Pay?

Though millions of Americans have embraced alternative medicine, many insurance policies still have not. But that's changing every day. American Western Life Insurance Company of Foster City, California, now covers an array of alternative therapies, including Ayurveda and massage, while HMOs such as Oxford Health Plans have started expanding their coverage, too. So does your insurance company cover alternative medicine? There's only one way to know: Give them a call.

How does it work? Let's say you have the flu. A homeopathic doctor would give you very tiny amounts of a potent homeopathic remedy, such as arsenic, that causes flulike symptoms such as diarrhea, cramping, and chills. The idea is that this will kick your immune system into high gear. The arsenic remedy itself won't make you sick because homeopathic remedies, which include a wide array of poisons, are so diluted that not one molecule of the original substance should remain.

Homeopaths will be the first to admit that they don't always know how their remedies work. But studies show that some homeopathic remedies do work. Those studies, however, the majority of which are foreign, have been criticized for poor design.

Right now, the most convincing evidence for homeopathy is for problems like diarrhea, flu, hay fever, recovery from surgery, headache, and menstrual and menopausal discomfort—and perhaps arthritis and other types of pain. Homeopathic remedies are regulated by the Food and Drug Administration and manufactured by drug companies under strict guidelines. Sales of these remedies are growing by more than 20 percent each year.

One big downside to homeopathy is that everyone responds differently to remedies, so it may take several months of experimenting to find the right treatment for a chronic problem. If you choose a homeopathic doctor, expect to be asked to get up close and personal: The average initial visit lasts up to 1½ hours and is as much a psychological profile about your fears and reactions to the environment as it is a medical history.

Qualifications: Look for a physician who is a Diplomate in Homeotherapeutics; a naturopath who is a Diplomate of the Homeopathic Academy of Naturopathic Physicians; or other practitioners who are certified in classic homeopathy.

Licensure: Three states require licensure (Arizona, Connecticut, and Nevada). Other states allow providers to practice homeopathy as a specialty under another medical license, as is the case with an M.D. or doctor of osteopathic medicine (D.O.) who practices homeopathy.

Cost: About $140 for the initial visit and $55 for follow-ups.

rage: Most insurance companies reimburse for homeopathy by an M.D. or D.O. Call your insurer to find out.

c Medicine: Prevention First

ledicine were an art form, naturopathy would be its mosaic. multifaceted practitioners are trained in an array of therapies including clinical nutrition, herbal medicine, homeopathy, Ayurveda, Chinese medicine, acupuncture, massage, and conventional care.

Naturopathic physicians (also known as naturopaths) pride themselves on first preventing disease. That means replacing bad habits like smoking with good ones like exercising. They also stress learning how to harness your body's healing powers through herbs, healthy living, and natural foods.

What you won't find in most naturopaths' offices are prescription pads (although some states do give them limited prescribing authority). If you should get sick, count on your naturopath to use every natural remedy at his disposal to help your body heal: Acupuncture, herbs, dietary changes, nutritional supplements, exercise, homeopathy, massage, and spinal manipulation may all be included in his healing arsenal. Individually, all of these remedies have evidence to back them up, but because naturopathy incorporates such a vast array of therapies, there are no studies to show how effective it is as a whole.

If you decide to try a naturopath, you may have to search a little for a practitioner, since there are only about 1,500 in the United States. Once you've found one, expect to spend at least an hour at your initial visit talking about all the factors that can affect your health, including exercise, diet, medical history, genetics, stress, exposure to pollutants, and emotional state. A naturopath will also use tests you'll recognize—x-rays, blood tests, and urinalysis, among others. When necessary, naturopathic physicians will refer you to M.D.'s and other health care professionals.

Qualifications: Find a licensed Doctor of Naturopathy.

Licensure: Licensing is required in 11 states.

Cost: $30 to $175 for the initial consultation.

Insurance coverage: Many companies cover naturopathic services. Call yours to be sure.

Osteopathy: Aligned for Health

If you're basically comfortable with conventional care but wish your physician relied a little less on prescription drugs and a little more on hands-on healing, a doctor of osteopathic medicine may be the way to go. Osteopathic physicians (also known as osteopaths) graduate from medical school, complete residencies, and pass certification exams just like M.D.'s. They can prescribe drugs and perform surgery. What D.O.'s have that M.D.'s don't is specialized training in osteopathic manipulation—techniques that osteopaths say can heal ligaments, muscles, and connective tissue.

Osteopaths believe that when it comes to health and healing, our musculoskeletal system gets short shrift. They say you can prevent and treat problems if your bones, vertebrae, ligaments, and tendons are lined up and working properly.

There's evidence that osteopathy may be effective for treating back and neck pain and injuries, plus headaches and menstrual cramps. It may also help with diseases like high blood pressure, arthritis, and digestive problems, though more research is needed in these areas.

Unfortunately, research on osteopathy's effectiveness in treating any one specific ailment is in short supply. Osteopaths also admit that some people have more success with osteopathic manipulation than others, so you should be prepared to give it three to five treatments before you decide whether or not it works for you.

Since D.O.'s have the same training as M.D.'s, you can see an osteopath for any problem for which you would call your family doctor. If you see a D.O., expect her to check the texture of your connective tissue, your posture, your range of motion, and other factors that reflect your skeletal health. She'll also take your medical history. And she may prescribe anything from prescription drugs and manipulation to at-home exercise as your treatment.

Qualifications: Look for a Doctor of Osteopathic Medicine.

Licensure: Osteopathic physicians are licensed in all 50 states.

Cost: $55 to $95 per session.

Insurance coverage: Osteopathic medicine is generally reimbursed the same as care from an M.D.

Traditional Chinese Medicine: Perfect Balance

In the eyes of traditional Chinese medicine (TCM), every person is a miniature universe. You are yin and yang—two complementary forces like day and night. And your body is the interaction of five universal elements: water, fire, wood, metal, and earth.

Fortunately, a river of life-giving energy known as *qi* flows through you, pulling all these elements together. When it does its job and the elements are in balance, you have good health, say practitioners of TCM. But when bacteria, an injury, or an unhealthy lifestyle throws these elements out of whack, you have disease—at which point a TCM practitioner's response will be to use acupuncture, medicinal herbs, massage, diet, and a movement meditation such as tai chi to restore balance and, consequently, health.

Since doctors can't find yin, yang, fire, or *qi* on an x-ray or in a test tube, TCM as a system is impossible to study by Western standards. What experts can study is the effectiveness of individual treatments like acupuncture, which has been extensively researched and found to be useful for a variety of conditions.

One major caution surrounding TCM: Don't use Chinese herbs, which you can buy in many Chinese markets, without asking a qualified practitioner about them first. Many can be dangerous if you take them improperly.

If you make an appointment with a TCM practitioner, expect to answer questions about everything from your sleeping patterns to the color and consistency of your menstrual flow. The doctor will listen to your voice and breathing, check your pulse, and inspect your skin, hair, and tongue.

Qualifications: Look for certification by the National Commission for the Certification of Acupuncture and Oriental Medicine or a Doctor of Oriental Medicine degree.

Licensure: Licensing varies widely.

Cost: $75 to $150 for the initial visit and $25 to $100 for follow-ups.

Insurance coverage: Insurance coverage varies widely.

part three

Disease
Defense

3

His and Her Health

Why Women Outlive Men

It's not an old wives' tale that women live longer than men. According to the latest figures from the National Center for Health Statistics, women still have the upper hand when it comes to longevity. Women born in 1975, for instance, can expect to live nearly 8 years longer than men born the same year. And although the gap has been closing slowly over the intervening years—it's down to 5.6 years for those born in 1997—women still live longer. Why?

"Women are more tuned in to their health than men and to any problems they might have," says Royda Crose, Ph.D., author of *Why Women Live Longer Than Men . . . and What Men Can Learn from Them.* "They notice when their bodies are out of whack and try to do something formally to correct the problems.

"Because of that," Dr. Crose continues, "they take better care of themselves. If they feel sick, they might take it easy that day. If the illness persists, they call their doctors. By contrast, men are raised to ignore pain or sickness and to work through it. They are applauded for denying their pain and discomfort—acknowledging it is perceived as a sign of weakness. By ignoring the symptoms until they worsen, men delay having a health professional examine them. Logically, the sooner you identify a disease, the greater your chances are of treating it and surviving it."

Women are also more knowledgeable about preventive measures, such as scheduling regular screening exams and following a healthy diet. There's plenty of evidence that a diet low in animal fat and protein and high in a variety of fruits, vegetables, and grains is critical to good health and longevity, says Dr. Crose. "If you follow such a diet, you can lower your risk of the leading causes of death, which are heart disease and cancer. Both men and women know this. Research shows, however, that men eat more meat, fat, dairy products, and eggs than women. By contrast, women eat more fruits, vegetables, grains, and low-calorie foods. The motivation may be to keep their weight in check, but the payoff is that women are living longer."

Other aspects of behavior typical to women—such as establishing social supports, role flexibility, and resilience—may also go hand in hand with better diet to help women live longer, adds Dr. Crose.

10

Is It
Menopause
or Isn't It?

E ver since Cathy was 18, her periods had come so regularly that she'd always been able to plan vacations around them. But now she's in her forties. And last month, her period arrived—off schedule—the day she flew off for a scuba diving adventure.

Cathy has entered perimenopause—a stage of life sometimes called the change before the change. She is one of millions of women between the ages of 40 and 55 who experience irregular menstrual periods and the other symptoms that come with the beginning of the end of their reproductive years.

But Cathy isn't stuck with her symptoms—and neither are you. There are many treatments, from drugs to herbs, that can make perimenopause smooth sailing.

Perimenopause is a distinct phase of a woman's life, doctors say, that usually spans about 4 years, but can last as long as 10.

"Perimenopause is a time when the abnormal becomes normal," says Patricia Y. Allen, M.D., founder and director of the New York Menopause Center in New York City.

"Your menstrual periods may be longer, shorter, heavier, lighter, closer together, or farther apart," says Dr. Allen, who is an assistant attending obstetrician and gynecologist at the New York Hospital-Cornell Medical Center. Also common are hot flashes and night sweats as well as insomnia, irritability, anxiety, forgetfulness, and fatigue.

Just because the symptoms are normal doesn't mean you have to put up with them, though. There are safe prescription drugs, delicious foods, herbal remedies, and even mind/body techniques that can help you better navigate your way through perimenopause. And there's a bonus: They can help during menopause, too.

Symptom 1: Irregular Periods

Who gets them: About 95 percent of perimenopausal women. In fact, an erratic period is considered the classic sign of perimenopause.

What causes them: Fluctuating levels of the female hormones estrogen and progesterone.

The natural solution: Certain chemical compounds in soy foods have an estrogen-like effect and may help relieve symptoms such as irregular periods for some. Aim for one serving of soy a day, such as a soy smoothie made with 1 cup of low-fat soy milk and frozen fruit whirled in the blender, or have 2 tablespoons of roasted soy nuts.

The medical solution: Talk to your doctor about taking low-dose birth-control pills (BCPs). Or try a prescription natural micronized progesterone, says Tracy Gaudet, M.D., executive director of the program in integrative medicine at the University of Arizona in Tucson.

Micronized progesterone is synthesized from soy beans or wild yams and matches your body's own progesterone. It's available by prescription in capsules called Prometrium. It works just as well as the commonly prescribed Provera—a synthetic progesterone called a progestin. But because Prometrium is exactly like the progesterone your body makes, it usually doesn't have the same side effects as synthetic progesterone does, such as breast tenderness, irritability, and bloating.

One caveat: Women should avoid taking BCPs if they smoke cigarettes, have had breast or endometrial cancer, have active liver disease or hepatitis, or have a personal or strong family history of strokes or blood clots. The estrogen in BCPs may aggravate existing health problems, cautions Dr. Allen.

Always report any unusual bleeding to your doctor; though it's usually just a perimenopausal symptom, it can signal something more serious, such as fibroids, endometrial polyps, a thyroid-hormone problem, or even cancer.

Symptom 2: Heavy Bleeding

Who gets it: About 75 percent of perimenopausal women.

What causes it: You're not ovulating regularly, so the uterine lining becomes thicker than usual.

The natural solution: Visualization—really! Relax with a few deep breaths, then close your eyes and picture your uterus, says Dr. Gaudet. Try to imagine the bleeding becoming less and less. Use the first image that comes to mind. "One of my patients visualized faucets throughout her uterus," says the Arizona physician. "She turned them tighter and tighter until the bleeding just stopped."

The medical solution: If bleeding remains a problem, see your doctor to figure out the cause and to ask about taking a natural micronized progesterone such as Prometrium, says Dr. Gaudet. Don't bother with over-the-counter progesterone creams for heavy bleeding: There's no evidence that they work. You should also get a blood test to make sure that you're not anemic.

Symptom 3: Hot Flashes

Who gets them: About 75 percent of perimenopausal women. Some women experience only mild, brief flushes while others suffer frequent, searing bouts of inner heat that make them perspire. (The worst hot flashes tend to occur 2 to 3 years before menopause actually occurs.)

What causes them: Dwindling estrogen. Low estrogen levels affect your body's climate-control center in the brain, upsetting its normal temperature regulation. Experts speculate that when estrogen levels take a dive, the center reads that event as a drop in body temperature. So it turns up your thermostat.

The natural solution: Try 40 milligrams of black cohosh a day. (Larger doses are unnecessary and may be unsafe.) It seems to act like estrogen in the body, says Dr. Gaudet. If you're not taking blood thinners, you should also take 400 international units (IU) of vitamin E daily. Try that dosage for a month, recommends Dr. Gaudet. If you still get flashes, boost it to 800 IU.

The medical solution: The medical options include low-dose BCPs.

Chill a Hot Flash in 60 Seconds

Heat surges pouring through your body can drive you nuts. Here are some simple strategies to smash the flash.

❖ Take several long, deep breaths and imagine yourself totally naked, sliding through soft, cold snow down the gentle slope of a mountain.
❖ Just breathe—deep belly breaths six to eight times a minute. Studies show that this alone can reduce hot flashes in some women.
❖ Suck on an ice cube.
❖ Drink a big glass of ice water.
❖ Keep a mini-fan handy for those heat waves.
❖ Take off any piece of clothing you can. Be creative: There are some things you can take off that no one else will notice!

Dong Quai Flunks Hot Flash Study

Dong quai (*Angelica sinensis*) is one of the most popular herbs in China, where it is used for the treatment of almost every gynecological ailment, including menopausal symptoms. Until recently, it had never been tested in the West.

In a study of 71 postmenopausal women with hot flashes, half took 4.5 grams of dong quai root daily for 12 weeks and half got a placebo (a worthless substitute). Although hot flashes decreased in both groups, there was no statistical difference between the dong quai group and the placebo group.

Symptom 4: Night Sweats

Who gets them: Almost anyone who gets hot flashes. Night sweats are simply hot flashes that occur at night while you sleep.

What causes them: Dwindling levels of estrogen.

The natural and medical solutions: The same things you do for hot flashes.

Symptom 5: Sleep Disturbances

Who gets them: About 70 percent of perimenopausal women.

What causes them: If you can't fall asleep, chances are the sense of uncertainty that often accompanies this time of physical transition has placed your sympathetic nervous system on the alert. If you wake during the night, it's a good bet that a hot flash roused you from sleep.

The natural solution: Use a mind/body relaxation technique every night before bed and when you wake during the night, recommends Dr. Gaudet. See "The Woman Doctor's Survival Guide for Perimenopause" on page 70 for more information on one such technique.

Women who train themselves to do a relaxation technique usually report that they're sleeping better within 3 weeks, says Ann Webster, Ph.D., a health psychologist who runs a clinic for perimenopausal and menopausal women at Beth Israel-Deaconess Medical Center in Boston.

If you're having a particularly difficult time sleeping, try taking valerian about 45 minutes before bed, suggests Dr. Gaudet. Try ½ to 1 teaspoon of tincture in water or juice. Also eliminate caffeine and alcohol after 5:00 P.M., says Dr. Allen.

Finally, don't forget the wonderful benefits of exercise. Regular exercise not only makes you feel and look better but also reduces stress and helps you sleep, says Dr. Webster.

The medical solution: Low-dose BCPs can boost declining estrogen levels and eliminate the hot flashes that disrupt sleep. Natural micronized progesterone taken 30 minutes before bed may promote sleep for some, says Dr. Allen.

Symptom 6: Irritability and Anxiety

Who gets them: There are no available figures, but the doctors who treat perimenopausal women say these emotional symptoms do occur, especially among women whose sleep is disturbed by night sweats.

What causes them: Fluctuating hormone levels, which can affect your general sense of well-being, or unresolved worries and concerns during this transition time.

The natural solution: Take a deep breath. Give yourself some breathing space, too, advises Dr. Gaudet. You need time to work out issues that emerge during perimenopause.

The Woman Doctor's Survival Guide for Perimenopause

HEALTH FLASH

Following just three simple strategies during perimenopause will make you less likely to have troublesome symptoms, says Tracy Gaudet, M.D., executive director of the program in integrative medicine at the University of Arizona in Tucson. Try these for relief.

Slip off the bonds of stress. Practice a mind/body relaxation technique twice a day, once in the morning and once at night. One of the easiest is an ancient technique in which you close your eyes, breathe in through your nostrils to the count of four, hold for a count of seven, and breathe out again through your nostrils for a count of eight. Repeat the sequence four times in a row.

Snack on flax. Flaxseed contains substances called lignan precursors that your body turns into weak estrogens. Added to your own dwindling supply, this may help balance your shifting hormones. Try 1 tablespoon of ground flaxseed on your cereal or salad. Grind it right before eating.

Hit the road. Walk, run, bike, or swim. Choose whatever type of pulse-accelerating exercise you like, but do some form of moderate-intensity exercise three times a week (or more) for 30 minutes at a stretch. No one understands just how exercise reduces perimenopausal problems, only that it does.

Is There Menopause after Hysterectomy?

Menopause may come earlier if you've had a hysterectomy but kept your ovaries. Some experts believe it may occur about 2 years sooner than normal because of changes in blood flow to the pelvis after surgery. So although you won't see menstrual cycle changes, you may still experience hot flashes and other typical menopausal symptoms. Without the absence of a menstrual period to help you know when you've reached menopause, a blood test to measure your estradiol and follicle-stimulating hormone levels can be useful.

Hormones aside, middle age is a topsy-turvy time when you may find yourself facing—and making—many changes in all parts of your life, from your career to your family to your relationships. Your kids may be gone or going, your career stalled or soaring, and your relationships stale or finally sparking. You also may find you're less tolerant of what once seemed like petty annoyances. After toting up your "years left," you may simply feel you don't want to put up with some things anymore.

If you're having a particularly stressful day, you may want to try the herb kava. Because of its potency, don't use it for everyday anxieties or to cover up problems that need to be addressed. And don't use kava in combination with alcohol, barbiturates, or other agents that depress the central nervous system. Look for a standardized product containing kavapyrones. Stay within the standard dose of 60 to 120 milligrams of kavapyrones or follow the label directions.

Symptom 7: Forgetfulness and Poor Concentration

Who gets them: About 50 percent of perimenopausal women—particularly those who are losing sleep because of night sweats, which can leave them feeling permanently jet-lagged.

What causes them: Fluctuating hormones or the craziness of the life transition.

The natural solution: "Learning to be mindful, focused, and in the present by paying attention to all of your senses is the best way of combating forgetfulness and poor concentration," advises Dr. Webster.

Another way to improve concentration and alertness is to use techniques that elicit the relaxation response: Close your eyes, take a deep breath through your nose, then exhale through your mouth. Focus your mind on a single word that has meaning to you, preferably a word related to your faith. Mentally repeat the word on every indrawn breath. If your mind wanders—which is guaranteed the first few times you do it—just gently bring it back to the word. After 10 minutes or so, open your eyes.

You might also want to consider using the herb panax ginseng, says Dr. Gaudet. Ginseng has an estrogen-like effect on the body. In Chinese medicine, it is used as a daily tonic to help balance some of the forces at work during perimenopause. Choose a product containing 4 to 7 percent ginsenosides and take a 100-milligram capsule once or twice a day.

Symptom 8: Tiredness

Who gets it: Nearly 50 percent of perimenopausal women.

What causes it: Changes in sleep patterns that are caused by hormonal fluctuations or night sweats. It's no wonder: Many women are waking up three or four times a night to cool themselves off. It's normal that they won't have any more energy the next day than they did when they got up at night with a newborn.

The natural solution: Take a brisk walk. Studies indicate that women who do some type of moderate-intensity exercise three times a week for 30 minutes at a stretch will have fewer symptoms and more energy during perimenopause, says Dr. Gaudet.

If you still need a boost, try ginseng, suggests Dr. Gaudet. But for a quick shot of energy whenever you need it most, try this breathing technique: Put one hand on your belly. Quickly breathe in and out through your nose, pushing your belly against your hand with each breath. Keep the breaths short and fast. It's just like panting during labor, except that this time you're using your nose instead of your mouth.

The medical solution: Always get checked out by your doctor if you're feeling fatigued. It may be a sign of anemia, especially if you've had heavy bleeding, or it could be a symptom of another medical condition such as a thyroid problem.

The New Breast Cancer Drugs: Are They for You?

11

P op a pill to prevent breast cancer? That dream edged closer to reality when two major studies found two drugs that could slash a woman's risk of breast cancer almost in half—or more.

In one study, tamoxifen (Nolvadex), a hormonal drug used for decades to treat breast cancer, reduced the incidence of developing breast cancer by 45 percent in women considered at high risk for the disease. Preliminary findings of the other study showed that raloxifene (Evista), recently approved by the U.S. Food and Drug Administration (FDA) to prevent bone loss in post-menopausal women, reduced the incidence of breast cancer by almost 60 percent in women considered at normal risk. Further, new drugs now being developed may be even better at preventing the disease that kills 43,500 women a year.

When those dramatic findings were announced, however, they raised as many questions as hopes. Perhaps you wondered: "Are these drugs right for me?" "Do they have any side effects?" "Can I get them now?"

Here's what the nation's leading experts on breast cancer and women's health have to say.

What Are These Drugs and How Do They Work?

Tamoxifen and raloxifene are what are called selective estrogen receptor modulators (SERMs). They're synthetic hormones that look enough like estrogen to fool some parts of your body into thinking they are. Like your body's own estrogen, they prevent your bones from thinning, as in osteoporosis. And more good news: They don't encourage cancer cells to grow as your body's own estrogen and the estrogen found in hormone-replacement therapy can.

Tamoxifen has been used in cancer therapy for more than 20 years to slow or stop the growth of breast cancer cells and to prevent recurrence of the disease. After years of research on hundreds of thousands of women, it has become the most widely prescribed drug for treating breast cancer.

Raloxifene, which just recently made its debut as an osteoporosis prevention drug, has fewer years of research behind it and fewer studies indicating its potential to prevent breast cancer.

SERMs prevent breast cancer by latching onto sites in breast cells called

Do You Need Tamoxifen?

The National Cancer Institute (NCI) in Bethesda, Maryland, has developed a computer program that can assist you and your doctor in weighing your need for tamoxifen.

After prompting you to answer a series of questions, such as your age and health history, the program calculates your estimated 5-year and lifetime risk of breast cancer and compares your risk with women who participated in the Breast Cancer Prevention Trial. It also provides information from tamoxifen research studies.

The result may be a suggestion that you discuss tamoxifen and other prevention options further with your doctor. More commonly, it may put you at ease, says Leslie G. Ford, M.D., associate director of the early detection and community oncology program in the division of cancer prevention at NCI. "Most women overestimate their risk of breast cancer," she notes.

The program, called The Breast Cancer Risk Assessment Tool, comes on a standard computer disk for PC or Mac and is available free by completing the Risk Assessment Tool order form on NCI's Web site at www.nci.nih.gov or by calling their toll-free number, (800) 4-CANCER (422-6237).

HEALTH FLASH

estrogen receptors and blocking estrogen from binding to those sites. Think of those receptor sites as a lock and estrogen as the key. In some women, putting the estrogen key into the lock fuels the cell growth that can cause cancer. These drugs also fit into that lock, but for a complex reason, they don't stimulate cell growth. That's why you'll hear them called anti-estrogens. Tamoxifen works in other ways, too, so it may help prevent tumors that aren't affected by estrogen. As D. Lawrence Wickerham, M.D., associate chairman of the National Surgical Adjuvant Breast and Bowel Project (NSABP) in Pittsburgh and conductor of the Breast Cancer Prevention Trial (BCPT) for tamoxifen, explains, "SERMs don't kill breast cancer cells in the traditional sense. But if you have cells that stop growing long enough, they just sort of go away."

Do These Drugs Have Serious Side Effects?

In some cases, tamoxifen and raloxifene do have serious side effects. Women who received tamoxifen in the BCPT (half of the 13,388 participants received the drug, and the other half received a placebo) doubled their chances of developing endometrial cancer, cancer of the lining of the uterus. They also had an almost three times greater chance of developing blood clots in their lungs or major veins—a risk similar to that of hormone-replacement therapy. Seventeen women who took tamoxifen developed clots in their lungs, and two died. Six women in the placebo group developed clots, but none died. Good news for women under 50: Tamoxifen did not increase the risk of these side effects.

No one yet knows for sure how long you need to take tamoxifen to prevent breast cancer. It's very likely that 5 years—the length of time the BCPT was designed to last—will provide the optimum benefits.

Raloxifene appears to have fewer side effects, based on short-term studies. It didn't promote endometrial cancer in the more than 7,000 postmenopausal women who took it, but it did cause a slightly increased risk of blood clots in the lungs, of a similar magnitude to that seen with tamoxifen.

Is Raloxifene the Better Drug?

We won't know which drug is better until we see the results of the head-to-head test of the two drugs that's now being planned. Bottom line: You'll have to wait and see.

If you'd like to enroll in testing, check out the NSABP Web site at www.nsabp.pitt.edu.

Are These Drugs for You?

If you're a premenopausal woman with significant risk factors, the answer may be yes to tamoxifen. It's definitely something you should discuss with your doctor. Even though tamoxifen is FDA-approved only for the treatment of breast cancer, she can still prescribe it for the prevention of breast cancer—something the FDA is also reviewing for approval.

If you're over 50 and at high risk for breast cancer, you may also reap the benefits of tamoxifen, but you have to weigh them against the increased risk for its uncommon but serious side effects.

Raloxifene is not approved by the FDA for any other use than to prevent osteoporosis in postmenopausal women. And as a potential cancer preventive, it has been tested only on postmenopausal women who have no significant risk factors for breast cancer. It's not recommended for premenopausal women because it hasn't been studied in this group, so its safety cannot be assured.

Who's at High Risk?

While there's no easy way to know for sure who's at the most risk for developing breast cancer, researchers use the following guidelines.

In the Breast Cancer Prevention Trial, only women at high risk for developing breast cancer were eligible to participate. This included women age 60 or older. (A woman's risk of breast cancer increases with age.) Also, women 35 to 59 were eligible based on an assessment of the following risk factors.

❖ Number of first-degree relatives (mother, sister, daughter) with history of breast cancer; a higher number equals greater risk
❖ Age at first delivery, if she had children
❖ Age at first menstrual period
❖ Number of benign breast biopsies or breast biopsies showing suspicious cell changes (atypical hyperplasia)
❖ Previous diagnosis with lobular carcinoma in situ, a condition that increases your risk of invasive breast cancer

For example, to qualify, a woman of 35 would need two or more first-degree relatives with breast cancer and would need to have had a benign breast biopsy herself. A woman of 45 would need only one first-degree relative with breast cancer and a benign breast biopsy herself, while a 55-year-old woman would need only one first-degree relative with breast cancer *or* a previous breast biopsy herself. Talk to your doctor about your individual risk.

Is There a Pill in Your Future?

One day, will every woman take an anti–breast-cancer pill along with her daily vitamin and calcium supplements?

These studies are too preliminary to make that prediction. "It's not something where there will be a simple guideline for everyone. It'll never be 'one size fits all,'" cautions Leslie G. Ford, M.D., associate director of the early detection and community oncology program in the division of cancer prevention at the National Cancer Institute.

But don't count it out either. "I think there are better drugs yet to come," says Clifford Hudis, M.D., acting chief of breast cancer medicine service at Memorial Sloan–Kettering Cancer Center in New York City. In fact, he's already working on a next-generation SERM that could be "a better anti–breast-cancer drug with all the benefits of raloxifene as far as helping to prevent osteoporosis."

Alternative to HRT?

Are these drugs a better choice at menopause than hormone-replacement therapy (HRT), which may cause breast cancer?

Taking estrogen, the key component in HRT, is still an effective strategy for preventing osteoporosis and possibly heart disease—both of which rank higher as health risks for the average American woman than breast cancer.

Estrogen is also effective in easing hot flashes and other menopausal symptoms, unlike the SERMs.

But Amy S. Langer, executive director of the National Alliance of Breast Cancer Organizations in New York City, believes these drugs, once tested thoroughly, could herald a new approach to managing menopause, because they give doctors a way to target your particular health risks. In the future, she says, your doctor should assess your individual risk for heart disease, osteoporosis, breast cancer, and other conditions and prescribe medications based on your own personal profile.

Are You at Risk for Skin Cancer?

W hen the freckle on Lisa Burton's upper arm started to change, she went to her family doctor. He said it was nothing. A few years later, when it developed into a sore that never healed, another doctor told her she had eczema.

It wasn't until 8 years later, when she saw a dermatologist and insisted on a biopsy, that Lisa learned that her freckle was actually a melanoma—skin cancer. Every year, more than 41,000 people are diagnosed with melanoma, and 7,300 people die from it.

Miraculously, even though more than a decade had passed since her symptoms first appeared, the diagnosis came in time to save Lisa's life. For that, she credits her own persistence.

It's a recipe that can work for you, too. To beat melanoma, consider the following suggestions.

See a Dermatologist

Studies have shown that dermatologists can identify melanomas with greater accuracy than other doctors. Yet only 40 percent of us take our skin complaints to these highly trained specialists.

Even doctors themselves recognize the problem. In a survey of 355 family physicians in the Toronto area, 56 percent said they lacked the confidence to

Heed the Warning Signs

You may be susceptible to melanoma and not even know it. Consider yourself at special risk if any of the following apply to you, says Thomas Fitzpatrick, M.D., professor emeritus of dermatology at Harvard Medical School.

❖ Moles that are atypical (just one doubles your risk)

❖ Moles that are numerous

❖ Red hair or freckles

❖ Inability to tan

❖ Sunburns (particularly severe ones before age 14)

❖ Family history of melanoma

identify melanoma. Nearly 80 percent said they would have trouble recognizing early or subtle lesions, and a shocking 72 percent didn't even know that an itchy mole can signal a malignancy.

You should see a dermatologist for a full-body screening at least once every 3 years between the ages of 20 and 40, and annually if you're 41 or older.

Check Your Skin

About half of all melanomas are initially discovered by the patient. It has been estimated that regular skin self-examinations reduce death from melanoma by 63 percent.

In fact, when confined to the upper skin layer, melanoma has a nearly 100 percent cure rate. Since melanoma can take anywhere from a couple of months to several years to grow deeper, take advantage of that window of opportunity by regularly checking your skin.

It's also important to listen to your gut feelings. If you have a suspicious mole that your doctor thinks is nothing, get a second opinion—fast. A good dermatologist can help you catch a melanoma in its curable stages.

Finding the Ideal Dermatologist

Look for 10-plus years of experience. As expected, dues-paying pays off. In a recent study, dermatologists who had 10 or more years of clinical experience showed an accuracy rate of 80 percent in diagnosing melanoma, higher than that of senior and junior trainees.

Listen for the right questions. To make an accurate diagnosis, the dermatologist should ask you questions like these: Have you noticed any new moles or a change in the size, color, shape, or sensation of a preexisting mole? Is there a history of skin cancer in your family? Do you tend to burn? What is your history with sunburns? Few or many? Severe or mild?

Expect the doctor to check every inch. Melanoma can occur on any part of your skin, including areas that rarely see the sun, such as the scalp and the bottoms of your feet. Studies have shown that patients who undergo full-body skin exams are 6.4 times more likely to have a melanoma detected than those receiving partial exams.

Pay attention to the ABCD checklist. The American Academy of Dermatology's ABCD checklist is the suggested tool for determining if a lesion is malignant. Moles with any one of these features have melanoma potential.

- ❖ Asymmetry (one half doesn't match the other)
- ❖ Border irregularity (ragged, notched, or blurred edges)
- ❖ Color variation (shades of tan, brown, and black—or even red, blue, or white)
- ❖ Diameter greater than ¼ inch (larger than a pencil eraser)

A recently proposed amendment to this rule includes "E" for elevation or enlargement. Other warning signs can include itching, bleeding, tenderness, or crusting of the mole's surface.

To prevent melanoma—or catch it early—follow these guidelines.

- ❖ Avoid sun as much as possible between 10:00 A.M. and 4:00 P.M.
- ❖ Wear a waterproof sunscreen with a sun protection factor (SPF) of at least 15 and full UVB/UVA protection.
- ❖ Check your skin regularly.
- ❖ See a dermatologist at least once every 3 years for a thorough head-to-toe skin check (annually if you're 41 or older).

Cancer Protection in a Pill?

Y ou've probably seen the claims: "New Cancer Fighter!" "Natural Cancer Fighter!" "May Help Prevent Breast Cancer!" They appear on the labels of all kinds of new products that can be purchased at health food stores and that claim to reduce your risk of cancer.

From humble beginnings—all contain active compounds extracted from everyday foods such as grapes, garlic, and grains—these pills have taken on scientific names. And they come with impressive-sounding scientific pedigrees.

But look more closely and you'll find that the research, though promising and credible, usually stops in the laboratory. While the compounds in these products have prevented or inhibited cancer in test-tube and lab-rat studies, few have ever been tested on people. And of those that have, at least one hasn't yet been proven to do for humans what it did for lab animals.

Have these products been hustled to market too quickly? Are they safe to take? Are the compounds they claim to contain better for you in their original packaging—as garlic, grapes, oats, apples, or grapefruit?

The top researchers in the field of cancer prevention sorted through the evidence. Here's what they discovered.

Garlic Compounds: Improvement with Age

Top food source: Fresh garlic, in any form.

The promise: "May afford protection against cancer."

The research: Aged garlic contains two sulfur compounds—S-allylcysteine (SAC) and S-allylmercaptocysteine (SAMC)—that slowed the growth of breast cancer cells in test-tube studies, says John Pinto, Ph.D., associate professor of biochemistry at Weill Medical College of Cornell University and director of the nutrition research laboratory at Memorial Sloan-Kettering Cancer Center in New York City. Garlic compounds have also suppressed the growth of human prostate cancer cells in test-tube studies, he says.

In other test-tube and animal studies, garlic has inhibited the growth of tumors of the colon, rectum, esophagus, skin, and stomach. Meanwhile, population studies in China, Italy, and the United States have found lower rates of colon and stomach cancers among people who consume raw or cooked garlic on a regular basis.

But SAC and SAMC are just two of 10 to 15 active compounds in garlic that may play roles in reducing cancer risk, Dr. Pinto says. All are made from raw garlic, and all form quickly after garlic's main component, alliin, is converted to the pungent, strongly scented allicin when a clove of garlic is cut or crushed. Allicin itself swiftly decomposes into many compounds, and these compounds quickly form still others. Among these, scientists are finding cancer-fighting potential.

"There's a big controversy among garlic supplement manufacturers and among scientists about which compounds are the key active ingredients in garlic that fight cancer," Dr. Pinto says. "The truth is, no one knows yet. It could be a combination of compounds, or it could be compounds we haven't even discovered yet. We do know that there's much more at work than SAC and SAMC."

One reason that aged garlic has garnered all the headlines is that it's used more often than fresh garlic in research. That's because aged garlic contains standard amounts of SAC and SAMC and lab animals will tolerate it more easily than raw garlic. Researchers have also studied this deodorized supplement because many consumers are put off by the taste, smell, and garlic-breath aftereffects of the real thing.

Will it work for you? Despite the many questions, researchers are pretty enthusiastic about garlic—whether fresh or in supplement form.

Supercharge Your Garlic

Get more cancer-battling compounds from your garlic: Let chopped or crushed garlic cloves stand at room temperature for about 15 minutes before cooking. This "rest" gives the potent compounds time to form.

"It's rare to come across a single food such as garlic that has been proven to provide considerable protection against the development of gastric and colon cancers in two kinds of studies—basic research and population studies," says Michael Wargovich, Ph.D., professor of pathology and director of basic research at the South Carolina Cancer Center at the University of South Carolina in Columbia. "I'd say it's important to get garlic—and other vegetables from the allium family such as onions and shallots—on a regular basis."

The safety factor: All garlic is safe.

The bottom line: Have some form of garlic every week or, better yet, every other day, Dr. Wargovich suggests. "We don't know how much is the right dosage, but population studies show that people who eat more garlic have more protection."

What kind of garlic? "Both fresh and deodorized aged garlic contain compounds that work against cancer in lab studies," says garlic researcher John Milner, Ph.D., head of the nutrition department at Pennsylvania State University in State College.

"If you want extra insurance or can't tolerate fresh garlic, take any deodorized garlic supplement," Dr. Pinto suggests.

Calcium D-Glucarate: Does It Work in Humans?

Top food sources: Apples, grapefruit, broccoli and other cruciferous vegetables, and bean sprouts.

The promise: Glucarate is the main ingredient in products advertised for women concerned with breast health and for former smokers. Marketing suggests that glucarate may help your body fight off breast cancer by regulating estrogen levels and may help prevent lung cancer by facilitating binding of carcinogens and tumor promoters with glucuronic acid to form glucuronides, which are then excreted from the body. This important process is called glucuronidation.

The research: While researchers at top cancer centers say glucarate may hold promise for reducing cancer risk, the evidence comes almost exclusively from test-tube and animal studies. And it hasn't been supported by human studies so far.

In several animal studies by biochemist Zbigniew Walaszek, Ph.D., conducted at the University of Texas M. D. Anderson Cancer Center in Smithville, rats fed glucarate after treatment with a cancer-causing agent developed fewer breast cancer tumors than rats who didn't get glucarate; some existing tumors also shrank. In other rat and mouse studies, glucarate inhibited all phases in the development of colon, lung, and skin cancers. Glucarate also slows prostate cancer in animals, says Dr. Walaszek, now a scientist at the AMC Cancer Research Center in Denver.

Glucarate seems to work, in part, by inhibiting the process that frees cancer-promoting hormones, such as estrogen and testosterone, from their inactive forms (glucuronides) and preventing the free hormones from being excreted to circulate in the bloodstream. "If you lower levels of these steroid hormones or increase levels of their inactive glucuronides, the growth of some cancers slows or stops," says Dr. Walaszek.

So far, however, this effect of glucarate has not been demonstrated in humans, says researcher Alexandra Simkovich Heerdt, M.D., director of the surveillance program for women at high breast cancer risk at Memorial

A Hot New Supplement for Men's Health

Selenium, a mineral found naturally in varying quantities in meat, dairy foods, and grains, cut the risk of lung, prostate, and colorectal cancers in half for those who took a 200-microgram supplement daily for 10 years.

Supplement takers—who were mostly men—also had about half the risk of cancer death and one-third the risk of getting any form of cancer compared with those who didn't receive selenium, says lead investigator Larry C. Clark, Ph.D., an epidemiologist at the Arizona Cancer Center in Tucson.

A newer study from the Health Professionals Follow-Up Study at Harvard University bolsters selenium's role in cutting prostate cancer risk. Researchers found that among 33,737 men, those with the lowest selenium levels in toenail clippings had twice the risk of men with the highest levels.

Since selenium levels in food aren't consistent (most Americans get about 100 micrograms a day), adding a supplement may sound like a good idea. But this "good guy" mineral has a dark side.

"The margin of safety for selenium is very narrow," says Bernard Levin, M.D., vice president for cancer prevention at the University of Texas M. D. Anderson Cancer Center in Smithville. Taking too much can be toxic. The evidence is that up to 200 micrograms a day from food is safe, and the amounts in most multivitamins are safe.

People with kidney disorders should not take additional selenium, Dr. Clark says.

If you're going to take a supplement, look for one with high-selenium yeast, as opposed to inorganic sodium selenite, suggests Dr. Clark. The yeast may be more active in the body.

HEALTH FLASH

Sloan–Kettering. In her study, women with a family history of breast cancer were given 10 grams of calcium D-glucarate a day.

"If it had been working, we would have found higher levels of estrogen and glucarate in their urine, indicating that more estrogen was being excreted from the body," Dr. Heerdt says. "But levels did not rise very much. Because of this, we did not proceed with the next level of human testing."

Still, Dr. Heerdt says, glucarate is promising; it just needs more research. "We may need a different form, a different dose, or a different way to deliver it," she speculates.

Answers may be on the way. Dr. Walaszek will begin a study of glucarate's effect on lung cancer risk in humans soon. He also plans to study breast cancer risk and glucarate intake in women.

Will it work for you? "For now, I would say calcium D-glucarate in the forms available is not effective at reducing breast cancer risk," Dr. Heerdt says. And until the results from the other studies are in, no one really knows if it will help other cancers either.

The safety factor: At the recommended dosage of 200 milligrams a day, the amount of glucarate in over-the-counter supplements seems safe, Dr. Heerdt says. "The women in our study got much more than that a day with no toxicity," she says. It's also not far from the amount you'd get every day from a fruit- and vegetable-rich diet.

The bottom line: "I tell my patients to eat a low-fat diet rich in fruits and vegetables, including citrus, which contain calcium D-glucarate," Dr. Heerdt says. "This kind of diet may reduce cancer risk, and it can lower heart disease risk, so you can't go wrong."

Inositol Hexaphosphate: Good Research but Not Enough

Top food sources: Whole grains, including rice, oats, wheat, and corn; nuts, seeds, and beans.

The promise: Advertising calls inositol hexaphosphate (IP6) "a natural cancer fighter" that can increase the activity of natural killer cells. The leading researcher claims that it transforms cancer cells into normal ones.

The research: Studies conducted in test tubes and on rats, mice, and human cancer cells implanted in laboratory animals back up the supplement-maker's claim. But so far, there have been no human cancer studies.

"In every cell line we tested, including breast, colon, lung, and liver cancers, IP6 showed that it can inhibit cancer," says lead IP6 investigator Abul Kalam M. Shamsuddin, M.D., professor of pathology at the University of Maryland School of Medicine in Baltimore.

Delicious Cancer Protection

One single serving of a food rich in beta-carotene every day could help you avoid breast cancer, suggests a new Swedish study of women over 50. Women who consumed at least 3.7 milligrams of beta-carotene a day from food—about half a carrot's worth—had up to 68 percent less risk than women who ate the least beta-carotene. Don't rely on beta-carotene supplements; most likely you need beta-carotene plus other compounds found in the same foods for cancer protection.

The 10 most delicious ways to get beta-carotene:

1. Sweet potatoes (9.5 milligrams in ½ cup baked)
2. Pumpkin pie (8.5 milligrams in ⅙ of an 8-inch pie made with canned pumpkin)
3. Baby carrots (6.2 milligrams in ⅔ cup)
4. Canned apricots (5.9 milligrams in four halves)
5. Spinach (4.7 milligrams in ½ cup steamed)
6. Spinach salad (3.1 milligrams in 1 cup raw spinach)
7. Cantaloupe (2.4 milligrams in 1 cup of cubes)
8. Tossed salad (1.9 milligrams in ½ cup red bell peppers plus 1 cup romaine lettuce)
9. Broccoli (0.8 milligram in ½ cup steamed)
10. Mangoes (0.8 milligram in 1 cup of slices)

In one study, only 10 percent of rats fed IP6 developed colon cancer, compared with 43 percent of rats who didn't get IP6. The treated rats also showed smaller and fewer tumors than the untreated ones.

"IP6 doesn't kill cancer cells. It tames them," says Dr. Shamsuddin, who also holds the patent for IP6's over-the-counter supplement formula. "It normalizes the uncontrolled cell growth that takes place in cancer. It prompts cancerous cells to revert to their normal function. It also boosts the ability of natural killer cells, called NK cells, which kill tumor cells."

IP6 research may help explain why high-fiber diets—and particularly diets that are rich in cereal grains such as corn and rice—are associated with lower cancer rates in large population studies. Human studies looking at IP6 and cancer are set to begin soon.

Will it work for you? The answer to this question remains unknown until human studies are conducted. "IP6 should be tested systematically in people," explains Lee Wattenberg, M.D., professor of laboratory medicine and pathology at the University of Minnesota Medical School in Minneapolis. "All one can say about IP6 now is that there are interesting animal studies. Whether or not it will be applicable to people is not defined."

The safety factor: Older studies found no untoward side effects in people given dosages of 8.8 grams of IP6 a day for up to 2 years. (The daily dose recommended on current IP6 supplements is 1 to 4 grams.) Some nutritionists have raised questions in the past, however, about whether consuming large amounts of phytate-rich foods (IP6 is also called phytate) might reduce absorption of calcium and iron. Dr. Shamsuddin says that in supplement form, IP6 has not blocked mineral absorption in lab animals. But no one has yet checked its effect on humans.

The bottom line: "It appears to be relatively safe," Dr. Wattenberg says, "but until someone does toxicity studies with the specific preparation of IP6 being offered for sale by the supplement makers, you cannot be sure about safety."

Others say that without human studies that clearly demonstrate both safety and a cancer-fighting benefit, a healthy diet (including whole grains) is the best route for now.

Resveratrol: Stick with Food

Top food sources: Grape juice, red wine (smaller amounts in white and rosé wines), and other grape products such as raisins; mulberries and peanuts also contain some resveratrol.

The promise: Resveratrol is advertised mainly as a supplement to promote cardiovascular health, but its cancer-fighting potential is often mentioned in educational literature supplied with the supplements. One manufacturer calls its resveratrol product "a new cancer fighter."

The research: When researchers at the University of Illinois at Chicago tested hundreds of plants in search of new cancer-prevention compounds, resveratrol—a substance found in abundance in grape skins—came up the clear winner.

So far, though, studies have been limited to test tubes and lab animals, says lead resveratrol investigator John Pezzuto, Ph.D., director of the program for collaborative research in the pharmaceutical sciences at the university.

Using resveratrol extracted from a Peruvian legume, and later a synthetic form, researchers have found that it inhibited the development or growth of skin and breast cancers in mice and defused colon cancer as well.

"Resveratrol seems to work at all stages of cancer development, from initiation to promotion to progression," Dr. Pezzuto says. "It also has an anti-inflammatory action, which may make it particularly effective against tumors of the gastrointestinal tract," he adds.

More laboratory studies of its effectiveness against breast, lung, and prostate cancers will take place soon, says Dr. Pezzuto.

Will it work for you? The answer is unknown. Human studies are at least 2 to 3 years away. Further, there are no population studies linking the consumption of resveratrol-rich foods with lower rates of cancer.

The safety factor: Resveratrol is probably safe in amounts up to 10 milligrams a day, roughly the amount you'd get from a fruit- and vegetable-rich diet, Dr. Pezzuto says.

"Very high doses in laboratory animals show no adverse effects, but toxicity studies should be performed before humans consume large amounts," he warns.

The bottom line: It may be safer and more effective to get resveratrol from food, says Bernard Levin, M.D., vice president for cancer prevention at the University of Texas M. D. Anderson Cancer Center. So enjoy a handful of red grapes or a glass of grape juice—or perhaps even raisins or some grape jam.

You may want to skip the wine or limit yourself to one glass a day, however. Long-term consumption may produce other adverse health effects. Women at high risk for breast cancer may want to stay with grape juice—one glass of wine a day raises lifetime risk by about 1 percent.

Survival Tactics for the Female Heart

Heart disease will kill twice as many women this year as all cancers combined. Surprised? The good news is that much of your risk for heart disease can be reduced or even eliminated by making simple, painless changes in your life. The process starts now!

One sunny afternoon, in the middle of her daily run, Mary noticed a squeezing sensation in her chest. She slowed her pace and the pain went away. But it kept returning, so she went to see her doctor. Since Mary was only 35, he said, she couldn't have a heart problem; she had probably pulled a muscle. Maybe she should tone down her workout for a while.

Mary did just that—and continued to whittle away her workout for more than 4 frustrating years. Finally, she told her doctor that if he didn't refer her to a cardiologist, she'd find one herself. That's how she wound up running on a treadmill at the Women's Heart Institute, part of the Cardiovascular Medical Group in Beverly Hills, where tests detected a dangerous constriction in her left anterior descending artery, which brings blood to the heart.

Despite her relative youth, Mary had lost 90 percent of the capacity of that artery. After having a procedure called angioplasty to reopen the artery and starting medication to prevent further damage, Mary was finally able to exercise without fear of dropping dead of a heart attack.

Here's an interesting question: If Mary had been *Martin*, would his internist have downplayed the significance of his chest pain for 5 years?

Know Your Risk

Do right by your heart by following these steps.

Look up your family tree. Does anyone in your immediate family have a history of heart disease or heart attack? Let your doctor know if your father or brother had a heart attack before he was 55 years old or if your mother or sister had one before she was 65 years old. That may put you at a higher risk for heart disease, according to the American Heart Association (AHA).

Know your risks. Do you eat a high-fat diet? Are you overweight or inactive? Do you smoke? Are you also on the Pill? Do you or does anyone in your immediate family have diabetes? Do you have high blood pressure or high cholesterol?

See the right doc. Monitor your cardiac health with an internist or general practitioner—beginning in your twenties. "Women shouldn't be going just to the gynecologist," says Marianne Legato, M.D., professor of clinical medicine at Columbia University College of Physicians and Surgeons in New York City. "Gynecologists are invaluable but are not likely to be trained in the latest information on testing and treatment of coronary disease." If your doctor dismisses your concerns or symptoms, don't hesitate to dismiss him.

Check your cholesterol. Have your cholesterol tested yearly. Knowing your total cholesterol count is not enough, however. Today, careful doctors order a full "lipid panel," which measures HDL (good cholesterol) and LDL (bad cholesterol) separately. An HDL level below 45 means increased risk.

Also in the panel will be triglycerides, the most common fat in the body. A woman's triglyceride count should be under 200. Some doctors also screen patients for a lipid called lipoprotein (a). "A high level is bad—it should be under 20," says Debra R. Judelson, M.D., director of the Women's Heart Institute in Beverly Hills. "A significant number of women in my practice have heart attacks in their thirties. About two-thirds of them had elevated lipoprotein (a)."

Check your blood pressure, too. Again, you should have your blood pressure checked regularly—especially if you have a history of heart disease—at least every 2½ years, according to the AHA.

Write it down. Keep a log of your weight, blood pressure, and cholesterol levels so you will be alert to negative changes.

And would he have waited that long before consulting a cardiologist? Probably not.

It Isn't a "Man's Disease"

Heart disease is the leading killer of American women, and women are twice as likely as men to die from a heart attack. Yet it's still seen primarily as a man's disease. The vast body of research on heart disease and its treatment was conducted, until very recently, on men alone. And many physicians don't realize that women who have heart disease—or even full-blown heart attacks—may present different symptoms, and get different results from diagnostic tests, than do men with similar conditions. As a result, when women are (eventually) diagnosed, they tend to be sicker, with worse prognoses, than men with cardiac problems.

Further, women don't even know they're at risk. According to a 1997 poll commissioned by the American Heart Association (AHA), 6 out of 10 women believe that cancer is the greatest threat to their health. But nearly twice as many women die from heart disease (505,440 in 1995, the last year for which figures are available) than from all types of cancer combined (256,844). Less than a tenth as many women die of breast cancer (43,800).

Even those women who religiously check their breasts each month and never miss a scheduled Pap test don't start thinking about heart disease until they're near menopause, when their doctors may suggest hormone-replacement therapy as a way to protect the heart. But heart disease starts much earlier—as early as the teens. And ignoring your heart in your thirties—by not eating right, not exercising, or by putting up with the stress of unfulfilling work or destructive relationships—may set you up for a deadly heart attack sooner or later.

New Heart-Protecting Antioxidant

Alpha-lipoic acid, also known as lipoic acid, is a powerful antioxidant that your body manufactures to help fight the free radicals that contribute to heart disease and some of the other ills of aging. Now for the first time, scientists have looked for lipoic acid in a variety of meats, fruits, vegetables, and beans. The result? So far, spinach is the top source of a lipoic acid precursor among foods that were tested.

Besides lipoic acid, every half-cup of cooked spinach brings you 15 percent of the Daily Value (DV) for beta-carotene, 25 percent of the DV for folate, 20 percent of the DV for vitamin C, and 16 percent of the DV for magnesium.

Perna Szabunio, a pharmacist from New York City, didn't believe she could have a heart attack at age 37—even though her brother had had angioplasty at 35 and she'd had high cholesterol for years. She recalls, "I had been cleaning the house all morning and had an uncomfortable tightness in my chest, throat, and neck. I thought I was having some sort of allergy attack, maybe a reaction to dust. After about 2 hours, I carried some laundry up from the basement and became breathless. That's when I knew something was wrong and called an ambulance."

Emergency medical technicians arrived minutes later to find Szabunio slipping into shock. They rushed her to the hospital, where prompt treatment helped to limit the damage to her heart. Szabunio, now 40, has already had cardiac procedures twice—an angioplasty to reopen her damaged coronary artery, then a second one to prop her arteries open with four springlike devices called stents.

The Heart under Siege

From birth to age 40, the average person's heart beats about 1,472,688,000 times. The heart muscle is responsible for performing the complex motions that pump blood into the lungs, throughout the body, and back again. In order to perform this essential task, the heart muscle itself must be maintained, and it has its own set of blood vessels—the coronary artery system—to bring it oxygen and food and to remove its wastes. Like all the body's blood vessels, the coronary arteries start out smooth and elastic. As we age, however, heredity, diet, and inactivity conspire to coat the arteries with plaque, a pasty substance made of cholesterol and other fats, calcium, and fibrin (a material the body uses to make blood clots).

This process begins as early as childhood. "While performing autopsies of accident victims throughout the 1990s, doctors found that 87 percent of Americans ages 14 to 35 had some plaque on their arteries, and 17 percent had significant coronary artery disease," says Debra R. Judelson, M.D., director of the Women's Heart Institute in Beverly Hills.

Almost all of us have some plaque—but the more that collects in your arteries, the narrower and less supple they become. The heart has to work harder to push blood through stiff, constricted passageways.

This is the beginning of heart disease. Eventually, your heart may begin to hurt, especially when you're exerting yourself or under stress. This condition, which women are more likely than men to experience, is called angina, and it can feel like tightness or squeezing in the chest; pain in the left arm, shoulder, neck, jaw, or back; or nausea, sweating, and shortness of breath. Consider it an invaluable wake-up call. A piece of plaque may break off, blocking a vessel that leads to the heart; that's called a heart attack.

The Female Heart before and after the Change

Women's hearts are two-thirds the size of men's, beat faster, and have smaller coronary arteries—all factors that should make them especially vulnerable to coronary artery disease and heart attacks. But what counterbalances those weaknesses is that during the childbearing years, women's hearts are protected by estrogen. This sex hormone helps prevent fats from attaching to blood vessel walls, thus keeping them elastic, and preserves the vessels' ability to carry extra blood in response to stress.

This is why the incidence of heart disease among women is fairly low until menopause slows estrogen production to a trickle. But estrogen's protective ability is not absolute, or all women would be completely safe until around age 55. In fact, by the time a heart attack strikes, being a woman offers no advantage.

Learn the Language, Spread the Word

According to Marianne Legato, M.D., professor of clinical medicine at Columbia University College of Physicians and Surgeons in New York City and author of *The Female Heart*, which first drew attention to the neglect of women's heart problems, the "classic" symptoms of a heart attack—uncomfortable pressure or squeezing in the chest; pain spreading to the shoulders, neck, or arms; chest discomfort along with lightheadedness, fainting, sweating, nausea, or shortness of breath—are the ones more likely to be experienced by men.

For reasons that have researchers stumped, some females have a different constellation of symptoms: pain in the upper abdomen, stomach, or chest; nausea or dizziness; difficulty breathing; unexplained anxiety, weakness, or fatigue; palpitations, cold sweat, or paleness. "Fifteen to 20 percent of women with heart attacks present unusual or atypical symptoms, such as upper back pain," Dr. Legato says. Women may experience the pain differently because their neurological wiring is different, making symptoms seem more diffuse.

"It's even a matter of vocabulary," observes Dr. Judelson. "We have to learn to describe symptoms in a way that makes doctors pay attention." Otherwise, you run the risk of having your symptoms ignored. If you sit quietly and say you'll be okay, more than likely you'll be waiting it out in the emergency room while cases that appear more urgent get immediate attention.

If you're having chest symptoms, Dr. Judelson advises, say, "I think I'm having a heart attack." That sends doctors into the rapid response mode that will enable you to receive lifesaving drugs, such as the clot-dissolving tissue plasminogen activator (TPA), which can reduce damage to heart tissue and increase your chances of survival.

Herbs That Help the Heart

Here are three herbs that can help both men and women fight heart disease.

Garlic. This herb has long been used to lower both blood pressure and blood lipids. Studies have shown that people who take garlic can reduce their systolic blood pressure by about 7 percent. Most of the clinical studies on garlic powder tablets, which are standardized to yield about 5 milligrams of allicin on a daily basis, show that you can reduce your levels of serum cholesterol by about 11 percent and triglycerides by about 12 percent. These reductions are positive steps toward helping to lower your risk of heart attack and stroke.

Not all recent trials have yielded such favorable results, however, and these have raised questions regarding the herb's effectiveness. The good news, though, is that you can still have confidence in garlic's value because recent clinical studies indicate that garlic helps to maintain the elasticity of the aorta in older men and women. Maintaining the flexibility of this largest artery is essential to healthy functioning of the entire circulatory system. In the long run, this activity alone may prove more essential to cardiovascular health than the actual cholesterol-lowering properties of garlic.

Red yeast. *Monascus purpureus*, or red yeast, which is cultivated on rice, contains several HMG-CoA reductase inhibitors related chemically to the popular statin prescription drugs. These protect by stimulating the formation of good (HDL) cholesterol and reducing the production of bad (LDL) cholesterol.

Clinical trials have shown that daily consumption of four 600-milligram capsules of a standardized red yeast product (called Cholestin) produced significant reductions in serum levels of both cholesterol and triglycerides.

The Food and Drug Administration tried to ban over-the-counter Cholestin because it felt that Cholestin's active ingredients were too closely related to those in the statin prescription drugs. An appeals court rescinded the ban. As of now, you can still buy Cholestin, but its status could change if the ruling is reversed.

Guggul. *Commiphora mukul*, or guggul, is an oleo gum resin from the trunk of a tree grown in India. There, a few studies have confirmed its ability to lower cholesterol and triglycerides in both small animals and humans. In one study, people were given 500 milligrams of gugulipid, one of the herb's active components, for 12 weeks. Cholesterol levels dropped by 24 percent and triglycerides dropped by 23 percent in 80 percent of the people studied.

Guggul appears to be safe, though it may cause stomach upset. (Pregnant women should never take it because it tends to stimulate uterine contractions.)

The Not-So-Silent Killer

Compounding the problem of misperceived symptoms is the fact that women are more likely than men to experience silent heart attacks. "These attacks are not called silent because they are asymptomatic," Dr. Legato says, "but because women and their doctors don't think of them as heart-related. Nothing happens until your heart muscle is impaired. Only then is it realized that that moment of back pain, indigestion, shortness of breath, or fatigue was, in fact, a silent heart attack."

Unfortunately, diagnosing heart disease in its early stages proves especially difficult for women. An electrocardiogram, or EKG, turns out normal in about 50 percent of people complaining of angina, even when they have heart disease. And an exercise stress test (an EKG done while you're exercising on a bike or treadmill) has a 40 percent false-positive rate for women, limiting its usefulness, while the false-positive rate for men is only 10 percent. More reliable stress tests such as echocardiograms and those that use x-ray–like tracers give better images of coronary blockages. They're more time consuming and expensive, though, so physicians may resist ordering them.

No One Is Immune

Who's at risk? The short answer: everyone. Lack of exercise, smoking, stress, and a diet high in saturated fat can set anyone up for heart problems. Many young women are at risk, even if they don't have dramatic symptoms like Perna Szabunio's.

Moreover, some of us are born with a predisposition for heart woes. "A woman whose father had a heart attack before age 50 or whose mother had one before age 55 has a 30 percent higher risk of developing heart disease," says AHA spokesperson Nieca Goldberg, M.D., chief of the women's heart program at Lenox Hill Hospital in New York City. (If these women had a family history of breast cancer, they could find a surveillance program at a local hospital, but so far there are no such programs for heart disease.)

Among African-American women, heart disease has reached critical levels: "It's now the number one killer of African-American women from age 25 on, and we really don't know why," says Dr. Judelson. The statistics are startling: The death rate from heart attack is more than 38 percent higher for African-American women than for Caucasian women. Women who take birth control pills and smoke also dramatically raise their risk of heart attack: Smoking 15 or more cigarettes a day while on the Pill increases your chance by 39 times.

What's Impotence Got to Do with It?

Of men who experience a form of impotence that's physically based, 70 percent have vascular disease, says John Mulhall, M.D., director of the Center for Male Sexual Health at Loyola University Medical Center in Maywood, Illinois.

What a man should do: Get a cardiac check (especially before getting a prescription for Viagra). "We have to consider that impotence may be a first sign of coronary artery disease," says Dr. Mulhall.

Another Good Reason to De-Stress

Stress is, of course, a fact of life. When you react strongly to stress, however, your body pumps adrenaline and harmful stress hormones into your system that elevate your blood pressure and increase your heart rate. Over time, these chemical reactions can contribute to coronary heart disease.

"Women with the highest life stress are those with dependent children and unrewarding work," says Dr. Legato. "Women with the lowest stress are unmarried, have no children at home, and love their work." Marriage reduces a man's cardiac risk but has no effect on a woman's, perhaps because it's usually the married woman who cooks, cleans, and looks after children long after punching out at work.

Unfortunately, people minimize the effects of stress overload. "If you're unhappy, be very sure you make your life what you want it to be before you stress yourself into heart disease," Dr. Legato says. A depressing or destructive relationship and an unsatisfying career are things you can change with significant rewards for your heart. "When you improve your circumstances," she says, "you improve your health in the future."

Turning the Tide

Luckily, awareness of women's heart aches is rising. Researchers are including women in more studies, as mandated in 1993 by the National Institutes of Health.

Moreover, a new study presented at a recent AHA meeting suggests that women with heart disease are starting to be treated more aggressively: During the mid-1990s, women made up 45 percent of patients receiving the most useful—and most expensive—diagnostic test for heart disease, the angiography (in which a substance is injected into the coronary arteries, making them more visible on an x-ray). This figure was up from 30 percent in the beginning of the decade. Women are starting to get the care they need.

Stop a Stroke before It Happens

Stroke is a time bomb that cripples or kills 731,000 men and women every year. Here's how to spot it and stop it.

Looking back to the days right before her stroke, Rusty Van Sickle says she never suspected what was happening to her. Neither did her family, friends, or co-workers. "Other people noticed that I had started having trouble with my speech and that I was having difficulty following their trains of thought," she says. But like the doctors who treated her in the hospital, none of them could believe that a young woman of 42 was having a stroke.

Unfortunately, Van Sickle's case is not unique. Although stroke is the third leading cause of death and the leading cause of disability in the United States, a recent study suggests as many as 43 percent of Americans can't even name one warning sign. Even more alarming, a second survey conducted by the University of Cincinnati stroke team found that nearly 40 percent of those who've already had a stroke can't identify a warning sign either.

These statistics are frustrating for Art Pancioli, M.D., the emergency department physician at the University of Cincinnati Hospital who led the first study. Many of his stroke patients have had dead-giveaway symptoms—no feeling on one side of the body, slurred speech, headache. But because people don't know what's happening, they don't seek help. By the time they do, the damage is done.

Don't let it happen to you.

Damage Report

If it doesn't kill you outright, a stroke can leave you brain-damaged, paralyzed, or unable to speak or think clearly. Think of it as a brain attack. The most common kind of stroke happens when a blood vessel leading to the brain becomes blocked. Typically, it's a vessel that's already narrowed as a result of fatty deposits known as plaque. Without blood, the brain is deprived of oxygen. This is known as an ischemic stroke, and it accounts for 84 percent of all brain attacks. (When this same process occurs in your coronary arteries, it can lead to a heart attack.) A less common kind of stroke occurs when a weakened vessel in the brain bursts. This is a hemorrhagic stroke, and it accounts for 16 percent of all strokes and is the most lethal.

As Rusty Van Sickle learned, strokes can strike at any time and at any age. But they happen more often as we get older. Every year, it's estimated that strokes end or irrevocably change the lives of 731,000 people in the United States. And the numbers are growing: New research suggests that by the year 2050, nearly a million strokes will occur every year in this country.

Do you know enough about your own stroke risk to avoid being a victim? Chances are you don't. Stroke risk seems to be one of medicine's best-kept—and most deadly—secrets. Studies show that Americans are not only ignorant of stroke's warning signs but don't even know what puts them at risk.

Yet 80 percent of all strokes could be prevented if people knew—and controlled—the risk factors. Here's what to do.

Warning Signs of a Stroke

HEALTH FLASH

If you experience one or more of the following symptoms, get to an emergency room as soon as possible. You may be having a stroke. If you can get to the hospital within 3 hours, you can be treated with clot-busting drugs such as tissue plasminogen activator, which improve your chance of making a full recovery.

❖ Sudden, unexplained weakness or numbness on one side of the body, possibly confined to one limb or one side of the face

❖ Sudden loss of vision or dimness, particularly in just one eye

❖ Trouble speaking, slurred speech, trouble understanding someone else's speech

❖ Sudden, severe headache with no apparent cause

❖ Dizziness, sudden falls (particularly when they occur with any of the other symptoms)

Lower Your Blood Pressure in 8 Weeks

Just 10 minutes of moderate activity, such as walking or taking the stairs, can help reduce blood pressure. According to a new study, when postmenopausal women with high blood pressure exercised for 10 minutes, three times a day, 5 days a week, their systolic (top number) and diastolic (bottom number) pressures dropped an average of eight and five points respectively after just 8 weeks. As a result, some women didn't require medication, and some blood pressures were brought down to normal. So aim for a short walk each morning, lunch break, and after dinner.

Another option: strength training. In another study, men and women ages 65 to 75 with borderline high blood pressure lowered their systolic readings by five points and diastolic readings by four points with strength training. For 6 months, they worked out 3 days a week and followed a weight-lifting program that targeted all the major muscle groups. To get started, consult a certified trainer.

Treat High Blood Pressure

More than 50 million Americans have high blood pressure. Worse, about half of them aren't doing anything about it, which puts them square in the stroke danger zone. If you have untreated high blood pressure, your risk of stroke is four to six times higher than someone whose pressure is normal, or under 130/85.

High blood pressure can lead to stroke in several ways. The excessive pounding of blood against the vessel walls can cause damage by stretching them like overinflated balloons. And like balloons, they can pop. The damage to your artery lining can also lead to atherosclerosis, in which your arterial walls harden and are clogged with fat and debris, explains Otelio Randall, M.D., professor of medicine at Howard University Hospital in Washington, D.C. It also creates a fertile environment for the development of blood clots, which can break off and sail through the blood vessels. If big enough, a clot can partially stop blood flow to the brain or lodge in an already clogged artery and cut off your brain's blood supply.

What's more, the higher your pressure and the longer it remains untreated, the sooner you might have a stroke. "If your blood pressure reading is slightly more than 130/85, your chance of having a stroke is less than someone with hypertension. But over 20 years, this high-normal blood pressure can still cause damage to your blood vessels," says Dr. Randall. "The higher your pressure is and the longer it remains high, the greater the chance of doing damage to your heart, brain, and arterial system."

If you have what's called mild hypertension (your systolic, or top number, is 140 to 159 and your diastolic, or bottom number, is 90 to 95), there's a good

**H
E
A
L
T
H

F
L
A
S
H**

Don't Ignore Ministrokes

They're called transient ischemic attacks—TIAs, or ministrokes. That "mini" is misleading, though. To Jack P. Whisnant, M.D., professor emeritus of neurology at the Mayo Clinic in Rochester, Minnesota, it's a stroke, albeit one of shorter duration.

TIAs are believed to be caused by a temporary blockage in a blood vessel: a clot that dissolves within a few minutes. Thus the ministroke lasts just minutes. One-sided numbness or weakness, slurred or impaired speech—all the classic symptoms of stroke—disappear as rapidly as they appeared.

You may be tempted to ignore a TIA. But don't. See your doctor immediately. At least 36 percent of all people who experience TIAs go on to suffer a stroke, most within a month of the ministroke, says Dr. Whisnant. Some people suffer a cluster of TIAs, which may increase their risk even more.

chance you can eat and exercise your way to lower numbers. Give these healthy habits 2 months to work before you and your doctor consider medication. If your systolic blood pressure is 160 or higher and your diastolic is more than 100, you still need to adopt the same diet and exercise habits. But healthy habits alone probably won't reduce your pressure to safe levels, cautions Dr. Randall. You may need medication. Diet and regular exercise, however, can help you reduce the dosage and the number of medications you take.

The American Heart Association's advice is to have your blood pressure checked at least every 2 years. If yours hasn't been checked for some time, make an appointment today.

Dash to the Produce Aisle

You may be able to lower your blood pressure simply by losing weight. Try switching to the same smart diet that protects you from heart attack: a fat intake at 25 percent or less of daily calories and lots of fruits and vegetables. You also should get moderate exercise, which can mean as little as a 30-minute walk most days, says Dr. Randall. In addition, reduce your sodium intake to a maximum of 1,250 milligrams per day. Although not everyone is sensitive to salt's blood pressure–raising ability, there's no way to predict who is.

The Dietary Approaches to Stop Hypertension Trial, a government-funded study, found that a diet high in fruits, vegetables, grains, and low-fat dairy products reduced high blood pressure as well as drugs did. Further, it dropped pressure points even though the study participants didn't do one other thing, such as lose weight, cut out sodium, or reduce their intake of alcohol.

Here's the dietary prescription that worked wonders for people with mild hypertension and lower (159/95 and under). Servings are based on an intake of 2,000 calories a day.

- ❖ 8 servings of grains
- ❖ 4 servings of vegetables
- ❖ 5 servings of fruits
- ❖ 3 servings of low-fat dairy products
- ❖ 2 servings of meat, poultry, or fish
- ❖ 1 serving of nuts
- ❖ 2½ servings of fats and oils

Prevent or Control Diabetes

Diabetes, which is on the rise, can double your risk of stroke. It increases the severity of atherosclerosis and may also encourage the formation of potentially deadly blood clots.

If you already have diabetes, keep it under control by following your doctor's diet and exercise advice and taking any medications you've been prescribed.

Diabetes prevention is stroke prevention: Get down to and maintain a healthy weight, exercise for at least 30 minutes 3 days a week, and eat a low-fat diet that is rich in fruits and vegetables and low in refined carbohydrates and sugars.

Stop Smoking

Smokers have about a 50 percent greater risk of having a stroke than nonsmokers. And if you puff away, you're not putting just yourself at risk—you may be harming your family and friends, too. A study by George Howard, Dr.P.H., professor of epidemiology at Wake Forest University in Winston-Salem, North Carolina, found that nonsmokers who are regularly exposed to cigarette smoke experienced a 20 percent increase in the rate of the development of atherosclerosis.

Smokers may drive up their own rate of atherosclerosis by as much as 50 percent, according to Dr. Howard's study.

"One way that smoking speeds up hardening of the arteries is by destroying the protective layer of cells inside artery walls, which is what causes them to harden," explains Dr. Howard. If you have high blood pressure or diabetes, you can do more than twice as much damage by smoking.

If you give up smoking, you won't wipe your arteries clean or stop atherosclerosis in its tracks. But you can greatly slow down its steady march, says Dr. Howard.

Lose Excess Weight and Keep It Off

Adding pounds, especially as an adult, can increase the risk of stroke in several ways, according to Kathryn Rexrode, M.D., a researcher in the division of preventive medicine at Brigham and Women's Hospital in Boston. As you gain weight, your blood pressure rises, and you increase your risk for high cholesterol and diabetes.

Who's More at Risk? Men or Women?

It has been said numbers don't lie. Maybe so, but they don't always tell the whole truth either.

Take stroke data, for instance. Research tells us that men get strokes 19 percent more often than women. At first glance, this should make women feel less at jeopardy—until you look at the whole picture. Despite their lower risk, in 1996 women made up over 60 percent of the total number of deaths from strokes. To add insult to injury, the American Heart Association's journal, *Circulation*, reported that more women than men are left physically and mentally disabled by strokes. Why?

The main reason seems to be that women live longer. "The simple fact is that the age group 85 to 94 is largely made up of women, and that's where the incidences of stroke are highest, most severe, and most likely to be fatal," says John R. Marler, M.D., a neurologist with the National Institute of Neurological Disorders and Stroke. This isn't just a magical occurrence for the over-83 set. As a woman's age increases, her risks of having a stroke and dying from one increase as well. These risks go up for men as they age, too, but other deadly forces like heart disease and cancer tend to take their toll first.

Considering the aging of baby-boomer women, there's real concern about a future stroke epidemic during the early third of the new millennium, says Dr. Marler. But you don't have to be a sitting duck. Keep your blood pressure under control via exercise, diet, regular check-ups, and hypertension medications recommended by your doctor. Don't smoke. "If you are over 50 and not currently taking aspirin or some other drug to prevent heart disease and stroke, ask your physician why not," says Dr. Marler. Although there may be good reason why you aren't using these heart helpers, it's wise to make sure your doctor has at least given them some thought.

A study conducted by Dr. Rexrode and her colleagues found that women who gained more than 44 pounds after age 18 were almost 2½ times more likely than slender women to suffer an ischemic stroke. Even a moderate weight gain—between 24 and 44 pounds—nearly doubled their risk. And it's not just women who need to worry about excess weight: Dr. Rexrode points out that previous research demonstrates similar risks in overweight men.

Losing weight and keeping it off should lower your stroke risk by improving your cholesterol levels and reducing your risk of diabetes, says Dr. Rexrode. Further, dropping just 10 pounds can significantly lower your blood pressure.

Lower Your Cholesterol

You already know that atherosclerosis can set you up for a stroke. A high-fat diet not only plasters your arteries with plaque but also plays a role in high blood pressure, obesity, and diabetes. So, not surprisingly, you can lower your cholesterol 5 to 15 points by changing your diet and exercise habits.

If diet and exercise alone don't lower your blood fats, talk to your doctor about cholesterol-lowering drugs. One class of those drugs, called HMG-CoA reductase inhibitors, has lowered stroke risk in preliminary studies.

Get Moving

Regular exercise will not only help you avoid these other risk-increasing conditions but also help prevent stroke altogether. Just 5 hours of exercise a week can drop your stroke risk by about two-thirds.

That's what Ralph Sacco, M.D., a neurologist at Columbia University College of Physicians and Surgeons in New York City, found when he compared 369 elderly people in northern Manhattan who had already had a first stroke with 678 stroke-free people. Those who exercised regularly had a 63 percent lower risk than those who didn't. They weren't running marathons, either. Most walked; others biked, did calisthenics, or gardened. It didn't matter what they did—just how long they did it. Those who did more rigorous activities or exercised for 5 hours a week or more showed the biggest benefits.

Just Do the Basics

If you do nothing else but control your blood pressure, Dr. Pancioli says, you could reduce your stroke risk significantly. Yes, it requires a commitment.

A Startling Connection to Suicide

Suicide is an unexpected side effect of stroke in many women under 60, says a Danish study. If you know someone who has had a stroke, make sure she's getting the kind of emotional support that will minimize this possibility.

You'll have to drop the excess weight, exercise almost every day, and eat a low-fat, plant-based diet. If you smoke, you'll need to break a stubborn habit. If you're on medication, you'll have to take it every day. It's hard, but it's worth it.

If you can't do it for yourself, Dr. Pancioli urges, do it for the people you love. Stroke is a killer and a crippler. More than most diseases, it's a family affair. "My stroke patients aren't afraid of dying," he says. "They're afraid of the disability, which is so tremendous for so many people. Stroke is demanding on everyone involved."

Don't Let "Bad" Genes Be the Death of You

Much of what determines your health and longevity is your genes, those tiny sets of human blueprints tucked inside every cell. You get them from your parents at conception, and for the rest of your life, they largely dictate who you are—from what color eyes you have to how well you fight off disease.

But if genes program who you are, can you rewrite the destructive programs that killed your forebears? The answer is yes.

Of the more than 4,000 different genetic diseases scientists have found thus far, the two most likely to affect us are heart disease and cancer. True, it's estimated that 90 percent of cancer and more than half of all heart disease is triggered by accumulated damage to our cells from things such as eating lots of french fries or smoking cigarettes. But the rest of it occurs because your parents passed you a set of genes in which one part of the genetic instructions to your cells was missing, altered, or out of whack.

In the case of cancer, for example, you may have inherited a gene that starts out producing replacement cells for basic body maintenance but then gets its accelerator stuck and keeps producing more and more cells.

Or you may have inherited a gene that is supposed to detect and repair mistakes made during cell production but can't seem to find the right tool. It fumbles around while mistakes pile up; cells forget what they're supposed to do, then multiply out of control.

Or you may have failed to inherit a gene that's supposed to identify and stop uncontrolled cell growth.

Heart disease is more complex, says gene researcher Herbert Schuster, M.D., professor of medicine at the Max Delbrück Center for Molecular Medicine in Berlin, Germany, and a pioneer in cardiovascular genetics.

Although some people inherit an altered gene that rearranges the heart's architecture or disturbs its rhythm, most heart disease is caused by the stealthy work of several gene variations that subtly alter cholesterol levels, blood pressure, fat storage, homocysteine metabolism, and other factors. Left unchecked, says Dr. Schuster, these conditions can evolve into high choles-

---

Know Your Risks and Options: Breast and Ovarian Cancers

Incidence: About 5 to 10 percent of all breast and ovarian cancers are triggered by inherited mutations.

Risk: At least 50 percent of women who have inherited BRCA1 and BRCA2 gene mutations will develop breast cancer; about two out of five women will develop ovarian cancer. It's estimated that one out of two Ashkenazi Jews—who represent 90 percent of the American Jewish population—with the BRCA1 mutation will develop breast cancer.

What you should do:

❖ If you suspect that you may carry one of these gene mutations, consult a physician trained in cancer genetics or a genetic counselor.

❖ Follow the screening guidelines explained in "Check It—Often" on page 110.

❖ Talk to your doctor about the pros and cons of tamoxifen to prevent breast cancer and birth control pills to prevent ovarian cancer. A recent landmark study found that the use of oral contraceptives for six or more years cut the risk of ovarian cancer in BRCA1 and BRCA2 carriers by 50 to 60 percent.

❖ Talk to your doctor about whether removal of the ovaries or breasts is right for you. The Penn Collaborative Prophylactic Surgery Study reported that removing the ovaries of women with the BRCA1 mutation reduced their risk of breast cancer by more than 50 percent. In the long term, says Tim Rebbeck, Ph.D., a breast cancer researcher at the University of Pennsylvania in Philadelphia, a woman's risk of breast cancer could be reduced by as much as 70 percent.

HEALTH FLASH

terol, high blood pressure, obesity, and other conditions that set the st~~ heart attack.

Few inherited diseases, however, are caused by a single defect in a single gene or group of genes, says Susan Nayfield, M.D., program director of epidemiology and genetics at the National Cancer Institute (NCI).

Often, one of your parents will pass on a common variation in a gene. It's well within normal limits—the gene can still do what it's supposed to do—and it may not affect your parent at all. But when that particular variation is combined with variations from your other parent, the gene may no longer work, leaving you prey to disease.

DNA Is Not Destiny

If you come from a family with heart disease, for instance, you can probably assume there's a genetic factor involved, according to Jan Breslow, M.D., professor of genetics and metabolism at Rockefeller University in New York City and a past president of the American Heart Association. But it's not 100 percent certain. What looks like a genetic trait carried through several generations could actually be nothing more than chance or even a coincidental clustering. After all, heart disease is the number one way we leave the planet—with or without a genetic boost.

Even if you did inherit an aberrant gene, that doesn't mean you're doomed, Dr. Breslow says. "You're not in total control," he admits. "But you can make things better for yourself—or worse. There's an old expression, 'Genes cock the gun; the environment pulls the trigger.' I think that's an apt description of what's going on."

Okay. So what should the millions of people whose genes place them at risk for heart disease or cancer actually do?

Doctors aren't sure. The genetic causes of disease haven't been mapped out as thoroughly as the globe. So the best doctors can do is suggest that you follow the nine steps that anyone might take to lower her risk.

1. Construct a family tree. Talk to as many family members as possible. Try to find out who was diagnosed with what and at what age. The earlier a disease occurs, the more likely there's an inherited gene involved. Building an accurate family tree can help you and your doctor assess your risks and determine appropriate preventive measures, says Anne Andermann, a researcher at the University of Oxford's Institute of Health Sciences in England.

   If many of your older relatives are gone, it's helpful to send for death certificates or obtain medical records to help fill in your family health picture, especially if you plan to get genetic testing. For death certificates, contact your state office of vital records or statistics.

‏c counselor. There are more than 1,700 genetic counselors ‏ountry, says Bea Leopold, executive director of the National Genetic Counselors in Wallingford, Pennsylvania. Each is help you evaluate your genetic risk and, along with other spe- ‏elp you develop a custom-tailored plan to minimize your risk. t have to have genetic testing done to see a counselor. To find a counselor near you, visit the society's Web site at www.nsgc.org and ‏click on "resource link."

3. Eat fruits and veggies morning, noon, and night. And in between, too, preferably in place of meat. Eating lots of plant-based foods has been linked to lower rates of heart disease and many kinds of cancer. You may have heard of the "five-a-day" rule promoted by the top cancer organizations. Well, five a day is where you should start, not stop, says Robert Smith, Ph.D., director of cancer screening for the American Cancer Society. If you consume more than 2,200 calories a day, strive for four or more servings of vegetables and three or more servings of fruit each day.

Know Your Risks and Options: Heart Disease

Incidence: Nearly 50 percent of all heart disease is triggered by a variety of inherited gene mutations.

Risk: Your risk depends on which genes you've inherited. If you've inherited the genetic mutation for familial hypercholesterolemia, for example, the odds are three out of four that you'll develop heart disease by age 60 if you're a man; they're one out of two if you're a woman. (Women's genetic risk for heart disease is equal to men's—women are just more likely to develop it after age 60 because of the protective power of estrogen.)

What you should do:

❖ If you suspect that you may carry a gene mutation, consult a physician trained in genetics or a genetic counselor.
❖ Follow the screening guidelines explained in "Check It—Often" on page 110.
❖ If diet and exercise don't reduce high cholesterol levels, talk to your doctor about cholesterol-reducing drugs called statins.
❖ If diet and exercise don't reduce high blood pressure, you and your doctor may want to talk about ACE inhibitors—drugs that counteract the effects of the gene that alters your body's fluid balance and sends your blood pressure soaring.

HEALTH FLASH

For example, the Women's Healthy Eating and Living Study reports that women with a family history of breast cancer had less damage to their DNA when they reduced the amount of beef and pork in their diets, ate three servings of fruit and five servings of vegetables, and drank 16 ounces of fresh vegetable juice a day.

4. Target saturated fat. Concentrate on reducing saturated fat to less than 7 percent of calories, says Dr. Breslow.

As for total fat, strive to keep your total fat intake to no more than 25 percent of calories. That's less than the amount recommended by many health organizations.

If, however, you know or suspect you're at special risk because of your genetics, talk to your doctor about which fat level is best for you. There are some inherited conditions in which a super low fat diet may actually have harmful effects on blood cholesterol.

So much of what we eat affects us differently depending on our genes, says Ronald Krauss, M.D., head of molecular medicine at the Lawrence Berkeley National Laboratory at the University of California at Berkeley. "Eventually," he adds, "we'll be able to custom-tailor diets to genetic traits."

5. Avoid smoke like the plague. "Avoiding smoke—including secondhand smoke—is a no-brainer," says Dr. Breslow. At least one study suggests that smoking can trigger the expression of a gene that may predispose people to heart disease. Even if you haven't inherited a gene for it, smoking is a major cause of heart disease and cancer.

6. Get addicted to endorphins. Exercise is a miracle drug that affects everything from the health of your arterial walls to their ability to forgive and forget molecular insults. It's prudent to accumulate at least 30 minutes of moderate-intensity activity a day, such as walking, jogging, or biking.

7. Get checked out early and often. Having a doctor frequently monitor known risk factors is important for those who know or suspect they have a faulty gene.

8. Volunteer for a clinical study. You might be part of the control group that gets the current treatment, says Dr. Smith. But you might also be part of the group that is getting a treatment that scientists think may be better than anything else available. And you could get your diagnostic tests for free or at reduced cost.

For a comprehensive listing of clinical studies by disease, check out the Web site of CenterWatch in Boston at www.centerwatch.com. Or contact the National Institutes of Health Clinical Center Patient Recruitment and Referral Line. Call (800) 555-1212 for their toll-free number.

9. Be aggressive. If you're at high risk for an inherited disease, you need to pull out all the stops, says Dr. Krauss. Lifestyle changes are probably mandatory. But sometimes, you might need certain drugs.

Check It—
Often

If disease runs in your family, here are some of the screening guidelines you should follow to increase your chances of living a long, healthy life.

Heart disease. Make sure you check detailed cholesterol and homocysteine levels, blood pressure, and weight regularly. General screening guidelines (no matter what your genetic predisposition) call for a cholesterol check—including the total/HDL ratio—every 5 years if normal, starting at age 20, every 4 months if abnormal. Your blood pressure should be checked every 2 years if normal, at your doctor's discretion if abnormal. (In some cases, you may want to check it at home regularly.) If you have a genetic flaw, you may need more frequent screening.

Very shortly, adds Jan Breslow, M.D., professor of genetics and metabolism at Rockefeller University in New York City and a past president of the American Heart Association, you'll be able to have something called an ultra-fast CT, an x-ray that can detect how clogged your arteries are by measuring the amount of calcium in artery walls.

Breast cancer. Those who believe they may have inherited a gene that puts them at risk for breast cancer should consider starting annual breast mammograms between ages 25 and 35, says Robert Smith, Ph.D., director of cancer screening for the American Cancer Society. Your doctor may order an ultrasound to go with it, especially if you have dense breast tissue. "Have a clinical breast exam once or twice a year and examine your own breasts monthly," adds Dr. Smith.

Ovarian cancer. Regardless of family history, get an annual Pap test and pelvic exam starting at age 18 or when you become sexually active. If you're at risk, talk to your doctor about a transvaginal ultrasound and the CA-125 blood test—two measures that are available but not consistently reliable or accurate.

Colon cancer. If you're at risk for hereditary nonpolyposis colon cancer, have a colonoscopy every 2 years starting between ages 20 and 25, then annually after age 35. Women at risk should also have endometrial cell samples taken during their yearly pelvic exams after age 30.

Prostate cancer. If your husband is at risk for familial prostate cancer, he should have a prostate specific antigen (PSA) test done annually, starting before age 50.

HEALTH FLASH

For example, if your cholesterol is maxing out and diet and exercise aren't lowering it, you may want to talk to your doctor about cholesterol-lowering drugs called statins. And if diet and exercise don't keep your blood pressure on an even keel, you may need to take an ACE inhibitor. (Lifestyle changes may make it possible for you to take very low doses of these drugs.)

If testing reveals genetic mutations that can lead to breast, ovarian, or colon cancer, there are drugs that may reduce your risk, such as tamoxifen in the case of breast cancer or aspirin therapy in the case of colon cancer. If your risk is very high, you may even want to talk to your doctor about having surgery to remove your breasts, ovaries, or colon before cancer has a chance to develop in them.

Yes, all these strategies have risks and some may seem drastic, says Dr. Nayfield. "But the risk of getting a disease determines the risk you take to prevent it. For someone with a very high risk, some of these strategies may be a reasonable trade-off."

17

How Old Are Your Bones?

Do you know the 10 hidden warning signs of osteoporosis? If you do, you can stop this crippler.

Unfortunately for Susan, ignorance was costly. For months, she suffered nagging back pain that wouldn't go away. Her gynecologist suspected osteoporosis, so he recommended a bone-density test. But her orthopedist (bone specialist) told her it was a waste of time, so she didn't get one.

"I thought if the orthopedic doctor said nothing is wrong, then nothing is wrong," recalls Susan, 61, who went back to skiing and tennis, her two passions.

But when the pain got worse, she contacted a few more doctors: first, a back specialist who found inflammation but didn't take it seriously, then a urologist who ruled out kidney stones, which she had had in the past.

Finally, her gynecologist talked her into the bone scan. The result? Susan had severe osteoporosis of the spine and osteopenia (low bone density) of the arms and hips.

How Osteoporosis Gets Overlooked

Susan's weak bones might have been diagnosed sooner if her doctors had paid attention to her history of kidney stones, which in certain cases can be a risk factor for osteoporosis, says Susan's current doctor, Marjorie Luckey,

The Most Common Risk Factors for Osteoporosis

According to the National Osteoporosis Foundation, these are the most common things that increase a person's risk of osteoporosis.

❖ Being female
❖ Being thin (less than 127 pounds for an average-size woman)
❖ Being Caucasian
❖ Smoking cigarettes
❖ Having a fracture as an adult
❖ History of fracture in a close relative such as a parent or sibling
❖ Inadequate physical activity
❖ Lifetime of inadequate calcium consumption
❖ Poor eyesight
❖ Poor health or frailty
❖ Recurrent falls
❖ Dementia
❖ Alcoholism

HEALTH FLASH

M.D., director of the Osteoporosis and Metabolic Bone Disease Center at the St. Barnabas Ambulatory Care Center in Livingston, New Jersey.

Her history of kidney stones, combined with her age, her back pain, and low intake of calcium—all warning signs of osteoporosis—should have signaled her orthopedist that she really needed that bone-density test.

Susan's story is not uncommon. The National Osteoporosis Foundation (NOF) estimates that more than 28 million Americans—80 percent of whom are women—have low bone density or osteoporosis and that half of all women will have an osteoporosis-related fracture in their lifetimes. What's going on?

Well, for one thing, osteoporosis is "nobody's disease," says Robert Lindsay, M.D., president of the National Osteoporosis Foundation. Since it doesn't "belong" to any one medical specialty, not enough doctors learn about the disease or test for it. Plus, advances in testing and treatment have come along so fast in the last decade that many doctors haven't kept up.

Add to that a long list of symptoms and warning signs—some, like kidney stones, so unusual many doctors haven't encountered them—and there's plenty of opportunity for missed diagnoses.

That may soon change. Late last year, for the first time, the National Osteoporosis Foundation issued guidelines to help doctors—no matter what their specialties—diagnose and treat osteoporosis. But if your doctor still isn't vigilant, *you* should be. Here are 10 of the most frequently overlooked warning signs that your bones are in trouble—and that should send you for a bone scan.

Hidden Warning Sign #1:
You're Thinner Than Normal

What most people think of as a plus really isn't: Low body weight puts you at increased risk for osteoporosis and fractures.

In fact, low body weight is probably the single most common important risk factor for osteoporosis and increased risk of fractures, says Steven Cummings, M.D., professor of medicine and epidemiology at the University of California, San Francisco.

The National Osteoporosis Foundation says you have low body weight if you're an average-size woman who weighs less than 127 pounds. If that sounds a little vague, think of it this way: You're potentially "osteoporosis thin" if you weigh less than you should for your body type.

According to Dr. Lindsay, the chief reasons you're more prone to fractures if you're thin are:

❖ You have less padding of muscle and fat to protect your bones.
❖ You have thin bones, too, which are more vulnerable to injury.
❖ You tend to make less bone-building estrogen after menopause.

Three Easy Steps to Stop Bone Loss

First, get 1,000 milligrams of calcium daily (1,500 milligrams if you're 50-plus or have low bone density). These foods make it easy to hit your target.

❖ 6 ounces sardines with bones—650 milligrams
❖ ½ cup Edy's or Dreyer's fat-free frozen yogurt—450 milligrams
❖ 1 cup Health Valley Fat-Free Soy Moo soy milk—400 milligrams
❖ 1 cup Light n' Lively cottage cheese—400 milligrams
❖ 6 ounces canned salmon with bones—362 milligrams
❖ 1 cup Dannon light yogurt—350 milligrams
❖ 1 cup Tropicana Pure Premium Plus calcium-fortified orange juice—350 milligrams
❖ 1 cup milk—300 milligrams

Second, get 400 international units (IU) of vitamin D daily. Or get 600 IU if you're 70-plus. Taking D will help you absorb calcium.

Third, exercise at least five times a week. Choose one of the following options for each exercise session.

❖ 1 hour of weight-bearing aerobic exercise such as walking
❖ 30 minutes of resistance training (such as weight lifting)
❖ Some combination of the two

If you're trying to be thin by dieting frequently, you're also at risk, Dr. Lindsay warns. When you lose weight, you lose fat, muscle, *and* bone. The first two may come back, but the bone may be gone forever.

Hidden Warning Sign #2: Your Backache Won't Quit

Persistent back pain that won't go away could be a sign that you have a spinal fracture, one of the symptoms of osteoporosis.

By the time Susan was finally diagnosed, her osteoporosis of the spine was so severe that she was close to suffering a spinal fracture. In fact, without treatment, she would be about "16 to 20 times more likely to have a spinal fracture within the next 5 years than the average woman her age," says Dr. Luckey.

Spinal fractures occur when the bones in your back become so weak that they fracture and collapse. This can happen without warning—even during ordinary activities such as bending over to pick up a newspaper.

The pain can be severe, requiring a long recuperation. But sometimes all you feel is a dull aching pain across the middle of your back and bottom of your shoulder blades. Unlike muscle pain, it doesn't go away with time and rest. Typically, the only way to ease the pain is to lie down, says Dr. Lindsay.

Having one spinal fracture puts you at greater risk for another and for hip fractures. Multiple fractures make it more likely you'll suffer chronic disability.

"If you are a post-menopausal woman, think you're getting a bit round-shouldered, and have back pain, talk to your doctor. Ask, 'Do I have osteoporosis?'" advises Dr. Lindsay.

Hidden Warning Sign #3: You're Shorter Than You Used to Be

A spinal fracture can steal inches from your height. When a bone in your back fractures, it literally collapses onto itself, causing you to shrink, explains Dr. Lindsay.

For some, loss of height happens gradually. For others, it happens quickly following an acute episode with sudden back pain that can be quite severe and disabling.

Multiple fractures can also cause the spine to form a C-like curve, causing the disfigurement known as dowager's hump. This can trigger pain in the ribs and abdomen as the lower ribs close in on the upper abdomen.

Not all height loss is caused by osteoporosis. As you age, the disks in your back lose their elasticity, causing your frame to shift downward. Gravity also takes its toll, and it's not uncommon to lose anywhere from $1/2$ to 1 inch be-

The Strength Test You Shouldn't Skip

Women of all races and ethnic backgrounds can have low bone density. After screening 48,270 women, researchers found low bone-mineral density (a major risk factor for future osteoporotic fractures) in 65 percent of Asians, 59 percent of Native Americans, 55 percent of Hispanics, 50 percent of Caucasians, and 38 percent of African-Americans, says Ethel Siris, M.D., medical director of the National Osteoporosis Risk Assessment research project.

Researchers don't know yet if low density means equal risk for osteoporotic fractures. But the evidence is strong that *all* women should take their bone statuses seriously.

To be safe, get your bone density tested in early menopause. (Start in your thirties or forties if you smoke or have a history of bone fractures, a family history of osteoporosis, a thin/small frame, or an inactive lifestyle.)

"If your doctor thinks your risk is lower because you're in a certain ethnic group and that you don't need a test yet, tell him about this research," Dr. Siris suggests.

The DEXA (dual-energy x-ray absorptiometry) test is the most accurate but also the most expensive. Newer devices cut costs significantly. Medicare now covers some bone densitometry testing, as do many health plans.

tween the ages of 60 and 80. "Any loss of height that's more than that, however, should be investigated," says Dr. Lindsay.

Hidden Warning Sign #4: You Break a Bone

Breaking a bone as an adult doesn't mean you have osteoporosis. But it could be a warning sign that your bones are weak, says Dr. Lindsay. In fact, someone who has had a fracture after age 40 is twice as likely to suffer a further osteoporotic fracture than someone who has not, he says.

"Obviously, the thing that causes a fracture is an injury of some sort, but if your bones are thin, then *any* injury is more likely to cause a fracture," Dr. Lindsay says.

Hidden Warning Sign #5: You Use Steroids

Many people with rheumatoid arthritis, asthma, lung disease, and other chronic illnesses rely on corticosteroids such as prednisone or dexamethasone for relief from their symptoms. And they work well. But taken over 2 to 3 months, they can also cause rapid bone loss that can lead to osteoporosis.

While steroid inhalers, usually used for asthma, can cause a small degree of bone loss and probably a small increase in your risk of fractures, steroids in pill form are the main bone robbers because they generally come in higher doses, says Dr. Cummings.

Steroids interfere with your body's ability to form new bone. They also interfere with the absorption of calcium by impeding the biochemical actions of vitamin D, explains Dr. Cummings.

Bone loss is most rapid in the first 3 to 6 months of treatment; taking almost any dose for more than 2 to 3 months can be harmful to your skeleton. Fortunately, the effects of 10 milligrams or less per day of a steroid can usually be offset in part by supplementing from the start of treatment with a daily dose of 1,500 milligrams of calcium and 600 international units (IU) of vitamin D, says Dr. Cummings.

For steroid doses greater than 10 milligrams per day, your doctor may recommend a more aggressive approach to stave off bone loss. At these doses, steroids can decrease bone mass by 10 to 20 percent and increase your risk of fractures by as much as threefold.

"Anyone who has been told by her doctor that she needs steroids and has to stay on them for whatever reason should ask, 'Is this going to affect my skeleton? And does this mean I need a bone-density test now to make sure I'm not already at risk?'" says Dr. Lindsay.

Hidden Warning Sign #6: You Have Thyroid Troubles

If you have hyperthyroidism, a condition caused by overproduction of the thyroid hormone thyroxine, you may want to schedule a bone-density test right away. Thyroxine speeds up the body's metabolism, so it breaks down bone faster than the body can make it, says Baha Arafah, M.D., an endocrinologist with University Hospitals of Cleveland and professor of medicine at Case Western Reserve University in Cleveland.

Ironically, having hypothyroidism (an underproduction of the thyroid hormone) can also put your bones in jeopardy, says Dr. Arafah. That's because

Chocolate-Covered Calcium

It's the latest—perhaps sweetest—way to get your daily dose. Chewy, fudgy squares of Viactiv deliver 500 milligrams of calcium apiece, about half of what premenopausal women need each day. For maximum absorption, have one after a meal or snack.

doctors may prescribe a synthetic version of thyroxine to treat hypothyroidism. When the prescribed dose is too high, the end result is the same: The body breaks down more bone than it builds.

Although bone loss can happen to anyone with too much thyroxine, women who have other osteoporosis risk factors, such as being peri-menopausal or postmenopausal, have even greater risk, notes Dr. Arafah.

If you're taking thyroxine, your doctor should be monitoring your dosage once or twice a year with a simple blood test; if not, ask for one, such as the Thyroid Stimulating Hormone (TSH) test.

Hidden Warning Sign #7: You're Being Treated for Endometriosis

Endometriosis is an often painful disease of the reproductive system in which pieces of the uterine lining break away through the fallopian tubes and implant themselves outside of the uterus.

Most doctors believe it's the treatment of the disease—not the disease it-self—that leads to osteoporosis, says John Bilezikian, M.D., director of the metabolic bone diseases program at Columbia-Presbyterian Hospital in New York City. The drug that doctors prescribe most often to treat endometrio-sis—gonadotropin-releasing hormone (GnRH)—essentially shuts down the reproductive system over time, thereby reducing estrogen levels. Bone breaks down more rapidly when estrogen levels drop, explains Dr. Bilezikian.

"It's an effective therapy for endometriosis, but when used long-term, it leaves women with an estrogen deficiency, and that's a big risk factor for os-teoporosis," says Dr. Bilezikian. That's why he recommends not taking the medication for more than 6 months.

Hidden Warning Sign #8: You Smoke

Perhaps the Surgeon General should add another warning to cigarette packs: If you smoke, you double your risk of suffering a fracture due to osteo-porosis.

Smoking harms bones in several ways. First, smokers tend to be thin, and thin frames usually mean thin bones. Smoking has also been linked with ear-lier menopause.

Smoking may also reduce your ability to absorb calcium. Further, if you started smoking at an early age, you may have put yourself at risk for osteo-porosis later in life—even if you kicked the habit as an adult, says Clifford J. Rosen, M.D., professor of nutrition at the University of Maine in Orono and

H
E
A
L
T
H

F
L
A
S
H

What about Men?

Men can develop osteoporosis as well as women, says Elizabeth Kunkel, R.D., Ph.D., professor of food science at Clemson University in South Carolina.

"Men lose bone mass in their forties at about the same rate as women," Dr. Kunkel says, "but because men have more bone mass to begin with, problems with osteoporosis won't show up until relatively late in life."

A complicating factor, suggests new research, is that low levels of estrogen—the female hormone that circulates naturally in men's bodies, too—can weaken a man's bones, raising the risk for fractures.

In one 8-year study of 382 men, researchers found that those with the strongest bones had the highest estrogen levels. In another, German researchers who tracked 300 men with osteoporosis for 5 years noted that 8 in 10 had low estrogen levels.

In the meantime, men at risk for osteoporosis—those who have small frames or are underweight—should follow the same bone-preserving strategies as women, says Eric Orwoll, M.D., professor of medicine and director of the bone and mineral unit at Oregon Health Sciences University in Portland.

These strategies include taking in 1,000 milligrams of calcium a day—roughly the amount in two glasses of milk and two servings of broccoli. Other calcium-rich foods to get plenty of include reduced-fat cheese and yogurt, soybeans, and green leafy vegetables.

director of the Maine Center for Osteoporosis Research in Bangor. That's because cigarette smoke is thought to damage bone cells and prevent new bone growth, and smoking at a young age coincides with the time of life when your body builds the most bone.

Hidden Warning Sign #9: You Have Kidney Stones

Studies have shown that kidney stones place some—but not all—people at higher risk for osteoporosis, says Dr. Luckey, who sees many patients with a history of kidney stones in her practice. People who are at risk are those who excrete too much calcium into their urine or who are advised to avoid calcium, she explains. When the body becomes calcium deficient in either of these ways, it dissolves bone to replenish its supply and keep the blood calcium levels normal.

Fortunately, only a minority of stone-formers are also calcium excreters, says Dr. Bilezikian. To find out if you're one of them, ask your doctor for the results of your urine calcium test, a simple urine test taken by some people with kidney stones.

If your urine calcium level is high, you may be at risk for osteoporosis. You and your doctor can then work out a plan—which may include cutting back on salt, drinking lots of water, and even taking extra calcium or prescription drugs under certain circumstances—to lower your risk.

Hidden Warning Sign #10: You Can't Drink Milk

Milk and other dairy products provide a major boost of bone-building calcium to American diets. Most American diets, that is. People who are lactose intolerant may not be able to stomach milk—literally.

Lactose is a natural sugar found in milk and other dairy products. Before the body can absorb lactose, an enzyme called lactase must break it down. If your body has little or no lactase enzyme, you have trouble absorbing lactose. The result: bloating, gas, and sometimes diarrhea.

Many people avoid these unwelcome symptoms by staying away from dairy altogether. And that's fine—as long as you're getting your calcium from other sources, including supplements, says Dr. Bilezikian.

Many people with lactose intolerance can eat yogurt and cheese, both of which are good sources of calcium. There's also good evidence that you can build up to as much as 3 cups of milk a day by starting with small amounts—$^{1}/_{4}$ to $^{1}/_{2}$ cup one to three times a day, taken with meals—and working up gradually.

Whip
Your Allergies
Now!

S ound familiar? Swollen eyes, drippy nose, stuffy sinuses, and sneezes. It's not a cold; it's allergies.

"People can't sleep, they can't think, they miss work, they get headaches," explains Gary Rachelefsky, M.D., associate director of the allergy immunology training program at the UCLA School of Medicine.

You could dose yourself with allergy medicine, as many women do, only to find yourself so groggy you can hardly stay awake or concentrate.

But there's no cause to suffer. Here's how to stop all the itching, dripping, wheezing, and sneezing.

Seasonal allergic rhinitis is the catchall term doctors use to refer to those stuffy-drippy-itchy-icky allergy symptoms that drive some 50 million of us nuts every year. No one really knows why some people develop an ultrasensitivity to pollens or mold spores, which are the primary causes of what we call hay fever. But if you're one of the unlucky ones, depending on where you live, you'll probably be developing symptoms caused by tree pollen in early spring, grass pollen in spring and early summer, and ragweed and other weed pollens in the fall.

Some years are worse than others. Unfortunately, once your defense system goes on the alert, it doesn't just shut down once the alert is over. It takes time before your body feels comfortable enough to holster its histamines and relax. In the meantime, here are some things you can do.

A Cure for Allergies Is on the Horizon

Do you find it impossible to imagine yourself going through an allergy season without your arsenal of drugs and tissues as your constant companions? Well, clinical trials for a drug that would short-circuit the body's allergic-reaction mechanism are currently underway. An antibody called IgE is what triggers the release of histamine, a chemical mechanism that causes the drippy nose, sneezes, and itchy eyes. The new drug is designed to intercept IgE before histamine gets out of the gate and, in effect, prevent the allergic reaction altogether.

"Instead of taking medication to treat the allergy symptoms, this may cure allergies by preventing them in the first place," says Gary Rachelefsky, M.D., associate director of the allergy immunology training program at the UCLA School of Medicine. It could be a few years before the drug is available.

Plan Your Day Wisely

Schedule outdoor activities for before breakfast or after dinner. Thermal currents and winds toss ragweed pollen and mold spores around in the air all day long, says Harold Nelson, M.D., a senior staff physician at the National Jewish Medical and Research Center in Denver. To minimize exposure, schedule outdoor activities such as yard chores and walks for before and after the wind whips things up—usually before 9:00 A.M. and around sunset.

Wear Cool Shades

Seasonal allergies can cause itchy, burning eyes, notes Gillian Shepherd, M.D., clinical associate professor of medicine at New York Hospital-Cornell Medical Center in New York City. But glasses can protect against flying pollen, and the more of your eye area they cover, the better. "Wear shades," she suggests. "Even better, wear wraparound or gogglelike sunglasses. They're designed to block glare from the sides, but they also block pollen."

Pray for Rain—And Get Wet

Heavy rains are wonderful because they wash pollen away, says Dr. Shepherd. Unfortunately, light rains may make everything worse. They break large clumps of pollen into tiny particles that are more likely to stay airborne longer. If you're staying indoors to avoid pollen, you may be able to make a break for it after a good downpour. If the weather won't cooperate, be sure to shower and wash your hair and, if you're a man, facial hair often—especially before going to bed—which will help reduce the amount of pollen you're carrying on your body. Wash your hands often during the day, too, and don't rub your eyes, adds Dr. Shepherd.

Pay Attention to Pollution

Air pollution makes seasonal allergies worse. "A number of studies have shown that if you are exposed to air pollution—especially ozone—you become more sensitive to lower levels of allergens such as pollens," says Dr. Shepherd. "No one knows why, but the presumption is that pollutants irritate the lining of the respiratory tract." So short of fleeing the big city, what can you do? Keep an ear on the news, says Dr. Shepherd. "If there's a pollution alert, that's a day to focus on indoor projects. You might also want to talk to your doctor about increasing your medication."

Filter the Air

Your home can be a refuge from seasonal allergies if you control the environment. The most important step is to use an air conditioner. That lets you keep the windows closed, says Dr. Nelson. "It recirculates the air instead of bringing in new air that's full of pollen."

Cleaning or changing the air conditioner's filter frequently during allergy season is helpful, too, adds Dr. Shepherd. She recommends high-efficiency particulate air (HEPA) filters to trap tiny allergy particles.

The same advice applies to your car, Dr. Nelson adds. Always drive with the windows up and the air conditioner on.

The worst possible situation in either case is to have the windows wide open with a fan going full blast. "That," says Dr. Nelson, "can keep pollen circulating in the air forever."

Minimize Mold

If you're allergic to mold spores, hold off praying for rain. Mold loves moist, humid conditions and dark places to hide, says Dr. Shepherd. Use a dehumidifier in damp areas such as basements, and use exhaust fans in high-moisture areas such as the kitchen and bathroom. Remove carpets and mats from

Cold or Allergy? How Can You Tell?

Runny nose, watery eyes, sore throat, cough—it could be a cold. Or is it an allergy? How do you know?

Confusing seasonal allergies with a cold or sinus infection is easy, says Gary Rachelefsky, M.D., associate director of the allergy immunology training program at the UCLA School of Medicine. "Both colds and allergies can cause sore throat, coughing, runny nose, sneezing, and nasal congestion." The big difference is the itching. With allergies, the nose and eyes are itchy. With colds or sinus infections, they're not.

There are other differences, too, says Dr. Rachelefsky. Colds frequently involve a low-grade fever, but allergies don't. Further, colds usually last for a week or so and go away gradually, while allergies can come one day and leave the next or last for many weeks.

If the problem is seasonal, that's another strong clue it's an allergy.

the bathroom as well and wash your towels, washcloths, and shower curtains frequently. It's also a good idea to keep houseplants to a minimum, adds Dr. Shepherd. Mold naturally grows on pots and potting soil.

Think Ahead

If the pollen count has been high for the past couple of days, you can pretty well predict that, barring a late-summer storm, tomorrow it's bound to be higher. So if your allergy medication is barely keeping you comfortable now, give your doctor a call. Ask whether you can head off even more discomfort by increasing your medication or perhaps boosting your medication's effect with a second product.

Go Natural

Every fall James A. Duke, Ph.D., author of *The Green Pharmacy*, encourages friends to come to his herb garden to pick some stinging nettle (*Urtica dioica*), which he says is good in freeze-dried form for allergic sniffling and sneezing. (From 150 to 300 milligrams of stinging nettle in capsule form is classified as safe.) He also recommends eating generous amounts of garlic and onions, which contain anti-inflammatory compounds such as quercetin; 60 to 240 milligrams of standardized ginkgo (*Ginkgo biloba*) extract a day, which interferes with a body chemical that triggers allergies; and the natural antihistamine vitamin C (1,000 milligrams a day through supplements and foods such as citrus fruits, bell peppers, broccoli, and watercress).

Choose Your Weapons

The old standbys for allergy relief—over-the-counter antihistamines or antihistamine/decongestant combinations—are still a good choice. But some allergy sufferers and allergists don't like the side effects: drowsiness, mental

The Female Side of Asthma and Allergies

Menstruation, pregnancy, and menopause. You associate cramps, morning sickness, and hot flashes with them, but did you ever make a connection with asthma and allergy complications? Maybe you should.

Some women with asthma experience flare-ups during their premenstrual and menstrual periods, says Ira Finegold, M.D., chief of allergy and clinical immunology at St. Luke's Roosevelt Hospital in New York City and past president of the American College of Allergy, Asthma, and Immunology. "It's not the majority of cases, but there seems to be a group of women whose asthma might be hormone-related." Bringing these types of flare-ups to your doctor's attention is important for asthma management.

Another large hormonal event in a woman's life—pregnancy—can also affect asthma. Roughly one-third of pregnant women with asthma are at risk of having their asthma get worse, says Dr. Finegold. Ironically, another third might actually see symptoms improve during pregnancy. The rest will probably experience no effect either way. No one is sure why this happens, says Dr. Finegold, but changes in the way a pregnant woman's body responds to inflammation in the lungs and bronchial tubes may be to blame.

Pregnancy can also affect a woman's allergies, says Dr. Finegold. In the first trimester, blood vessels—including those in the nose—become more active and engorged. As a result, stuffiness increases. Some women might not even notice it, but those with allergies might turn into sniffly, stuffy, suffering ladies for the duration.

If you use any kind of allergy treatment, it's important to tell all your doctors (including your allergist, obstetrician/gynecologist, and primary-care physician) as well as your pharmacist if you become pregnant—or even if you're trying to conceive. Some medications are not safe for your baby, but other options are available. Injections and vaccinations, for example, are safe to use, notes Dr. Finegold. "If you are receiving allergy injection treatments or allergy vaccinations before you become pregnant, you can continue with them during pregnancy," he says.

And then there is menopause. Women who are not on estrogen-replacement therapy can suffer from a dry, irritated nose, says Dr. Finegold. For some women, the nasal tissue dries out and shrinks during menopause, and complications such as infection and discomfort may arise. Hormone-replacement therapy may help, as might using a hormone nasal spray, he says.

dullness, and driving impairment. That's why experts recommend that those who don't tolerate or get relief from these older antihistamines should consider the following newer nonsedating products. People with more severe allergies should also consider these new products, since some experts find that they are more effective than the older antihistamines in some people.

- ❖ Nonsedating prescription antihistamines
- ❖ Nonsedating prescription antihistamine/decongestant combinations
- ❖ NasalCrom, an over-the-counter nonsteroidal nasal spray
- ❖ Prescription steroidal nasal sprays (which some doctors think may be the most effective allergy fighters of all)
- ❖ Astelin, a prescription antihistamine nasal spray

Work with your doctor to determine which medication is best for you, says Dr. Rachelefsky. And don't be shy about trying two or three different medications before you find one that works. Often, trial and error is the only way to do it. "There's no way of knowing in advance which one is best," he says.

Give Hypnosis a Whirl

If you're the type who likes to try new things, use your mind for allergy relief. A few studies have found that some people can reduce their allergy symptoms under hypnosis. Does this mean that allergies are psychosomatic? No, but the study results add to the evidence that your mind controls more of your physical responses than anyone had guessed.

To find a person near you who is trained in medical hypnosis, send a business-size self-addressed, stamped envelope to the American Society of Clinical Hypnosis, 2200 East Devon Avenue, Suite 291, Des Plaines, IL 60018, and you'll receive a list of medical hypnotists in your area.

Power over Pain: The Female Advantage

W hen it comes to how men and women handle pain, why are some men the big babies? Painstaking new research suggests that because women tend to experience a greater number of painful events in their lives and because they feel pain more keenly than men, they become better than men at coping with and managing pain.

"For women, their experience with pain is something that happens on a regular basis, through painful menstrual cycles and childbirth. You either deal with the pain or it becomes a debilitating situation," says M.A. Ruda, Ph.D., chief of the cellular neuroscience section at the National Institute for Dental and Craniofacial Research. "For men, their typical experience with pain is an injury that happens traumatically and only occasionally. So their need to develop coping strategies is not so necessary on a regular basis."

Although in the course of their lives women feel more pain than men, women ironically have lower thresholds for pain, meaning the same stimulus can hurt a woman more than a man, according to Karen J. Berkley, Ph.D., of the neuroscience program at Florida State University in Tallahassee. Also, women are statistically more likely to be the victims of a variety of highly painful diseases, such as irritable bowel syndrome, fibromyalgia (achy pain and stiffness in muscles, tendons, and ligaments), and disorders of the temporomandibular joint in the jaw.

How Women Cope

Research shows that women tend to be better at dealing with pain than men. Here are some reasons.

Breathing. Women learn the value of breathing techniques in childbirth-education classes. By focusing on your breathing during a painful episode, you can relax yourself and take your mind off your pain.

Support. Women tend to seek more support during times of pain. They are more likely than men to join support groups and seek out supportive friends and relatives.

Alternative therapies. Just as they are more likely to join support groups, women are more likely than men to pursue alternative therapies such as meditation, biofeedback, and acupuncture.

Attitude. For some reason, women seem to have more of a positive attitude about dealing with pain—they take it less personally and tend to have less lingering antipathy than do men about a spell of pain after it ends.

Even injuries seem to hurt women more than men: Studies show that women appear to feel the pain of traumatic injury more acutely than men.

Hormones, Society, and Culture All Play a Role

As for why women feel pain more keenly than men, scientists aren't completely sure, Dr. Ruda says, although hormones play a role. "We now know that hormones act as receptor sites in the nervous system and can actually affect how the nervous system responds," she says. Scientists also have learned that hormones can modulate the activity of certain genes that are involved in the body's pain sensor system, and they also know that the nervous system of a man is built somewhat differently than a woman's. But details are sketchy, and the unknown outpaces the known.

Society and culture may also play a part. In a world where it's okay for girls to cry, but not boys, males and females are conditioned from infancy to react differently to pain. They also may describe their pain differently, depending on who's listening: Researchers have found that in pain-measurement studies, men who are subjected to painful stimuli act far more stoically when the researcher who asks them to describe the pain is an attractive woman. The men, they found, are more likely to complain to another man.

For women, the adage "practice makes perfect" seems to apply when it comes to pain. Because they feel pain more frequently, women appear to be better able to handle it, according to Francis J. Keefe, Ph.D., professor in the department of psychology at Ohio University in Athens.

Dr. Keefe and his team studied women and men with osteoarthritis, a common age-related condition in which joint cartilage and bone degenerate, causing stiffness and pain. They found that even though women with osteoarthritis appear to feel more pain than men, they coped better than the men in the study. "Women used more pain-coping strategies," Dr. Keefe says. For example, women are more likely than men to go to a doctor or health clinic, talk with others about their pain, join a support group, or experiment with alternative pain-relief strategies such as biofeedback, acupuncture, or meditation, some of which have been scientifically proven to reduce pain in some people.

Further, men showed a much greater carry-over effect—that is, they were in a grumpier mood the day after a bout of intense pain than were the women. "These results suggest that while women may experience more intense pain than men, they may be better able to limit its emotional consequences," Dr. Keefe says. In other words, women tend to take pain less personally than men and don't hold a grudge the next day.

You Can Ease Your Partner's Pain

HEALTH FLASH

A wife may be more sensitive to her husband's pain than he is to hers, suggests a recent study of 19 osteoarthritis patients conducted at Duke University Medical Center in Durham, North Carolina. Watching tapes of the patients performing a variety of tasks, women were more accurate in detecting the level of pain reported by their husbands than vice versa.

"It may be that women are more tuned in to picking up social cues in people than men are," says Francis Keefe, Ph.D., professor in the department of psychology at Ohio University in Athens and one of the researchers in the study. But either sex can help the other deal with chronic pain, he adds. If your spouse suffers from chronic pain, he suggests you try the following tips.

Recommend relaxation. Remind your partner to take deep breaths and relax one muscle at a time from scalp to toes.

Say "whoa!" Encourage your spouse to pace his or her activity and to take frequent breaks.

Listen. Rather than suggesting solutions, ask questions and let your partner vent about the pain.

Develop a pain game plan. Map out your spouse's pain cycles together to help you predict when one is about to hit so you can prevent or alleviate it.

Get help. Psychologists specializing in communication are especially good at helping couples through the problems that occur as a result of chronic pain.

Pain Relievers Work Better on Women

Researchers have discovered another difference between the genders: Certain pain-relieving drugs appear to help women more than men. At the University of California, San Francisco, researcher and professor of nursing Christine Miaskowski and her colleagues evaluated the effectiveness of several pain-relieving medications on men and women who'd had their wisdom teeth removed by the same surgeon. The researchers found that a family of medications known as kappa opioids, prescription analgesics that are commonly administered for postsurgical dental pain, eased pain better and for longer periods of time for women than for men.

Although there's no research on whether other medications, such as over-the-counter pain relievers, work differently for men or women, gender-related pain research could put a whole new spin on how a doctor prescribes medication. Not only might women and men need different amounts of medication, but doses may vary for an individual woman.

"In the future, a major aspect of our diagnostics and treatment for women may be based on a timeline of where a woman is in life—before puberty, puberty, childbearing years, menopause, beyond menopause, or on hormone-replacement therapy," Dr. Ruda says. "All of those things, and for that matter, what phase of the menstrual cycle you're in, are likely going to contribute to the dosages of drugs or what drugs it would be better to take at different times."

For now, though, researchers are continuing to study the ways in which men and women feel pain differently.

Lyme Disease: Prepare— Don't Panic

Sally was concerned. She had several of the symptoms of Lyme disease—joint pain, fatigue, and headaches—but her blood test was negative. Could she have Lyme disease anyway?

"It's unlikely," says Mary Jane Minkin, M.D., a board-certified obstetrician/gynecologist in New Haven, Connecticut, and clinical professor at Yale University School of Medicine. "But Sally isn't the first person to express concern to me about having Lyme disease in spite of a negative blood test.

"While it's especially important to be aware of the warning signs of the disease—a skin rash around the site of a tick bite, headache, fever, fatigue, and muscle or joint pain—Lyme paranoia, as I call it, is not warranted. Even in high-risk areas such as Connecticut, where I live, the chance of developing Lyme disease after a tick bite is only 1 to 2 percent," Dr. Minkin says.

"Many patients come in with relatively nonspecific symptoms, believing they have Lyme disease," says noted Lyme researcher and rheumatologist Robert Schoen, M.D., clinical professor of medicine at Yale University School of Medicine. They may have another illness that needs treatment, but they also may be quite healthy and experiencing fatigue, headaches, and muscle aches simply because of stress and overwork, he adds.

So what's the bottom line? If you have a negative test for Lyme disease,

The Easy Way to Remove a Tick

Removing a tick within 24 hours of attachment means there's much less risk of infection. Here's the best way to go about it: Take a pair of tweezers with very thin ends and grasp the tick as close as possible to your skin (at its mouth parts). Pull the tick straight out using firm and steady pressure. Don't jerk or twist it. Try not to squeeze the body, or you may inject the contents of the tick into your skin. After removal, disinfect the skin and wash your hands with soap and water.

pursue further testing to determine the true cause of your symptoms. Even if they're caused by stress, they're very real and can be treated.

Take Precautions

The fear of Lyme disease is understandable. This debilitating condition, caused by an infection with a bacterium called *Borrelia burgdorferi*, can be transmitted to people when they are bitten by a tick carrying it. If you live in an area where Lyme disease is a risk, your best bet is to avoid getting bitten. The best way to do that is to take the following precautions.

- ❖ Avoid tick-infested areas.
- ❖ Wear long-sleeved shirts and pants outdoors.
- ❖ Trim the grass and clear away leaves and brush from around your house to discourage ticks from hanging out.
- ❖ Use insect repellent that works on ticks and follow the instructions carefully.
- ❖ When you come indoors, check yourself for ticks and remove them as soon as possible.

Consider the New Vaccine

The good news on the Lyme front is the approval by the Food and Drug Administration (FDA) of the Lymerix vaccine, the first vaccine to prevent Lyme disease. It can reduce your chance of becoming infected by about 80 percent.

People who live in or plan to visit tick-infested areas should consider getting the vaccine. (Check with your local or state health department if you're not sure about a certain area.)

The vaccine is given in a series of three shots. After the initial dose, you receive a second shot a month later and the final one 12 months after the first injection. (An accelerated schedule is being considered by the FDA.) Side effects include some redness and swelling where the injection is given and possible flulike symptoms. The cost of the series of shots is about $150.

Even if you've had Lyme disease in the past, you're still a candidate for vaccination since you can get it again. Lymerix is only approved for people ages 15 to 70, since that's the age group included in the experimental studies. Women who are pregnant should not be vaccinated. In studies of the vaccine, women were advised to wait 3 months after finishing the series of vaccinations before becoming pregnant.

Don't forget that it's not just you and your immediate family who need protection against Lyme disease. If you live in an area where the deer ticks that cause the disease are prevalent, make sure that your pet gets a vaccination also.

part four

Healing with Food, Herbs, and Nutrition

4

His and Her Health

What Your Food Cravings Mean

You just got home from work, and you're starving. You want to reward yourself for surviving another day. Research shows that if you're a woman, you'll reach for something chocolate. If you're a man, you'll probably see red—red meat, that is.

"Women crave carbohydrates, especially simple sugars, such as chocolate, cake, pastries, candy, cookies, and ice cream," says Janet Zalman, president of the Zalman Nutrition Group in Washington, D.C., and specialty advisor for the National Women's Health Resource Center. "They also crave white bread, white rice, and regular pasta as opposed to the more complex, denser carbohydrates like whole-wheat pasta, brown and wild rice, and whole- or multi-grain breads.

"On the other hand, men crave more fatty, salty, protein-rich foods, such as steaks, roasts, hamburgers, cheese, nuts, french fries, and potato chips," Zalman says. "Their first choice when they're cooking for themselves or when they go out to dinner is a thick, juicy steak and some fries on the side."

What's causing these cravings? Nix the myth that your body craves something it needs. These foods are all big sources of fat, sugar, and salt, and our Western diet provides us with plenty of them. According to Zalman, stress is the number one culprit behind cravings for both women and men. "As our lifestyles become more and more frantic, people are increasingly stressed. After eating a high-carbohydrate meal like pasta and garlic bread, your body releases the amino acid tryptophan. This gets converted into serotonin, which is the 'feel-good' brain chemical. High levels of serotonin have a calming effect. When under stress, women don't reach for carrots; they reach for chocolates. Eating this way is self-medicating because it changes your brain chemistry."

Men use food as ammunition against stress. Their thinking: "I worked hard all day, and I want a reward. Now." They like to ingest a lot of calories very quickly. "Women will prepare a salad, have some fish, and add a little rice. Men think of a meal that's quick and easy to prepare but that's dense in calories, such as steak and fries," says Zalman.

How can you curb those cravings? Follow these tips.

❖ Ask yourself why you're craving the food. What did you have for breakfast or lunch that has put your body out of balance? Are you under stress?

❖ Strive to eat a healthy diet. Consume low-fat protein, such as fish, chicken, pork, egg whites, and low-fat dairy. Add plenty of fruits, vegetables, and whole grains. Fat should come from olive or canola oil and fish high in omega-3 fatty acids, such as salmon, swordfish, or tuna.

❖ When you're faced with a craving, reach for a healthier version of the food in question. "If you crave chocolate, skip the candy bar and whip up a warm drink made from unsweetened cocoa powder, skim milk, and a little vanilla extract," advises Zalman. "This chocolaty drink has no fat or sugar, yet it's satisfying. I call it Zalman's Healthy Hot Chocolate Fix."

❖ Participate in some form of aerobic exercise every day, such as walking, bicycling, or swimming. "Exercise helps your body and your mind release stress," notes Zalman. "It will also help your body metabolize glucose more effectively."

21 What Men Eat: A Woman's Guide

How can your guy pack away so much more than you? Three couples wrote down everything they ate for 3 days. Here's how their diets compare, with a nutritionist's assessment of each one.

Danielle and Ben—She Diets, He Doesn't

Danielle DiMarco, 29 (5'6", 123 pounds). "I'm really conscious of what I eat. Everything is either fat-free or light. When we go to the grocery store, we have to buy separate cheese, cream cheese, salad dressing—even separate creamer for our coffee. Before we were married, we never ate the same things. Now we feel bad if we don't eat together. But our eating habits are totally opposite. I usually don't eat breakfast, and Ben has two bagels with gobs of cream cheese. He tends to snack more; he'll buy potato chips and then snack on them during the day. (He works at home.) He'll eat a whole bag of tortilla chips at one sitting if I let him. He also drinks a lot of soda pop. When we go out to dinner, he either eats my leftovers right there or takes them home and eats them later.

"I love to exercise. I hop on the treadmill for half an hour, and I run—I don't walk. Then I do a step class. I might go half an hour early and do weights. When I can't get to the gym, I do it at home. I have to do some type of activity every day. Before our wedding, I kept a journal of my workouts.

What They Ate: Danielle and Ben

Danielle

Day 1
Breakfast: 1 cup tea with skim milk and honey
Lunch: Orange; 1 pretzel; water
Dinner: 1 cup sesame chicken; small baked potato; small applesauce; 1 glass lemonade

Day 2
Breakfast: Small bag Frosted Mini-Wheats; sugar-free low-fat hot chocolate
Lunch: Apple; 5 small pretzel pockets; water
Snack: Two tortilla chips and salsa just for taste
Dinner: Small salad with fat-free dressing; gnocchi with 2 meatballs; water

Day 3
Breakfast: 1 cup cranberry juice
Lunch: Orange; cinnamon cappuccino
Dinner: Small piece of fat-free chicken broccoli pie; water

Ben

Day 1
Breakfast: 2 bagels with cream cheese; coffee (black); cranberry juice; water
Lunch: Burger King Whopper; large fries; large soda
Snack: Half a can of nuts
Dinner: 3 slices sausage-and-pepperoni pizza; salad with blue cheese dressing; 10 wings; Pepsi; water

Day 2
Breakfast: 3 scrambled eggs with cheese; 2 bagels with butter; water
Lunch: Salsa and half a bag of tortilla chips; frozen broccolini dinner; water
Snack: Half a bag of tortilla chips and salsa
Dinner: 2 helpings of spaghetti and meatballs; 3 slices of Italian bread with butter; Pepsi

Day 3
Breakfast: Full bowl of Total cereal; banana; coffee (black)
Lunch: Potato soup; pasta with mushrooms, chicken, and cheese; water
Dinner: 3 slices pepperoni pizza; 10 bite-size pizza rolls; handful of pistachio nuts; salsa and chips

Now I write in my calendar what I did the day before. I do take one day off—if I didn't, my body would be dead."

Ben DiMarco, 27 (5'10", 190 pounds). "I think my eating dates back to high school wrestling. To get down to my weight class, I'd basically starve every week to lose 15 pounds. As soon as my team weighed in, we'd hoard ourselves. Now, whenever I get a chance, I eat like a pig. Danielle eats less than half the food I do. She tells me that when we eat dinner, I don't look at her—I only pay attention to my food. I come from a family where everybody ate a lot. If Danielle and I go out, I'll eat almost all of the appetizer myself, then the salad, my meal, and the other half of hers. My big problem is that I don't stop when I'm full. My work environment is tough. When I'm out with clients, it's hard for me to just get a salad. When I'm at my home office, I'll do 2 or 3 hours of work and I'll have to run and see what's in the refrigerator.

"I've been too busy with my business to work out. I have things that are more important—like big jobs, big money, meeting deadlines. Those are things that are a priority to me because our economic well-being is what I have to worry about."

The expert's assessment: "I hope Ben has good genes!" says nutritionist Phyllis Roxland, R.D. "His low-fiber and high–animal protein/fat diet, combined with lack of exercise, puts him at increased risk for several diseases. Here are a few things he could add to his diet: a bowl of minestrone soup, a veggie burger with tomatoes, pasta with red clam sauce, a black bean burrito with salsa. And he should get rid of the hot wings, fast-food burgers, and pepperoni pizza. Also, I always recommend a daily multivitamin and mineral supplement—just to provide a margin of safety.

"At first glance, Danielle's diet seems very spartan and restrictive, but her low calorie intake (less than 1,000 a day) is apparently adequate for her: She's not underweight, and she's able to do plenty of exercise. Her protein intake is borderline, because she doesn't consume any high-protein foods for breakfast or lunch. (Maybe she could have a bowl of minestrone soup with Ben.) Her calcium intake could also use a boost; if she doesn't want to add dairy, some green leafy vegetables—other than spinach, whose oxalates interfere with the absorption of calcium—would help."

Nancy and Eric: He Diets, She Doesn't

Nancy Chwatt, 35 (5'5", 105 pounds). "We're total opposites. Eric is definitely a much more disciplined person than I am. I eat whenever I can, when I get to it. Between taking care of two kids and working part-time, sometimes I don't get to it. He'll stand in front of the mirror and check himself out in the morning, watching the improvements in his body. I get dressed and I'm out

What They Ate: Nancy and Eric

Nancy

Day 1
Breakfast: Coffee with whole milk; blueberry muffin (shared with daughter)
Lunch: 1 slice cheese pizza; 1 piece chocolate cake
Snack: 1 small bag Ruffles potato chips; diet peach Snapple
Dinner: Pork lo mein, Pellegrino

Day 2
Breakfast: Bagel with cream cheese and bacon; instant coffee with whole milk
Lunch: taco; guacamole with chips; jelly doughnut
Dinner: 1 piece of lasagna; half a Ring Ding; Pellegrino

Day 3
Breakfast: Bagel with olive cream cheese; cappuccino; grapefruit juice
Lunch: Half a chicken salad sandwich; chicken nuggets her daughter didn't eat
Dinner: Three-quarters of a box of Kraft macaroni and cheese mix

Eric

Day 1
Breakfast: Egg-white omelette; bialy; mango juice; water; acidophilus capsule
Lunch: Organic shell steak with salad
Snack: 2 bananas; water
Dinner: Steamed chicken and broccoli; shrimp in black bean sauce; brown rice; wonton

Day 2
Breakfast: Egg-white omelette with turkey and lite Swiss cheese; English muffin; acidophilus capsule
Lunch: Tuna on rye with tomato and canola mayo; water
Dinner: Stew with organic chicken, potato, carrots, and organic turkey sausage

Day 3
Breakfast: Organic pancakes with pure maple syrup; water; acidophilus capsule
Lunch: Roasted chicken and coleslaw; water
Dinner: Organic banana and other organic fruit; water

of there. I'll eat whatever is around and easiest. If I'm out and hungry, I'll just get a hot dog on the street. Eric would never put that in his body.

I wish I did eat more healthfully. But I've never had to worry about my weight, so I don't think twice about it. We never eat the same meal. Right now, I'm making him dinner—organic chicken and vegetables—and I'm probably going to order Mexican food. All I've had today is pizza and then some chocolate caramels and coffee. In restaurants, I usually order dessert, and he won't even taste it. I wish I exercised. I haven't for over a year. It doesn't fit into my life right now. I always tell Eric I want to come back as him."

Eric Chwatt, 37 (5'10", 150 pounds). "As poor as Nancy's eating habits are, I never say anything to her. She's very thin, and I always tell her she needs to eat more. I try to eat wholesome meals. I've started giving up sugars because I was feeling sluggish. I'm not eating any desserts or simple carbohydrates. I can't go a day without breakfast because my body can't handle it—I get lethargic.

"I do what I do just because I feel better and I have more energy. Nancy already has all that energy. The longest I've taken off from exercise is 5 days. In the back of my mind, exercise helps me get all the toxins out of my system. The kids are always sick from school and play groups. I find when I exercise as hard as I do and take steams afterward, I sweat it out and I'm able to fight off the bugs that the kids are passing around. Nancy belongs to a gym but hasn't been there in a while. I bought her prepaid training sessions, but she hasn't had a chance to use them."

The expert's assessment: "Nancy had no fruits or vegetables at all (except for things like the jelly in her doughnut, grapefruit juice, and the olives in her cream cheese)!" says Roxland. "Her fiber intake for the day was half of a gram. The recommended daily allowance is 20 to 30 grams. Her diet is low in every nutrient. There's also a problem with the type of fat she eats: It's either saturated animal fat from meat and dairy or hydrogenated fat from processed foods, such as chips and pastry. I realize she's pressed for time, but maybe she could grab a handful of nuts and some fresh or dried fruit instead of a doughnut, for example.

"Eric's diet is certainly varied and adequate with respect to all nutrients. His concern about salt, preservatives, and pesticides might not be necessary, but it doesn't hurt. Acidophilus is usually prescribed for certain intestinal conditions or if someone has been on long-term antibiotic therapy. But again, it won't hurt. The one change I would make (because Eric is obviously concerned about health) would be to replace animal proteins with vegetable proteins such as beans, tofu, and veggie burgers."

Elissa and Justin: Neither Diets; Both Eat Well

Elissa Comsudi, 25 (5'6", 120 pounds). "Justin and I really are in sync about our eating. From our very first date, we've spent a lot of time in restaurants

What They Ate: Elissa and Justin

Elissa

Day 1
Breakfast: Banana; coffee (with cream and sugar)
Lunch: Half a chicken burrito (with rice, black beans, sour cream, salsa, cheese, guacamole, lettuce, and tomatoes)
Dinner: Stir-fry chicken with onions, mushrooms, snap peas, broccoli, and rice

Day 2
Breakfast: Banana; latte
Lunch: Minestrone soup; Caesar salad; corn muffin
Snack: Half a bag of Skittles
Dinner: Calamari in tomato sauce; porcini mushroom ravioli; red wine
Snack: Shared Häagen-Dazs coffee ice cream, added chocolate chips

Day 3
Breakfast: Banana; coffee (with cream and sugar)
Lunch: Half of a leftover chicken breast; mashed potatoes
Snack: Small yogurt
Dinner: 3 slices pepperoni-and-mushroom pizza

Justin

Day 1
Breakfast: Honey Nut Cheerios with banana and milk
Lunch: Burger King Broiler chicken sandwich; large fries; Coke
Dinner: Clam soup and salad

Day 2
Breakfast: McDonald's Egg McMuffin; hash browns; Honey Nut Cheerios with milk
Lunch: Chicken burrito (with rice, sour cream, cheese, guacamole, salsa, lettuce, tomatoes)
Snack: Apple
Dinner: Calamari in tomato sauce; seafood ravioli; red wine

Day 3
Breakfast: Honey Nut Cheerios with milk; water
Lunch: Spinach salad with almonds, artichoke hearts, sprouts, tomatoes, and honey vinaigrette dressing; roll
Dinner: 3 slices pepperoni-and-mushroom pizza

bonding over food. We like to make a huge deal out of the meal, enjoying the food, thinking about what we want to order. We also think about where we want to eat the next night. We eat out a lot together in restaurants. We'll usually share an appetizer, then each eats what the other has ordered. Justin is more of a sweet dessert person. His favorite is dumping chocolate chips in coffee Häagen-Dazs ice cream. That was a nice creative dish that he introduced me to! Unlike Justin, I never can finish a dessert. I'll have a couple of bites, and then he'll wind up polishing it off. I eat a lot of food for a woman, but he still beats me. When we're not together, I tend not to make such a big deal about food. For dinner, I'll just make pasta with some cut-up tomatoes or have the other half of the burrito left over from my lunch. I admit, I do have to have a sugar fix almost every day—my favorites are Gummi snacks or Starbursts or Skittles.

"Justin and I both exercise, but we view it very differently. It has been more of a priority for him than it is for me. He feels very strongly about getting to the gym and lifting some weights or swimming. My exercise is usually walking to and from work. I like to exercise, but I don't feel like I'm going to die if I don't make it to the gym."

Justin Cheen, 27 (6', 185 pounds). "We both really enjoy eating. We like everything from dining at a fine restaurant to going out for fast food. The only thing that's really different is that Elissa eats faster than I do. Also, I like a lot of fish, but she doesn't.

Since we share everything, I'm glad she is adventurous and orders cool things. Elissa tends to get these cravings, so when it comes to consulting over the menu, she tells me what she's craving and we see if that jives with my stomach. I wouldn't be happy if we went to dinner and she picked at a salad. She can eat, but I eat more than she does. That's one of the advantages I have: If we go out to dinner, we'll order a bunch of stuff, and I get to eat off her plate, so that's nice. If we're not eating, we'll spend our time talking about eating. For some reason, it's really enjoyable. It's been like that since our first date."

The expert's assessment: "This is a perfect blend of nutritional adequacy and fun!" says Roxland. "Elissa and Justin's diet obviously includes some high-fat, high-sugar, empty-calorie food, but there's plenty of room for the 'good stuff,' too. With the exercises they're both doing, they seem to be in good calorie balance. Power to the chocolate chips!"

The Top 10 Super-Healing Foods

Every second of your life, your cells are bombarded by thousands of dangerous particles called free radicals. In a split second, they can alter your DNA in ways that cause cancer. Or they can change LDL cholesterol so it sticks to artery walls. Free radicals can even damage collagen and make skin wrinkle-prone. Over time, changes like these add up, and they accelerate the aging process.

Fortunately, you can fight back. The trick is to load your diet with antioxidants—the natural enemies of free radicals—by eating lots of fruits and vegetables. The more antioxidants you have on board, the more free radicals you can neutralize before they harm you.

The following super foods are loaded with antioxidants as well as other disease-fighting nutritional powerhouses that can help you live healthier and longer.

1. Beans

Healing powers: Beans contain a healthy dose of fiber and can help lower cholesterol, stabilize blood sugar, and reduce breast cancer risk.

Best bets: Black-eyed peas, chickpeas, kidney beans, and limas each pack 7 grams of fiber or more per half-cup. Rinse canned beans to reduce sodium.

2. Berries

Healing powers: Berries contain fiber, vitamin C, and an antioxidant called ellagic acid, which is helpful for preventing cataracts, cancer, and constipation.

Tip: To get the most nutrients, buy or pick berries at peak freshness and eat them raw. Cooking berries destroys some vitamin C.

3. Broccoli

Healing powers: Broccoli contains two powerful cancer-fighting compounds as well as fiber and beta-carotene, which ward off heart disease, certain cancers, and cataracts.

Best bets: Broccoli that's dark—almost purple—has the most beta-carotene. Lightly steaming it helps release healing compounds; overheating can destroy nutrients.

4. Carrots

Healing powers: Carrots contain rich stores of the antioxidant beta-carotene, which improves night vision and protects against heart disease, cancer, and macular degeneration (the leading cause of blindness in older adults).

Tip: Trim greenery off carrots before storing to prevent the leaves from leaching nutrients from the roots. Juicing or lightly cooking carrots helps release the beta-carotene. Eat carrots with a little fat to boost absorption.

5. Fish

Healing powers: Fish contains omega-3 fatty acids—a type of fat that helps prevent heart disease, may fight colon and breast cancers, and may protect you from depression.

Best bets: Try fresh or canned salmon (not smoked), mackerel, rainbow trout, tuna, whitefish (fresh, not smoked), sardines, and pickled Atlantic herring. Also choose canned white (albacore) tuna packed in water, but look for the most grams of fat per serving; the more total fat, the more omega-3 fats.

6. Milk

Healing powers: Milk contains calcium, which helps strengthen bones, prevent osteoporosis, and lower blood pressure and cholesterol. It may also protect against certain cancers.

Stay Young with the Miracle Berry

Want to stay young, live longer, and keep your mind sharp? Make blueberries a habit! These scrumptious berries have emerged as nature's number one source of antioxidants. Calorie for calorie, they are the single most ferocious food in your supermarket, capable of zapping the free radicals responsible for so many diseases.

In tests at the USDA Human Nutrition Research Center on Aging at Tufts University in Boston, blueberries beat out 39 other common fresh fruits and vegetables in antioxidant power—even such heavyweights as kale, strawberries, spinach, and broccoli. Much of that power comes literally "out of the blue"—from the anthocyanin pigments that give blueberries their deep blue hue.

With a mere ½ cup of blueberries, you can just about double the amount of antioxidants most Americans get in one day.

Perhaps the most miraculous potential of blueberries: There's a possibility that they can actually reverse the mental decline that accompanies getting older, says James Joseph, Ph.D., a USDA scientist who studies the effects of aging on the brain.

Two varieties of blueberries are generally available. The most plentiful are hybrid cultivated blueberries, grown throughout the United States. Wild blueberries from Maine and eastern Canada are available frozen. Wild blueberries are smaller, and their flavor is more intense. They also hold up better in baking. (When baking with frozen blueberries, lightly dust the unthawed berries with flour before stirring them into the batter.)

Blueberries are heavenly in muffins, pies, and other baked desserts. Mildly heating blueberries does not cause loss of antioxidant power, says Ronald Prior, Ph.D., head of the USDA Phytochemical Laboratory at Tufts University. Other ways to enjoy these blue wonders: Sprinkle them over your cold breakfast cereal, stir them into oatmeal, add them to tossed salads and fruit cups, serve them with low-fat milk and sugar, scatter them over light ice cream, or blend them into smoothies. For a special breakfast treat, spread softened light cream cheese on a warm toasted English muffin and top generously with blueberries.

Best bets: Buy nonfat milk; for thicker consistency, add nonfat milk powder. Also, choose cartons. Translucent plastic jugs admit light, which destroys some nutrients.

7. Nuts

Healing powers: Nuts contain antioxidants called flavonoids and other compounds that protect against heart disease and help lower cholesterol. Ellagic acid and omega-3 fats in walnuts may help prevent cancer.

Best bets: Some good choices are peanuts, almonds, and walnuts, but don't exceed your desired daily fat intake. Sprinkling chopped, toasted nuts on cereals or salads is a good way to control portions.

8. Onions

Healing powers: Onions contain compounds that lower cholesterol, thin the blood, and prevent hardening of the arteries (all helping to prevent heart disease). These compounds may also help ward off gastrointestinal cancers.

Best bets: Red and yellow onions have the highest flavonoid content; white onions have the least.

9. Oranges

Healing powers: Oranges contain vitamin C, which aids healing, boosts immunity, and helps the body absorb iron. They also contain pectin, which helps lower cholesterol and control blood sugar.

Tip: Don't peel off the white spongy layer just beneath the skin; it contains half of the fruit's pectin. And stock up on juice concentrate; it's as nutritious as fresh juice.

10. Tomatoes

Healing powers: Tomatoes contain two antioxidants—lycopene and vitamin C—that protect against heart disease and cancers of the prostate and lungs.

Tip: For maximum nutrition, buy ripe tomatoes, not pale ones. The best sources of lycopene are processed tomato products such as tomato paste and spaghetti sauce. To make the lycopene in fresh tomatoes more absorbable, cook them in a little oil.

Painless Ways to Love Those Veggies

While most women eventually outgrow their childhood loathing of vegetables, some of us never quite reach that nutritionally mature state. Sure, we'll choke down a broccoli floret or two—if it happens to come with dinner. But sauté some spinach on our own? You have to be kidding. Why waste time and calories on veggies, when you can save on both and stockpile nutrients by popping a vitamin?

Glad you asked. Truth is, you can compensate for an underdeveloped diet by popping a daily vitamin supplement. But while that pill may provide your daily value of vitamins and minerals, eating a diet that's bereft of beans or even beets means you're missing daily doses of two other critical nutrients—phytochemicals and fiber.

Phytochemicals shield vegetables from viruses, bacteria, and fungi, and they do much the same in us, offering protection from cancer, heart disease, and other debilitating conditions. As for fiber, unless you're swallowing your daily vitamin with a glass of Metamucil, you're probably not getting as much as you need to lower your cholesterol level and your risk of colon cancer.

To keep you on track, here's a sneaky, five-point plan for slipping the green stuff into your diet without causing your tastebuds too much shock. Follow it, and you'll reap the benefits of eating vegetables as efficiently as possible.

Make the Most of Every Bite

Don't worry about eating three to five servings of vegetables a day. It's not the quantity as much as the nutritional quality of your choices that counts. If you pick and prepare your produce wisely, you can eat fewer vegetables because every mouthful will be nutritionally packed. Here are a few ideas.

Skip the fresh and go for frozen. If your produce is stashed in the fridge for more than a few days, most fresh vegetables lose a substantial amount of nutrients. That's why frozen vegetables make just as much sense.

"Vegetables are usually frozen within a few hours of harvest, so the nutritional quality can actually be better than fresh," says Diane Barrett, Ph.D., associate professor of food science and technology at the University of California, Davis. As for canned veggies, they're fine if you're stocking a bomb shelter, but the heat of the canning process destroys B vitamins. Better to skip them.

The Top Fiber-Filled Vegetables and Fruits

Eating the recommended 20 to 35 grams of fiber a day doesn't mean you have to eat like a rabbit—just choose the produce that packs the most punch. Here are the 20 that contain the most fiber.

Vegetables	Serving	Grams of fiber
Acorn squash, cooked	1 cup	9
Black beans, cooked	½ cup	8
Lima beans(large), cooked	½ cup	7
Pumpkin, canned	1 cup	7
Artichoke, cooked	1 medium	6
Chickpeas, cooked	½ cup	6
Great Northern beans, cooked	½ cup	6
Kidney beans, cooked	½ cup	6
Parsnips, cooked	1 cup, slices	6
Yams, cooked	1 cup	5

Fruit	Serving	Grams of fiber
Avocado	1 medium	10
Blackberries	1 cup	8
Raspberries	1 cup	8
Apple	1 large	6
Seedless raisins	1 cup	6
Figs	3 medium	5
Guava	1 fruit	5
Papaya	1 medium	5
Pear	1 large	5
Blueberries	1 cup	4

Pick a rainbow assortment. When you do buy fresh produce, opt for the most brightly colored vegetables you can find, since vibrant hues usually mean more vitamins, says Anne Dubner, R.D., a nutrition consultant and spokesperson for the American Dietetic Association. This means that you should go easy on light green items like iceberg lettuce, celery, and cucumbers—and load up on carrots, tomatoes, sweet red peppers, and sweet potatoes. Or go for darker shades of green like spinach and romaine lettuce, which packs nearly seven times the vitamin C and twice the calcium of its paler cousin iceberg.

Relish them raw. Want to ruin perfectly good produce? Just add hot water. "When you boil vegetables, the water-soluble B and C vitamins are drawn into the water," explains Dr. Barrett. In fact, anywhere from 33 to 90 percent of a boiled vegetable's vitamin C typically ends up at the bottom of the pot—along with a lot of its taste.

Dip them. Store a bag of washed and cut vegetables in a plastic bag in your refrigerator. (If you don't have time to chop them yourself, just swing by the supermarket and raid their salad bar.) When you want a snack, skip the nachos and use your salsa to garnish the veggies instead. Or use your favorite low-fat version of onion dip, cheese spread, or salad dressing. Just make sure you pick brightly colored vegetables like sugar snap peas, carrots, sweet red peppers, and broccoli. Celery sticks simply won't cut it.

Flash 'em. "Flash boiling" is one of the fastest and healthiest ways to cook vegetables. Just bring a pot of water to a rolling boil, add your veggies, count to 10, then drain them. You'll soften the vegetables a bit (which makes it easier for some people to get them down) but preserve much of their vitamin and mineral content. Steaming, stir-frying, and microwaving also preserve nutrients while cooking vegetables fast.

Are You Eating the Wrong Carbohydrates?

That English muffin you had for breakfast? The soft pretzel you ate for lunch at the mall? The plateful of pasta and Italian bread you had for dinner? And those crackers before bed? They're all high in complex carbohydrates—so they're just what the Food Guide Pyramid ordered, right?

Well, surprisingly enough, not quite. The trouble is, almost all of the complex carb foods we healthy eaters have been gobbling up lately are made from refined grains, which are stripped of their nutritious bran and germ, instead of whole grains as nature made them. In 1994, the average American ate 199 pounds of grains, but only 10 pounds of that were whole grains.

So in essence, we're eating a ton of white bread—or its equivalent in pasta, crackers, pretzels, and more. And here's the problem: To your body, refined complex carbs like these are virtually the same as sugar. True, your white bread is fortified with important vitamins and minerals such as iron and folic acid and contains a smidgen of protein and fiber. But for the most part, refined carbs are "sweet nothings": thousands of sugar molecules strung together that are rapidly absorbed by your body—a source of calories for energy but not much else.

Think of it this way: Every slice of white bread you eat is like eating three or four vitamin-fortified marshmallows. A cup of pasta? Eight marshmallows. And this "all-marshmallow" diet could make a big difference in your health.

Based on interviews with experts including Walter Willett, M.D., head of the nutrition section of Harvard University's School of Public Health, it seems that diets high in refined carbohydrates are actually harmful. "We're seeing that whether you eat lots of refined grains or whole grains can make a major difference in your risk of several diseases," he says. Those diseases include the following:

Heart disease. Iowa women who ate two or more servings of whole-grain foods every day had 30 percent less risk of death from ischemic heart disease than women who ate three servings a week or less. An earlier study found that for each 10-gram increase in whole-grain fiber per day, men had a 30 percent decrease in heart attack risk.

Diabetes. In a study of 65,000 nurses by Dr. Willett and his colleagues, the ones who ate the most white bread and other refined carbohydrates and the least whole-grain cereal fiber had 2½ times more risk of developing type 2 diabetes over 6 years of follow-up.

Colon cancer. In Italy, people who ate the most whole grains had half as much colon cancer as those who ate the least whole grains over 13 years of follow-up. Diets higher in whole-grain fiber help prevent chronic constipation, which itself has recently been linked to double the risk of colon cancer.

Breast cancer. Though some studies find no connection, a recent study in Italy discovered that women with breast cancer ate more bread, cereal, cakes, and dessert—all of which, the researchers pointed out, are usually made in Italy from refined grains. Diets high in wheat bran have been linked to lower rates of breast cancer.

"It would be nice if refined grains were protective or at least neutral," says grain expert Joanne Slavin, R.D., Ph.D., of the University of Minnesota, St. Paul. "But some of the new epidemiologic studies aren't positive at all for refined grains."

Whole Grains Are Loaded

Compared with refined carbs, whole grains carry nutrients by the truckload. That's because they retain invaluable parts of the grain kernel called the bran and the germ. It's these "extra" nutrients that may protect you from illness.

Here's how some of these nutrients work.

Fiber. This helps to fight constipation. It's fermented by bacteria in the colon to a fatty acid that arrests the growth of colon cancer cells in test tubes. Wheat fiber lowers levels of estrogen in women, which may reduce breast cancer risk. Soluble fiber such as oat bran lowers cholesterol.

Antioxidants. In whole grains, antioxidants—vitamin E, phenolic acids, phytic acid, tocotrienols—keep free radicals in check, which helps prevent heart disease, cancer, and diabetes.

Lignans. These are precursors to weak forms of estrogen in the body and are linked to lower rates of breast cancer.

The Wonders of Whole Wheat

In a grain of wheat, 80 to 90 percent of all micronutrients are located in the bran and germ, the parts stripped away to make white flour. Here's how whole-wheat flour stacks up against the white stuff.

- ❖ Fiber—4 times more
- ❖ Copper—2 times more
- ❖ Magnesium—6 times more
- ❖ Potassium—3 times more
- ❖ Selenium—2 times more
- ❖ Zinc—4 times more
- ❖ Vitamin E—20 times more

In addition, whole-wheat flour has substantially more:

- ❖ Lignans
- ❖ Phenolic acids
- ❖ Phytic acid
- ❖ Tocotrienols

Trace minerals. Trace minerals, such as zinc and selenium, help beef up the immune system and participate in antioxidant reactions. Whole grains are stuffed with hard-to-get minerals.

Is the Pyramid Wrong?

It appears that the Food Guide Pyramid is incorrect. After all, it advises you to eat 6 to 11 servings—not whole-grain servings—of bread, cereal, rice, and pasta a day as the mainstay of a healthy diet. The critical suggestion—"To get the fiber you need, choose several servings a day of foods made from whole grains"—gets lost in the fine print.

In fact, Dr. Willett thinks that the Food Guide Pyramid is "highly misleading," and he wants to see it redesigned to recommend whole-grain foods specifically—in big print.

How Many Servings Are Enough?

Clearly, the correct number of servings is more than the current average—only about 1 person in 10 eats even one whole grain a day. The American Dietetic Association suggests three a day. "Three are key" is their poetic guideline.

But other experts think that's too conservative. "I would go much higher," says Dr. Slavin. "If we could get more whole grains in the diet, people would have long-term gains in their health."

One scientist who anticipated the potential harm from diets too full of refined carbohydrates was John Weisburger, M.D., Ph.D., honorary senior member of the American Health Foundation in Valhalla, New York. "Back in 1978, when the FDA tried to ban saccharin, I noted that the American people would be better off if the FDA banned white bread," he says.

The Bottom Line

Whole grains look too important to ignore. Start now to replace at least half—or more—of your refined carbohydrates with whole-grain carbohydrates. Here are seven easy ways to increase your intake of whole grains.

1. Instead of white or "wheat" bread, eat whole-wheat. "Any bread you buy should be whole-grain," says Moshe Shike, M.D., head of cancer prevention and wellness at Memorial Sloan-Kettering Cancer Center in New York City. To find whole-grain bread, read the ingredient list: The first ingredient must include the word "whole." If it doesn't, the bread was made using mostly refined flour. Words such as "unbleached," "stone-ground," "enriched," and "wheat" may sound good, but they don't mean whole-grain.
2. Start the day with a high-fiber cereal. "It's what I do, and I highly recommend this to everybody," says Dr. Shike. Look for a cereal with at least 7 grams of fiber per serving, he suggests. If the first ingredient is wheat bran or oat bran, that's as good as a whole grain—since so many nutrients are linked to the bran. If you prefer oatmeal, rolled oats and steel-cut oats are whole grains.
3. Use whole-wheat pasta instead of regular. Look for the word "whole" in the first ingredient. If you don't like one brand, try another. A variety of shapes are available, from fusilli to angel hair to alphabet-shaped. Most supermarkets have at least one or two kinds.
4. Instead of white rice, try Texmati, wehani, or brown rice. Or use bulgur (cracked, partly cooked wheat kernels), wheat berries (whole-wheat ker-

Don't Go by Color

When choosing a loaf of bread, don't assume that beige or dark brown ones like rye and pumpernickel are whole-grain. "The color of bread means nothing. Usually, it's just dye," says grain expert Joanne Slavin, R.D., Ph.D., of the University of Minnesota, St. Paul. Read the label to find out what's really in there.

Put These in Your Cart

There are hundreds of whole-grain products on the shelves. Here are a few great examples to get you started.

Bread. Wonder 100 Percent Stone-Ground Whole-Wheat Bread, Thomas Sahara 100 Percent Whole-Wheat Pita Bread, Mestermacher Organic Whole Rye Bread, Martin's 100 Percent Stone-Ground Whole-Wheat Sandwich Rolls, Cedars Whole-Wheat Roll-Up Mountain Bread

Cereal. Kellogg's Original All-Bran, General Mills Fiber One, Post Raisin Bran, General Mills Multi-Bran Chex, Post Shredded Wheat 'n Bran, Kashi Seven Whole Grains and Sesame

Pasta. Hodgson Mill Whole-Wheat Spaghetti, Bionaturae Organic Pasta 100 Percent "Stone-Ground" Whole-Wheat Semolina Chiocciole, De Boles Whole Wheat Penne

Rice and other grains. Kraft Minute Brand Instant Brown Rice, Success Rice 10 Minute Brown and Wild Mix, Lundberg Wehani Naturally Aromatic Brown Rice, Wolff's 100 Percent Pure Roasted Buckwheat Kasha

Snacks. Health Valley Roasted Garlic Crackers, Triscuit Reduced-Fat Baked Whole-Wheat Wafers, Wasa Original Hearty Rye Crispbread, Health Valley Healthy Biscotti Amaretto Cookies, Tree of Life Fig Bars, New Morning Organic Whole-Wheat Honey Grahams

nels), kasha (whole buckwheat), Kashi (a mix of whole grains), or quinoa (a South American grain). Splurge on wild rice for special occasions.

5. Look for whole-grain snacks. These are the toughest to find, says Dr. Slavin. But supermarkets usually have whole-grain rye crispbread, woven whole-wheat crackers, whole-wheat crackers, and popcorn.

6. Check out natural food and health stores. They offer whole-grain varieties of crackers, graham crackers, cookies, muffins, bagels, pretzels, pizza shells, pitas, wraps, English muffins, and many shapes of pasta.

7. Bake with whole-wheat flour. Substitute whole-wheat for all or part of the white flour in a recipe—start with ¾ cup whole-wheat for each cup of white. Whole-wheat flour gives a denser texture and a hearty, nutty flavor.

Foods That Add Years to Your Life

S tock your cart with fruits and vegetables, and cut your cancer risk in half! Yes, that's right: Eating fruits and vegetables actually helps keep cancer at bay. And now a major new study confirms more dramatically than ever the power of produce. Researchers in America and Germany reviewed more than 200 diet studies from around the world, and they found consistent evidence that people who rate high on the produce-consumption scale rate low on the cancer-developing scale. In fact, folks who eat lots of fruits and vegetables have about half the risk of developing a broad range of cancers, compared with people who eat few of these foods.

What's more, one of the study's authors, Kristi Steinmetz, R.D., Ph.D., a nutritional epidemiologist in Forchheim, Germany, says she believes that some of the studies she looked at may even have underestimated the threat of cancer. So in real life, eating your broccoli and bananas may have a greater effect on reducing cancer risk than previously thought.

Which Foods Are Real Winners?

The new study found that the strongest protection against cancer may come from garlic, onions, legumes, carrots, green vegetables, cruciferous vegetables (broccoli and its relatives), tomatoes, and citrus fruits. But Dr. Steinmetz emphasizes that these particular foods are also the ones people eat most often; other varieties of produce might be just as protective but wouldn't show up in studies because they're uncommon. Like most nutritional experts, she believes that all produce is likely to be helpful and healthful.

No wonder. Fruits and vegetables deliver a legion of substances believed to fight cancer.

- ❖ Beta-carotene and essential vitamins like folate and vitamin C
- ❖ Fiber
- ❖ Dozens of natural cancer-fighting substances called phytochemicals—like lycopene in tomatoes and ellagic acid in strawberries

Fortunately, this latest study also confirms that you don't have to martyr yourself to reap the benefits of produce. (Nobody's making you eat 12 bowls of raw kale a day.) Raw produce may provide a slight edge over cooked in some cases, Dr. Steinmetz says, but your main concern should be getting enough servings, raw or not.

How Much Do You Need?

This part's really simple: The National Cancer Institute's official dietary guideline is a minimum of 5 servings of fruits and vegetables a day. (For men eating the median 2,270 calories a day, the minimum is 7 servings.) Sadly, only one in four Americans really follows this advice. The average American eats— at most—3.3 servings of fruit and vegetables per day (not counting potato products like french fries). Women probably average even less than that.

Dr. Steinmetz's study shows just how much we stand to gain from bringing up that average consumption of fruits and vegetables. "There is no doubt in my mind that Americans can substantially improve their long-term health outcomes if they'll simply get in the habit of eating vegetables and fruit more often," says Peter Greenwald, M.D., director of cancer prevention and control at the National Cancer Institute.

What (Exactly) Is a Serving?

For starters, the ideal breakdown of the "five a day" is this: two servings of fruits and three of vegetables. And though this may sound like a lot to someone who tends to be more carnivorous, it's really pretty easy to achieve. Simply have a banana on your cereal and a glass of orange juice in the morning, and you've hit your fruit requirement. Eat a 2-cup salad for lunch and a helping of broccoli with your dinner, and you're done with the vegetables, too. Here's how to measure a serving.

H
E
A
L
T
H

F
L
A
S
H

Foods That Block Breast Cancer

Recent studies have linked each of the following foods to fighting the illness women fear most: breast cancer.

Wheat-bran cereal. Women who ate a daily ½-cup serving of All-Bran—that's 10 grams of fiber from wheat bran—saw drops in their estrogen levels. Experts think high estrogen levels stimulate breast cancer.

Canola oil. This vegetable oil is rich in an omega-3 fat. A UCLA study is testing whether omega-3's can prevent recurrence of cancer in breast cancer survivors, partly because women from countries with the least breast cancer have more omega-3 fats in their tissue. Other top sources of omega-3's: salmon and white (albacore) tuna.

Carrots and spinach. Compared with women who ate carrots or spinach more than twice a week, women who never ate them had twice the risk of breast cancer.

Yogurt. In a test-tube study, yogurt slowed the growth of breast cancer cells, even if the yogurt's active bacterial cultures were removed first. So any yogurt—not just the kind with live and active cultures—may be protective, for reasons yet unknown.

❖ 1 cup of raw leafy greens (spinach, romaine lettuce, kale)
❖ ½ cup cooked, canned, or raw vegetables (sliced carrots, broccoli pieces)
❖ ½ cup cut-up raw, cooked, or canned fruit (cubed melon, applesauce, pineapple rings)
❖ 1 medium fruit or vegetable
❖ ¾ cup (6 ounces) fruit or vegetable juice
❖ 2 tablespoons dried fruit (raisins)

20 Easy Ways to Get Your Five a Day

For women who say they don't have time for fruits and vegetables, we've assembled 20 tips requiring almost zero extra time or effort. If you incorporate just a few of these tips into your daily diet, you'll meet your produce needs with ease.

1. Give canned soup a boost. Add a cup of frozen peas, string beans, or carrot slices. You instantly increase its veggie content.

2. Stock up on low-sodium tomato juice or vegetable-juice cocktail. Keep a few 6-ounce cans in your desk at work, in the car, and in your briefcase. Each counts as one instant serving.

3. Add extra vegetables to casseroles. After all, you're already chopping up broccoli, carrots, or whatever. It takes just seconds more to slice twice as much as the recipe calls for.

4. Doctor up pasta sauce. Add extra chunks of cooked zucchini, onions, mushrooms, peppers, or shredded carrots.

5. Add fruit to chicken salad. Add chopped apples, grape halves, pineapple cubes, or diced mango. Shoot for half chicken, half fruit.

6. Tune up your tuna. Add lots of chopped celery and onion or jicama—a mild, slightly sweet, crunchy vegetable similar to a water chestnut. Aim for half tuna, half vegetables.

7. Indulge your salsa cravings. Each ½ cup counts as one serving, since most are tomato-based. Try the fruity varieties like mango salsa, too.

8. Make breakfast a breeze. For easy grapefruit in the morning, keep a jar of grapefruit sections on hand.

9. Satisfy cravings for sweets with dried fruit. Only 2 tablespoons equals one serving. Beyond raisins, consider dried cranberries, cherries, or papayas.

10. Veg-up your macaroni and cheese. Cook a box of frozen mixed vegetables to add to your mac and cheese recipe. If you're in a cafeteria, take small side dishes of noodles, steamed broccoli, and carrot slices and combine them for a similar effect.

11. Munch an apple in the car. This fruit is perfect for dashboard dining—no drips or crumbs.

12. Keep single-serving cans of fruit cocktail on hand. Or open a can of tropical fruit cocktail and transfer it to single-serving containers for quick take-along snacks.

13. Look for Just Vegetables or Fruit Munchies snack mixes. The former packs a healthy dose of freeze-dried corn and peas and pieces of tomato, carrot, and bell pepper. It's crunchy, lightly sweet, preservative-free, and addictive. The fruit snack is a tart-sweet mix of freeze-dried apples, raisins, blueberries, sour cherries, mango, pineapple, and raspberries. Both are available in health food stores.

14. Top your pizza with double the vegetables. If you don't order double when you ask for a vegetable topping, sometimes all you get is a token sprinkling.

15. Order extra vegetables when dining out. If your entrée doesn't come with a vegetable side dish or two, order one à la carte.

16. Swap side dishes for salads. If your entrée includes a salad, ask if it's mostly iceberg lettuce, which isn't as nutrient-rich as most leafy greens. If the answer is yes, ask to trade it in for a vegetable, applesauce, or fruit cup.

17. Ask for a fresh-fruit appetizer. Many restaurants offer sliced in-season fruits for before or after your meal. Another appetizer idea: Order the vegetable of the day.
18. Use the salad bar to make a vegetable sandwich. Fill a sandwich roll or pita half with shredded carrots, chopped peppers, tomato wedges, sprouts, and more. Top with a splash of olive oil or balsamic vinegar, if available.
19. Cater with crudités. When you're asked to bring a contribution to parties or family dinners, become famous for the beautiful sliced-vegetable trays you bring, complete with low-fat dip.
20. Take a heaping helping. This one is so obvious it's often overlooked: Instead of taking a ½-cup serving of vegetables, go ahead and take a full cup. It's only a few more bites, and you'll rack up two servings at one meal.

Really Satisfying Low-Fat Snacks

T he world of snack foods has changed since the days when rice cakes were supposed to supply munching pleasure without unnecessary calories. Companies have improved upon their initial attempts at low-fat fare and have come up with stuff that not only keeps us slim but actually tastes pretty good as well. Heck, even some of the new rice cakes are in the running.

Here's the latest and greatest in the world of low-fat edibles.

Crackers

Reduced-Fat Wheat Thins. If they were good enough for Sandy Duncan, count us in! 18 crackers, 120 calories, 4 grams total fat, 29 percent calories from fat

SnackWell's Snack Crackers. Go for the Salsa Cheddar variety. 32 crackers, 120 calories, 2 grams total fat, 13 percent calories from fat

Harvest Crisps. Bits of Romano and Parmesan cheeses coat these herbed crackers. Italian Herb: 13 crackers, 130 calories, 3.5 grams total fat, 23 percent calories from fat

Reduced-Fat Cheez-Its. Whether you opt for the big or the small size, these are the best cheese-flavored crackers around. And they're baked, so they have 40 percent less fat than the original ones. 29 small crackers (or 15 big crackers), 140 calories, 4.5 grams total fat, 29 percent calories from fat

Cookies

SnackWell's Bite Size Cookies. These little guys are tiny, but they have a strong, crunchy texture and rich flavor. Double Chocolate Chip: 13 cookies, 130 calories, 4 grams total fat, 27 percent calories from fat

Barnum's Animal Crackers. Relive your childhood. 9 crackers, 130 calories, 4.5 grams total fat, 31 percent calories from fat

Reduced-Fat Nilla Wafers. As good as the originals but healthier. 8 wafers, 120 calories, 2 grams total fat, 17 percent calories from fat

Reduced-Fat Oreos. Twist 'em open and enjoy—guilt-free. 3 cookies, 130 calories, 3.5 grams total fat, 23 percent calories from fat

Chips

Baked Lay's. The gold standard for low-fat potato chips; just 16 percent of the fat of typical chips. KC Masterpiece Barbecue: 11 chips, 120 calories, 3 grams total fat, 12 percent calories from fat

Baked Tostitos. These salty mini-tortillas are so similar to regular Tostitos that you won't know the difference. Salsa and Cream Cheese Bite Size: 14 chips, 120 calories, 3 grams total fat, 23 percent calories from fat

Baked Munch 'ems. The ridged texture of a potato chip with the crunch of a cracker. Savory Original: 41 crackers, 130 calories, 4.5 grams total fat, 31 percent calories from fat

Air Crisps. Thin, crispy, and definitely habit-forming. The best flavors: Original Potato, Barbecue Potato, and Ritz Cracker. Barbecue Potato: 22 crisps, 120 calories, 3.5 grams total fat, 29 percent calories from fat

Snack Mixes

Chex Mix. They've packaged the classic party mix recipe: Crunchy Chex cereal, pretzels, crisp bagel chips, and more. Available in four flavors. Traditional: 2/3 cup, 130 calories, 4 grams total fat, 27 percent calories from fat

Cheez-It Reduced-Fat Party Mix. You might not know what all the pieces are, but eat them anyway. 1/2 cup, 130 calories, 3 grams total fat, 23 percent calories from fat

Popcorn

Quaker Popcorn Cakes. Four-inch butter, caramel, and Monterey Jack cheese cakes. Low enough in calories so that you can actually eat enough to satisfy your hunger. So tasty you'll satisfy your tastebuds. Fat-Free Monterey Jack: 1 cake, 40 calories, 0 gram total fat

Orville Redenbacher's 100 Percent Popcorn Mini Cakes. Popcorn crunch with great flavors such as sour cream and onion, chocolate peanut crunch, nacho, and barbecue. Truly tasty. Sour Cream and Onion: 8 cakes, 60 calories, 1 gram total fat, 17 percent calories from fat

Orville Redenbacher's Butter Light Popping Corn. The best of the microwave popcorns. $5\frac{1}{2}$ cups, 110 calories, 2.8 grams total fat, 25 percent calories from fat

Pretzels

Baked Rold Gold. Be it a stick, twist, or bite-size bit, these are king. Tiny Twists: 18 pretzels, 100 calories, 0 gram total fat

Goldfish Pretzel Snack Mix. Regular twists, along with the pretzel fish and crunchy pretzel sticks. Go ahead and steal them from your kids. $\frac{1}{2}$ cup, 100 calories, 0 gram total fat

Superpretzel Baked Soft Pretzels. Yum. Doughy. 1 pretzel, 190 calories, 0 gram total fat

Candy

SnackWell's Chocolate Chews. These caramel-like chocolate chews are the best of SnackWell's line. 7 pieces, 160 calories, 3 grams total fat, 17 percent calories from fat

Hershey's Sweet Escapes. The Crispy Caramel Fudge and Crunchy Peanut Butter bars are good but far too small to be satisfying. Crispy Caramel Fudge Bar: 80 calories, 2 grams total fat, 25 percent calories from fat. Crunchy Peanut Butter Bar: 90 calories, 3 grams total fat, 28 percent calories from fat

Starburst Fruit Twists. They look like licorice twists but come in orange, strawberry, lemon, and cherry. 4 twists, 140 calories, 1 gram total fat, 7 percent calories from fat

Trolli Gummi Bears. Fat-free from the start, this jelly candy now comes in countless shapes. Classic Bears: 18 pieces, 130 calories, 0 gram total fat

Jelly Belly Jelly Beans. 39 flavors in one can, including chocolate pudding, buttered popcorn, and pink grapefruit. 25 pieces, 100 calories, 0 gram total fat

Milky Way Lite. If you haven't tried one, you're missing out. 1.6-ounce bar, 170 calories, 5 grams total fat, 29 percent calories from fat

Miscellaneous

Quaker Chewy Low-Fat Granola Bars. Some granola bars pack lots of useless calories and fat into each bite—but not these. S'mores: 1 bar, 110 calories, 2 grams total fat, 18 percent calories from fat

Baked Bugles. Great as a snack or as finger puppets for the kids. Original flavor: 1¹/₂ cups, 130 calories, 3.5 grams total fat, 23 percent calories from fat

Quaker Fat-Free Mini Rice Cakes. Even though they're rice cakes, they taste good. Apple Cinnamon: 5 cakes, 50 calories, 0 gram total fat

Breyer's Smooth and Creamy Low-Fat Yogurt. There are a lot of good low-fat yogurts on the market nowadays, but this is one of the best. Orange Vanilla Cream: 8 ounces, 230 calories, 2 grams total fat, 7 percent calories from fat

Dannon Light Duets Fat-Free Yogurt. This is another one of the good ones. Cherry Cheesecake: 6 ounces, 90 calories, 0 gram total fat

Jell-O Fat-Free Snack Pack pudding cups. Just like the regular stuff, except it's made with skim milk. Chocolate: 4 ounces, 90 calories, 0 gram total fat

Fruit Snacks

Newtons Fat-Free Cobblers. Unexpectedly habit-forming. The moist, chewy apple-cinnamon variety is great. Apple Cinnamon: 1 cookie, 70 calories, 0 gram total fat

Fat-Free Newtons. The new cranberry, raspberry, and strawberry flavors add some versatility to this perennial fave. Strawberry: 2 cookies, 100 calories, 0 gram total fat

Fruit by the Foot. Like a fruit roll-up but with a funnier name. Strawberry: 3-foot roll, 80 calories, 1.5 grams total fat, 13 percent calories from fat

Frozen Treats

Starburst Fruit Juice Bars. The Tropical Fruits pack features Mango Melon/Tropical Punch, Citrus/Tropical Punch, and Orange/Strawberry-Banana flavors. 1 bar, 20 calories, 0 gram total fat

Klondike Fat-Free Big Bear Ice Cream Sandwich. Looks a bit strange but tastes good. 1 sandwich, 190 calories, 0 gram total fat

Yoplait Double Fruit Nonfat Frozen Yogurt Bars. Flavors: strawberry, peach, and cherry. 1 bar, 45 calories, 0 gram total fat

Tropicana Fruit Juice Bars. Flavors: orange, raspberry, and strawberry. 1 bar, 25 calories, 0 gram total fat

Edy's Fruit Bars (east of the Rockies); Dreyer's Fruit Bars (west of the Rockies). Flavors: strawberry, peach, lime, raspberry-kiwi. 1 bar, 90 calories, 0 gram total fat

The Smart Fat Makeover

If your motto is "fat is bad," here's a shocker: Some fat is turning out to be very healthy. So healthy, in fact, that you probably need more—especially if you've been holding it to a bare minimum.

Specifically, you need more smart fats, which are omega-3 fats, from foods such as salmon and walnuts, and monounsaturated fats, from delicacies such as olive oil, almonds, and avocados.

Omega-3 fats are essential to the diet because the human body can't make them, and they seem to protect you from a whole army of diseases that are on the rise. Research shows that people who eat more omega-3 fats and monounsaturates get less cancer, heart disease, depression, asthma, even Alzheimer's disease. Smart fats can help control diabetes and high blood pressure, too.

Make no mistake, though: Too much total fat—more than about 25 percent of calories—is still a bad idea. You want to limit saturated fats and trans fats. And you want to curb the omega-6 fats, such as corn oil.

Omegas in a Capsule

If you don't like fish, experts say getting up to 1 gram of omega-3's per day from fish oil capsules is safe. Most capsules have about 0.3 gram of EPA and DHA. Concentrated products have almost 1 gram per capsule.

But, finally, there's fat so healthy you can go for it! Try these easy tips to automatically get the right balance of fats in your diet—especially more delicious smart fats—starting now.

Reel In the Fish, Bring On the Flax

Only recently have we discovered that the smart fats play critical roles throughout the body. Further, if you don't eat fish two times a week, chances are you get only about one-fifth of the omega-3's you need!

Where you get omega-3's: There are two sources: fish, which provides eicosapentaenoic acid (EPA) and docosahexaenoic acid (DHA), and plants, which have alpha-linolenic acid (ALA). Foods with high EPA and DHA are salmon, mackerel, sardines, herring, anchovies, rainbow trout, bluefish, caviar, and white albacore tuna. Foods with ALA are canola oil, flaxseed, flaxseed oil, walnuts, walnut oil, and dark green, leafy vegetables. In your body, ALA is only partially converted to the much more powerful EPA and DHA.

Your goal: There's no RDA for omega-3's, though one is being considered. Omega-3 expert Penny Kris-Etherton, R.D., Ph.D., distinguished professor of nutrition at Pennsylvania State University in State College, recommends at least 0.5 gram total of EPA and DHA per day. (In England, the government recommends 1.25 grams per day.) For ALA, she recommends about 1 gram per day minimum.

Incredible Omega-3's

Science has uncovered roles throughout the body for omega-3's. Here are a few of the ways omega-3's may help.

Prevent heart attack deaths. Omega-3's help heart muscles beat in a steady

The Most Luxurious Health Food

Celebrate New Year's Eve or any festive occasion with caviar, and you'll get a burst of omega-3 fats for your heart. Just 1 tablespoon of caviar has 1 gram of omega-3's—more than what's in half a can of white tuna. Yet it has only 40 calories and a total of 2.8 grams of fat.

Serve your caviar on toast points. Or get fancier with one of these suggestions. Halve small cooked potatoes and serve them warm or cold topped with caviar and low-fat sour cream. Spoon caviar over potato pancakes, stuffed baked potatoes, seafood salad, or scrambled eggs.

rhythm. Maybe that's why studies show that men who eat more fish have fewer fatal heart attacks.

Fight depression. Scientists wonder why some patients with depression have lower levels of one omega-3 fat, DHA; we do know that nerve cell membranes in the brain are composed mainly of DHA at the point where one cell "talks" to another.

Quench pain. Omega-3's can help tone down rheumatoid arthritis pain and severe menstrual cramps because they dampen out-of-control inflammatory processes.

Fight breast cancer. In studies, women with breast cancer have lower levels of omega-3's in adipose tissue.

Eight Ways to Get More Omega-3's

1. Eat fatty fish twice a week. That way, you'll average about 0.5 gram of EPA and DHA per day.
2. Most salmon, including the farm-raised kind, is rich in omega-3's. Most restaurants have a salmon entrée—an easy way to get omega-3's. A serving of salmon the size of a deck of cards (about 3 ounces) will bring you almost 2 grams of DHA and EPA. Take home what's left and use it for salmon burgers the next day. Be aware that smoked salmon and lox aren't good choices. During processing, they lose most of their fat, including omega-3's.
3. Buy cans of water-packed white tuna with the highest fat content. (Fat can range from 0.5 to 5 grams per serving. The more total fat, the more omega-3's.) Be aware that light tuna has less omega-3's. Make tuna salad using fat-free mayonnaise or mayonnaise made from canola oil. A 3-ounce serving of tuna averages 1.1 grams of DHA and EPA. (Restaurant tuna is mostly yellowfin, which isn't a high omega-3 fish.)
4. Order pizza with anchovies. Five anchovies have 0.4 gram of EPA and DHA.
5. Make a mini-meal of sardines with whole-wheat toast. Two sardines have 0.36 gram of DHA and EPA.
6. Use canola oil for baking and cooking. Buy mayo, margarine, and salad dressing made with canola oil. One tablespoon of canola oil has 1.3 grams of ALA.
7. Make salad dressing from walnut oil and red wine vinegar. One tablespoon of walnut oil has 1.4 grams of ALA.
8. Sprinkle ground flaxseed on cereal or yogurt. Flaxseed is the plant with the highest ALA levels by far. One tablespoon of flaxseed has 2.2 grams of ALA. You can buy flaxseed at health food stores or natural food supermarkets such as Fresh Fields.

Open the Olives, Crack the Nuts

In Mediterranean countries, monounsaturated fat from olive oil reduces the risk of heart disease and possibly breast and colon cancers. Unfortunately, in America we get about one-third of our monounsaturates from a different source—meat, which means we also get artery-clogging saturated fat. What we need is less meat and more monos from heart-healthy sources.

Where you get monos: Olive oil, olives, canola oil (also a good source of omega-3's), most nuts (almonds, cashews, pecans, pistachios), avocados, peanuts, and peanut butter are good sources.

Your goal: Aim for up to 15 percent or more of daily calories. The American Heart Association recommends up to 15 percent, but some heart experts recommend even higher levels.

Trash the Trans Fats

A pervasive presence in processed foods and fast foods, trans fats have been found to raise LDL cholesterol levels and lower levels of HDL cholesterol. There's also a possible link to breast cancer.

Where you get trans fats. They're in fried fast foods and processed foods (margarine, cookies, crackers, frozen entrées) that have partially hydrogenated oil as an ingredient.

Your goal. Eliminate them if possible, but set a maximum intake of 1 gram a day.

To accomplish this goal, follow these strategies.

❖ When you shop for crackers, cookies, frozen entrées and desserts, and snack cakes, choose products without partially hydrogenated oils in the ingredients list. Don't assume all health food store products are trans-free; check the label.

❖ Switch to trans-free margarines, such as any fat-free margarine or Country Morning Blend Light, Brummel and Brown Spread Made with Yogurt, Promise Ultra Spread, and Spectrum Naturals (sold in natural food stores).

❖ At the drive-up window, order a small, plain hamburger or grilled chicken sandwich without mayo instead of a fried fish fillet sandwich or chicken nuggets.

❖ Skip the french fries. Instead, order a baked potato without sour cream and butter.

HEALTH FLASH

Seven Ways to Get More Monounsaturates

1. Dress salads in olive oil. Buy salad dressing made with olive oil or make your own. (Bonus: A dressing with fat means that you absorb more protective carotenoids from your vegetables.)
2. Sprinkle 1 tablespoon of toasted, chopped nuts a day on cereal, yogurt, stir-fries, casseroles, rice dishes, or cream soups.
3. Dip crusty bread in olive oil.
4. Opt for olive oil in cooking. Though you can find special high-mono sunflower and safflower oils (called high-oleic), they're not good substitutes for olive oil, since they lack the disease-fighting phytochemicals that olive oil contains.
5. Savor peanut butter—in moderate amounts (1 to 2 tablespoons).
6. Appreciate avocados. Stop passing up this delicious treat. One-quarter of an avocado packs 4.5 grams of monounsaturates.
7. Add punch to salads and casseroles with chopped olives.

Go Back to "Flintstones" Fats

Omega-6 fats in vegetable oils such as corn oil are essential—our bodies must have some of these polyunsaturated fats. But we've gone overboard and need to cut back.

Experts think humans evolved on a diet of equal portions of omega-6 and omega-3 fats. Today, because we eat so much corn, soybean, and cottonseed oil, we get 10 to 20 times more omega-6's than the Stone Age person. In your body, that hinders the work of omega-3's. It lowers LDL cholesterol but also can reduce healthy HDL cholesterol. Some research hints that it could also encourage breast cancer.

Where you get omega-6's: Vegetable oils made from corn, cottonseed, safflower seed, sunflower seed, and soybeans contain the most.

Note: Soybean oil has more healthy omega-3's than many oils, but it also has very high levels of omega-6's.

Your goal: Omega-3 expert Artemis P. Simopoulos, M.D., author of *The Omega Diet*, recommends aiming for no more than four times as much omega-6 fat as you get of omega-3 fat, or about 6 grams a day. Don't worry if that sounds complicated—these tips can make it happen easily.

Three Ways to Tame Omega-6's

1. Top strategy: Margarine and mayonnaise are often made from soybean or other oils that are high in omega-6's. Look for brands made from canola oil.

2. Make or buy salad dressing with olive oil. Bottled salad dressings are often made from a base of soybean oil.
3. Use olive or canola oil for cooking or baking instead of corn, safflower, or sunflower oil.

Smart Switches

All fats are high in calories—nine calories per gram. To avoid gaining weight when you add smart fats to your diet, use them to replace a fat that's not so good for you.

Instead of 3 ounces broiled sirloin (229 calories, 14.2 grams fat)

Choose 3 ounces roasted Atlantic farmed salmon (175 calories, 10.5 grams fat)

Smart fat payoff: +1.8 grams omega-3 fats (DHA and EPA), −3.5 grams saturated fat

Instead of topping salad with ¼ cup shredded Cheddar cheese (114 calories, 9.3 grams fat)

Choose 1½ tablespoons chopped toasted almonds (125 calories, 11 grams fat)

Smart fat payoff: +4.5 grams monounsaturated fat, −4.9 grams saturated fat

Instead of sautéing in 2 teaspoons corn oil (80 calories, 9.1 grams fat)

Choose 2 teaspoons canola oil (83 calories, 9.4 grams fat)

Smart fat payoff: +3.3 grams monounsaturated fat, +0.8 gram omega-3 fats (ALA), −3.4 grams omega-6 fat

Instead of topping pizza wedge with 11 pepperoni slices (55 calories, 4.8 grams fat)

Choose 5 anchovies (42 calories, 1.9 grams fat)

Smart fat payoff: +0.4 gram omega-3 fats (DHA and EPA)

Instead of spreading bread with 2 teaspoons butter (68 calories, 7.7 grams fat)

Choose 2 teaspoons olive oil (80 calories, 9 grams fat)

Smart fat payoff: +4.4 grams monounsaturated fat, −3.6 grams saturated fat

Home Remedies from Your Spice Rack

You can ease an upset stomach, stop a toothache, cool off menopausal symptoms, and much more with herbs you'll find right in your own kitchen.

Healing herbs grow everywhere—in your backyard and deep in the Amazon rain forest, high on remote mountain ridges and in sun-baked deserts, in shady woodlands and even in the sea. Some, such as dandelion, are often scorned as weeds; others, such as red clover and oats, are common farm crops. Still others, such as thyme and cayenne pepper, may be sitting in your kitchen spice rack right now.

Though you may have thought of them as cooking ingredients only, there are herbs in your spice rack that can ease a variety of conditions, from bad breath to urinary tract problems. Here are easy home remedies that use the healing power of the spices that flavor your best meals.

Bad Breath

Chew on some cardamom. Cardamom, a popular spice in Arabian cuisine, is rich in cineole, a potent antiseptic that kills the bacteria that cause bad breath, says James A. Duke, Ph.D., former ethnobotanist with the U.S. Department

When to See the Doctor

If you have a serious illness or suffer from asthma or allergies, talk to your doctor before treating yourself with herbs. Never substitute herbs for your prescription medication unless you have your doctor's okay. If your symptoms don't improve within a week or if you have a bad reaction, discontinue use.

of Agriculture and author of *The Green Pharmacy*. You can buy whole cardamom in specialty herb shops and some supermarkets. To freshen bad breath, discard the pods and chew on a few seeds, then (discreetly) spit them out.

Drink some peppermint tea. The aromatic oil that gives peppermint its distinctive flavor and smell is a potent antiseptic that can kill the germs that cause bad breath. Drink a cup of peppermint tea whenever you feel the need. Use 1 tablespoon whole dried leaves (or 2 tablespoons fresh leaves) or a tea bag per cup of hot water and steep for 10 minutes.

Toothache

Stun the pain with cloves. Rub a drop of essential oil of clove directly on an aching tooth, suggests Ellen Kahmi, R.N., Ph.D., of Oyster Bay, New York, an herbalist and host of the nationally syndicated radio show *Natural Alternatives*. "If you don't have oil of clove handy, just wiggle a whole clove, pointed end down, next to the tooth," she adds.

Open sesame. According to Dr. Duke, sesame contains at least seven pain-relieving compounds. Boil 1 part sesame seeds with 3 parts water until the liquid is reduced by half. Cool the resulting decoction and apply it directly to the tooth.

Heartburn

Speed digestion with turmeric. Bitter herbs help stimulate the flow of digestive juices, moving food along and preventing acid buildup. So spice up your food with the bitter herb turmeric, which is the base of most Indian curries, says David Frawley, O.M.D., a doctor of Oriental medicine and director of the American Institute of Vedic Studies in Santa Fe, New Mexico. If simply flavoring your food isn't enough to stop the burn, he suggests two or three turmeric capsules ($\frac{1}{2}$ to 1 gram each), available at health food stores, before a meal.

Gas

Destress with peppermint. Stress can trigger a gas attack. Fortunately, the smell of peppermint tea can calm your nerves as the active ingredient you sip travels to your gastrointestinal tract. Have a cup of peppermint tea in the morning and a cup at night or more often. Sip slowly and smell the tea as you relax.

Indigestion

Grate some ginger. For best results, grate fresh ginger and mix 1 to 3 teaspoons in 1 cup of hot water. Steep for 10 to 15 minutes and then strain (or use a tea ball). You can also buy and use premade ginger teas.

Diarrhea

In an emergency, use cinnamon tea. If your diarrhea is so frequent that you risk dehydration and you need to quickly stop the flow, prepare some cinnamon tea. Cinnamon is a natural astringent that will dry up your bowel. Mix 1 tablespoon ground cinnamon into 1 cup of hot water. Steep for 10 to 15 minutes. Use cinnamon this way only for short periods of time—chronic diarrhea requires medical attention.

Nausea and Vomiting

Pair cinnamon with ginger. If food poisoning has double-whammied you with vomiting and diarrhea, make a ginger-cinnamon tea, says Douglas Schar, a practicing medical herbalist in London and editor of the *British Journal of Phytotherapy*. The ginger will stop your nausea while the naturally astringent cinnamon dries up your stool. Mix 1 teaspoon ground cinnamon with ½ teaspoon grated fresh ginger and add them to 1 cup boiling water. Steep for 10 to 15 minutes; strain and drink.

Out of ginger? Substitute peppermint. Although not as effective as ginger, peppermint can decrease nausea in a pinch. Pour hot water into a cup with 1 tablespoon fresh peppermint leaves. Let steep for 5 to 10 minutes; keep it covered to keep the oils from escaping. Then strain and drink.

Headache

Sip some rosemary. "A good herbal preventive for some vasoconstrictor migraines is rosemary, because it can help keep blood vessels dilated," says Lisa

Home-Grown Healing Herbal Brews

Creating an herbal tea for medicinal purposes isn't much different than preparing one for culinary enjoyment. Further, the ritual itself of brewing an herbal tea can make you feel better. Heating the water, holding the warm cup in your hands, and inhaling the fragrant steam can be tremendously comforting.

If you can boil water, you can brew herbal tea. Bring 1 cup of water to a boil. Crush the herb leaves or flowers (see below for amounts) and place in a dry teapot. Add the boiled water. Cover and let steep for the amount of time listed below (the average time is 10 minutes). Place a strainer over your teacup and pour. Drink as needed up to three times a day.

The following are all herbs you can grow yourself. The amounts given are for dried herbs or flowers. To use fresh, double or triple the amount.

❖ Basil helps soothe stomach ulcers. Use 1 teaspoon of leaves; steep for 10 minutes.
❖ Dandelion acts as a diuretic. Use 1 to 2 teaspoons; steep for 10 minutes.
❖ German chamomile soothes stomach upset, gas, and cramping. Use 1 to 2 teaspoons of flowers; steep for 10 to 15 minutes.
❖ Lemon balm reduces anxiety, restlessness, and migraine headaches. Use 1 to 2 teaspoons; steep for 10 minutes.
❖ Passionflower reduces insomnia and restlessness. Use 1 teaspoon; steep for 10 minutes.
❖ Rosemary eases digestive upset. Use 1 teaspoon of leaves; steep for 15 minutes.

Alschuler, N.D., a naturopathic physician and chairperson of the department of botanical medicine at Bastyr University in Bothell, Washington. Use 1 teaspoon rosemary per cup of hot water.

Make ginger part of your plan. "Ginger inhibits a substance called thromboxane A_2 that prevents the release of substances that make blood vessels dilate," says Tieraona Low Dog, M.D., a physician at the University of New Mexico Hospital in Albuquerque. In other words, it can help keep blood flowing on an even keel, which is essential in migraine prevention. Grate fresh ginger into juice, nosh on Japanese pickled ginger, use fresh or powdered ginger when you cook, or nibble a piece or two of crystallized ginger candy daily.

Sinus Pain or Pressure

Choose thyme. If your sinus secretions are clear or white, you need a warming, drying herb such as thyme, says David Winston, founder of

Herbalists and Alchemists, an herbal medicine company in Washington, New Jersey. Thyme is strongly antiseptic and is a traditional remedy for respiratory infections. Drink a cup of thyme tea—made by steeping 1 to 2 teaspoons dried thyme in 1 cup of boiling water for about 10 minutes—three times a day.

Insect Bites and Stings

Cool the itch and squelch the swelling with mint. A tiny drop of peppermint essential oil rubbed into the center of a bite or sting can bring quick, long-lasting relief, says Sharol Tilgner, N.D., a naturopathic physician and president of Wise Woman Herbals in Eugene, Oregon.

"Peppermint makes the area feel cool, so you don't feel like scratching," Dr. Tilgner says. "At the same time, it increases blood flow to the area, which helps to quickly carry off the little bit of venom the insect has deposited under the skin surface as well as the chemicals your body has produced in reaction to the venom. That means less swelling and less itching."

Remember to wash your hands after applying the oil, and don't use essential oils near your eyes because they can be irritating. Don't use this remedy on large venomous bites, such as those from a poisonous spider or snake, which require immediate medical attention.

Menopausal Night Sweats

Get some help from sage. Garden sage can help reduce or sometimes even eliminate night sweats. To make a sage infusion, place 4 heaping tablespoons of dried sage in 1 cup of hot water. Cover tightly and steep for 4 hours or more. Then strain and drink.

Motion Sickness

Give ginger a thumbs-up. For some people, fresh ginger works better than dimenhydrinate, the active ingredient in over-the-counter motion sickness medications such as Dramamine. The ginger works by controlling the symptoms of motion sickness or by dampening impulses to the brain that deliver messages about equilibrium. You need to give ginger time to kick in, says Lois Johnson, M.D., a physician in private practice in Sebastopol, California. To be on the safe side, do one of the following 1 hour before your trip: Take two 500-milligram ginger capsules; grate 1 to 3 teaspoons fresh ginger into 1 cup

Stay Away from These!

These are herbs you *don't* want to use as home remedies.

Coltsfoot as a cough suppressant. It's a possible carcinogen (cancer-causing agent).

Comfrey for anything internal. This herb contains toxic pyrrolizidine alkaloids (PAs). The American Herbal Products Association recommends that herbal products containing PAs be given the following label: "For external use only. Do not apply to broken or abraded skin. Do not use while nursing."

Germander for weight loss. One germander species, *Teucrium chamaedrys*, may cause liver damage.

Sassafras as a tonic. It contains safrole, a suspected carcinogen.

Yohimbe as an aphrodisiac. This African herb stimulates the central nervous system, increasing blood pressure and causing rapid heartbeat (and sometimes nausea).

HEALTH FLASH

of water, steep for 10 to 15 minutes, then strain, and drink; or place 60 drops of ginger extract on a teaspoon and swallow.

Colds and Flu

Warm up in the kitchen. To take the chills out of your cold, make a beeline to the kitchen and fix yourself a traditional herb and spice remedy, suggests David Hoffman, a fellow of Britain's National Institute of Medical Herbalists and assistant professor of integral health studies at the California Institute of Integral Studies in Santa Rosa. Combine 1 ounce (by weight) sliced fresh ginger, one broken-up cinnamon stick, 1 teaspoon coriander seeds, three cloves, one lemon slice, and 1 pint water. Simmer for 15 minutes and then strain. Drink a hot cupful every 2 hours.

Congestion

Break it up with horseradish. Another timeless herbal remedy for respiratory ills is horseradish. If you've ever inhaled its pungent vapors, it's easy to understand why. "The best way to get horseradish into your system is to just eat it. A teaspoonful on some crackers should help clear you right up," says Ed Smith, founder of the Herb-Pharm in Williams, Oregon.

Cough

Give it thyme. Thyme is a good herb to clear a congestive cough because it not only acts as an expectorant and an antiseptic but also relieves bronchial spasms, says Smith. You can prepare thyme tea, which you can drink up to three times a day when you're sick, by steeping 1 to 2 teaspoons dried thyme leaves in 1 cup boiling water for 10 minutes, says Varro E. Tyler, Sc.D., Ph.D., dean emeritus of the Purdue University School of Pharmacy and Pharmacal Sciences in West Lafayette, Indiana.

Urinary Tract Problems

Go with parsley. Parsley is an excellent diuretic, says Dr. Tyler. This herb contains myristicin and apiol, compounds that are thought to help increase the output of urine by increasing the flow of blood to the kidneys. To make a tea, pour boiling water over a few sprigs of crushed fresh parsley or 1 teaspoon dried parsley. Let steep for 10 minutes, then strain and drink.

Sagging Energy

Get an energy boost. Try peppermint or spearmint tea for a pick-me-up.

Hot Tips for Cold-Related Ills

Warm up cold hands and feet. Mix 1 tablespoon cornstarch and 1 tablespoon ground red pepper. Sprinkle into your gloves or socks.

Soothe a raw throat. Cover 1 teaspoon dried sage or thyme with boiling water. Let it steep, covered, for 10 minutes, strain, and gargle.

Herbs
and Drugs
That Don't Mix

C an herbs cause problems with other medicines you take? Maybe. We now know that some herb-drug combos have the potential for problems. Here's the latest information.

Herbs and Antidepressants

Since St. John's wort became renowned as the herb for people with the blues, many people have wondered whether it interacts with drugs they may already be taking for depression.

The answer? Experts simply don't know whether it's safe to combine St. John's wort with any prescription tricyclic antidepressant, including Tofranil and Elavil, because no one really knows how this herb works. It's what's known as an atypical antidepressant. It may work like Prozac and other similar drugs. Best advice: Don't take St. John's wort with any antidepressant drug unless, of course, your doctor recommends it.

Another caution: Never take ephedra (also called ma huang) with monoamine oxidase (MAO) inhibitors like Nardil and Marplan—in fact, avoid ephedra altogether unless you're under the care of a practitioner experienced in using herbs.

The Next Herbal Superstars

New research reveals herbs for arthritis, varicose veins, indigestion, even herpes, according to herb expert Varro E. Tyler, Sc.D., Ph.D., dean emeritus of the Purdue University School of Pharmacy and Pharmacal Sciences in West Lafayette, Indiana. Here are some to be on the lookout for.

Artichoke: protects your liver and heart, eases indigestion. New studies show that extract of artichoke leaves is not only useful for treating indigestion but also has liver-protective and cholesterol-reducing properties. Two clinical studies have now verified the herb's digestive action. German Commission E (that country's equivalent of our FDA and the world's leading authority on herbs) has approved artichoke preparations for dyspeptic complaints.

Devil's claw: holds promise against arthritis. This South African herb enjoyed considerable popularity 20 years ago as a treatment for arthritis. The herb is once again gaining some popularity as an anti-inflammatory that reduces pain and allows additional joint flexibility for people with rheumatoid complaints.

Horse chestnut: the varicose vein remedy that works. About 20 percent of the U.S. population suffers from varicose veins. Happily, seven clinical studies with standardized extract of horse chestnut seeds showed quite favorable results in 558 patients. The German Commission E determined that doses of 250 to 312.5 milligrams of the extract taken twice daily are safe and effective.

Lemon balm: an effective treatment for herpes. Herpes simplex type 1 virus causes cold sores or fever blisters, and herpes simplex type 2 virus is primarily responsible for genital herpes and its painful lesions. Concentrated water extract of lemon balm has been clearly demonstrated to have antiviral activity against both. It can help speed the healing of painful lesions. The extract is sold in a 70:1 concentration in a cream base that is applied locally two to four times daily to the affected area. It can greatly reduce the severity of the lesions by speeding the healing process.

Sea buckthorn: anti-aging balm for the skin. Sea buckthorn oil is commonly applied to the skin in Russia and China to reduce inflammation, relieve pain, promote tissue regeneration, and reduce age-induced skin wrinkling. It is an ingredient in beauty lotions.

HEALTH FLASH

Herbs and Anticoagulants

Some popular herbs lengthen the time it takes for blood to clot, usually by hindering the ability of the platelets to clump together. Most often, this anti-clotting action is a good thing. But if you take anticlotting herbs in combination with anticoagulant drugs, you may become susceptible to too much bleeding because your blood lacks the ability to clot.

Herbs with clot-preventive qualities include garlic, ginkgo, ginger, and feverfew. Use clot-preventive herbs only after checking with your doctor, if you take anticoagulant drugs—whether it's over-the-counter aspirin or the potent prescription drug warfarin (Coumadin).

If you undergo surgery, your surgeon will usually tell you to stop taking anticoagulant drugs a few days before the procedure. But he may not inquire about anticoagulant herbs. So ask whether you should avoid herbs like garlic, ginkgo, ginger, and feverfew before surgery. In fact, it's a good practice to discuss everything you take—herbs, drugs, and supplements—with your doctor.

Herbs and Certain Diuretics

Both herbal stimulant laxatives and certain diuretics can potentially cause potassium loss, especially if they're used to excess over prolonged periods. Used properly by themselves, neither poses a serious problem. But combine the herbs with the popular type of diuretic drugs called thiazide diuretics, and you may have trouble.

Uncorrected, potassium loss can lead to hypokalemia, a serious condition that causes confusion, muscular weakness, and irregular heartbeat. In some cases, it can even make you stop breathing.

Thiazide diuretics are commonly used to treat high blood pressure and the edema (swelling from fluid buildup) associated with congestive heart failure. Such drugs include Diuril, HydroDiuril, Naturetin, and Saluron.

Potentially potassium-draining stimulant-laxative herbs include aloe, cascara sagrada, and senna. Licorice can also contribute to potassium loss, so avoid it as well if you take thiazide diuretics.

Get Enough Potassium

One way to avoid potassium loss with laxatives and diuretics is to eat food high in potassium—legumes such as kidney beans, skim milk, fruits, and vegetables. Each of these contains about 500 milligrams of potassium: 1 cup of prune or orange juice, 1 banana, 1 white potato, 7 prunes, and 4 figs.

Melatonin in Herbs?

Since melatonin has been found in plants such as St. John's wort and feverfew, many people wonder if they can be taken for insomnia instead of melatonin tablets.

Unfortunately not. Although a few studies have identified melatonin in a variety of plant sources, it's always at extremely low levels. The greatest amounts were found in Baikal skullcap, which contained 7.11 micrograms per gram. Amounts were even less for feverfew and St. John's wort. Many physicians recommend a dose of 3 milligrams of melatonin for its sleep-inducing effects. To obtain this amount, it would be necessary to consume about 1 pound of the Baikal skullcap herb and 2 pounds of the other richest herb sources.

Herbs and Sedatives

Herbs that sedate or tranquilize, like kava and valerian, are liable to enhance the effects of drugs that also sedate or tranquilize. This could cause problems such as prolonged drowsiness, loss of coordination, or trouble driving. Fortunately, some of the older drugs—heavy-hitter sedatives such as secobarbital and phenobarbital—that are most likely to produce these effects are rarely prescribed these days. More common now are the benzodiazepines, including Valium, Librium, Halcion, and Dalmane. Unfortunately, these may also interact badly with certain herbs. To be safe, don't take kava or valerian with any sedative or tranquilizing drugs.

Other Herb-Drug Interactions

Many different, less significant interactions can occur between herbs and drugs. For example, if you take them at the same time, herbs containing lots of mucilage (a gelatinous substance) may slow the absorption of any drug you take orally. Such herbs include aloe, flaxseed, marshmallow root, and slippery elm bark. To avoid this problem, simply take the herb and the drug several hours apart.

As we gain more experience using medicinal herbs, it's likely that we'll discover other interactions. In the meantime, it's smart to consult a qualified medical practitioner (one with clinical herbal experience) if you have any doubt about the compatibility of herbs and the drugs you take.

part five

Maximum Weight Loss with Minimum Effort

5

His and Her Health

Gender Differences in Weight Loss

"I have my mother's hips. I'll just have to accept that," says a man mocking women in a TV commercial touting low-fat breakfast cereal. The truth is that men and women do have different views on body image—and weight loss. When they go on a diet, they even lose weight differently, as one recent study showed. If you're a woman, that's a good thing.

German researchers enrolled 16 men and women in a 4-month weight-loss program. The men consumed 1,500 calories a day, while the women were given 1,200 calories a day for the first 3 weeks of the study. Both the men and the women were instructed to exercise for 30 minutes five times a week. At the end of the program, the men lost more visceral fat, which is located around the abdomen, while the women lost more fat under their skin over their entire bodies.

"Most men have more visceral fat than women, which is probably why they were able to lose more of it," explains Susan Zelitch Yanovski, M.D., director of the obesity and eating disorders program at the National Institute of Diabetes and Digestive and Kidney Diseases, a branch of the National Institutes of Health (NIH). "Visceral fat, or fat in the upper body or stomach area, is more dangerous because it has been linked with an increased risk of heart disease. Women tend to have more fat around their hips and thighs. The good news is that this fat appears to be less likely to travel throughout your body wreaking havoc like visceral fat. It may be less likely to break down to free fatty acids and travel to the liver, which increases your risk of heart disease and diabetes."

Another difference between the sexes is motivation. "Women want to lose weight so they look better for themselves, to boost their self-esteem," says Dr. Yanovski. "They also feel pressure to stay thin so that they conform with society's ideal standards. On the other hand, men often don't want to lose weight, even when they should. Men are often in denial. Their doctors and their wives may tell them to lose weight, but they aren't as concerned. Some men lose weight to boost athletic performance."

According to Dr. Yanovski, it's important for women to realize that they're different from men, and that it's okay. Women's bodies are designed to hold fat around their hips and thighs because that's important for reproduction, especially breastfeeding.

Here are some sensible recommendations for achieving and maintaining a healthier body weight from the Centers for Disease Control and Prevention, the American College of Sports Medicine, and the United States Department of Agriculture.

- ❖ Engage in at least 30 minutes of moderate-intensity physical activity, such as brisk walking, gardening, bike riding, or strength training, on most—preferably all—days of the week.
- ❖ Vary your exercise so that you won't lose motivation and get bored, but stay consistent. For example, you might play tennis one day, ride your bike the next day, and go for a brisk walk the third day.
- ❖ Follow a low-fat, high-fiber diet that includes a wide variety of fruits, vegetables, and grains.

Diet Scams: How to Avoid Getting Taken

S orting the legitimate weight-loss claims from the crackpot kind can be a full-time job. Just ask the staff of the Federal Trade Commission's Operation Waistline. Workday after workday, these selfless public servants scan newspaper, magazine, Internet, and late-night TV advertisements for weight-loss scams masquerading as "breakthroughs."

"In a typical week, there may be as many as a dozen new advertisements," reports Richard Cleland, assistant director of service industry practices at the Federal Trade Commission (FTC).

Some recent Operation Waistline finds: ads for weight-reducing insoles ("Just slip them inside your shoes, and they melt away pounds while you walk!") and an appetite-suppressing seaweed.

Sounds fishy, you say?

"I'll look at some of these and think, 'Nobody's going to believe this,'" says Cleland. "But I'm continually surprised. People buy this stuff."

But while there's plenty of flimflam to be fooled by, there are also many programs and products on the market that really can help you lose weight.

To save you the chore of sifting the good from the good-for-nothing, the staff at Operation Waistline and several top weight-loss experts identified some of the more notable—and notorious—weight-loss breakthroughs and

The Best Hunger Remedy

Hunger can be the downfall for many dieters. If it is for you, focus your weight-loss efforts more on exercise and less on cutting calories.

Exercise doesn't increase hunger or make you eat more—despite what you might think, explains John Blundell, Ph.D., chairman of psychobiology at the University of Leeds in England. But skipping meals or drastically cutting calories does. In a recent study, women cut calories by eating a very low calorie breakfast one day. Another day, through exercise, they burned off the same number of calories that had been trimmed from the breakfast.

When they ate less, they were hungrier and ate more at lunch compared with when they had exercised. This suggests that an exercise-induced calorie deficit may be easier for people to maintain. "According to earlier research, even two intense exercise sessions per day did not make people eat more," says Dr. Blundell.

scams of late. What follows is an at-a-glance guide to what works and what doesn't.

The Smart Way to Lose

Indulge your appetite. That's right, eat more often than usual, and you're likely to bid a permanent farewell to excess pounds. Proof: A study of nearly 800 dieters in the University of Pittsburgh School of Medicine's National Weight Control Registry (a listing of people who've lost 30 or more pounds and kept them off for a year or longer) found that successful losers eat frequent small meals and never go hungry.

The flip side: If you ignore hunger, you'll hit your body's starvation alarm, warns James Chenoweth, M.D., an exercise and weight-loss specialist in Ann Arbor, Michigan. Your body thinks you're in the midst of a famine. So it turns down your metabolism.

To keep your metabolism revving, consume at least 1,500 calories a day, suggests Dr. Chenoweth. You'll lose weight more slowly than you would on a 500-calorie-a-day deprivation diet—but only at first. And, in reality, not all that slowly: You should be able to drop 1 or 2 pounds a week, assuming that you exercise. In fact, you shouldn't lose more than 2 pounds a week, says

Five Ways to Burn More Fat

Scientists have discovered why some people can eat anything they want without gaining a pound. They burn off the extra calories through everyday activities—walking, fidgeting, climbing stairs, doing household chores, and maintaining posture—a process that researchers call nonexercise activity thermogenesis (NEAT).

Researchers suspect that you can train yourself to increase NEAT. It's probably something you do unconsciously, but if you make it a conscious action, you could do more of it, says Michael Jensen, M.D., one of the study authors and professor of medicine at the Mayo Clinic in Rochester, Minnesota. Here are five effortless ways to train your body to burn more calories.

❖ Every time the phone rings, stand up before answering it.
❖ Whenever a commercial comes on TV, do something that gets you moving—take the garbage out, put in a load of laundry, pick up the newspaper.
❖ Set your watch timer to beep every 30 minutes or so. When it goes off, tap each foot 10 times.
❖ Put on music when you're doing the dishes, ironing, or folding clothes—and bop to the beat.
❖ Pick a cue word when you're at the movies or in a meeting. Whenever the speaker says that word, rotate each ankle five times or shift the way you're sitting.

Michael Steelman, M.D., chairman of the board of the American Association of Bariatric Physicians and an obesity specialist in Oklahoma City. Lose weight by deprivation, and you're more likely to regain it—fast.

Eat whenever you want. Like the people listed in the registry, those in a Scandinavian study ate whenever they were hungry, but they rarely ate anything high-fat. Danish researchers recruited 43 volunteers who'd recently lost about 28 pounds apiece and divvied them up into two groups. The scientists gave one group information on eating the low-fat, high-carbohydrate way—lots of whole grains, fruits, and vegetables—and told them to eat whenever their stomachs rumbled. They put the other group on a formal weight-maintenance plan that dictated how many servings of various foods they could have in a day. Six months later, the group that listened to their bellies had regained just half a pound each. The others? They'd added back an average of 9 pounds.

What if you're hungry at night? No problem. It's perfectly okay to eat after 7:00 P.M. According to a study of 7,000 people, dining late won't sabotage your waistline. The study found that people who ate more than 64 percent of their calories after 5:00 P.M. were no more likely to gain weight over a 10-year period than those who ate less than 25 percent of their calories after 5:00 P.M.

The Wrong Way to Lose

High-protein diets. High-protein diet books—often celebrity-endorsed—continue to top bestseller lists, much to the dismay of the American College of Sports Medicine, the American Dietetic Association, the Women's Sports Foundation, and the Cooper Institute. These organizations released a joint statement advising dieters against taking the high-protein route—but not on the grounds that such diets don't work. They do work—in the short run. But that's only because they're so incredibly stingy with calories. Unfortunately, that's not all these diets skimp on. As a rule, high-protein diets are too low in carbohydrates to be good for you. Carbohydrates—namely fruits, vegetables, and whole grains—tend to be high in nutrients, explains Dr. Steelman. So shortchanging yourself on carbohydrates means shortchanging your body of key vitamins and minerals.

In addition, losing weight on a high-protein diet may set you up to quickly regain lost pounds, says Ralph Carson, R.D., Ph.D., a nutritionist in Huntsville, Alabama. "When you're starved for carbohydrates, you become ravenous for them," he says. "I've had patients on high-protein diets who are so ravenous for carbohydrates when they go off their diets that they eat much more than usual, and they regain lost weight extremely fast."

Gadgets That Help

Elliptical exercise machines. These machines let you run to your heart's content without wounding your sensitive knees. Working out on one of these machines is like pedaling a bike while standing up—but the foot and leg motion is elliptical instead of circular. (Ask a trainer at your gym for pointers on using one.) The smooth, rolling action exerts little impact, so the machines are safe even if you have joint problems or injuries. "You get a workout similar to what you'd get with running or stairclimbing, but with low impact," says Dr. Chenoweth, who's a fan of these machines. At-home versions by HealthRider and NordicTrack are already on the market.

High-tech scales. You probably know that your body composition is a better indicator of your fitness than your weight. But do you even know what your body composition is? Until recently, you had to schlepp to a gym or a doctor's office to get these numbers. Now you can check your stats in the privacy of your own bathroom. A new generation of high-tech scales calculates your percentages of body fat and lean tissue by sending a painless mild electrical current through you. How fast the current flows depends on your composition. Healthy ranges of body fat for men ages 18 to 29 are 14 to 20 percent; for men over 30, 17 to 23 percent. For women ages 18 to 29, healthy ranges are 17 to 24 percent; for women over 30, 20 to 27 percent.

Rating the Big-Four Diet Programs

According to the Calorie Control Counsel in Atlanta, up to 15 percent of Americans turn to commercial weight-loss programs—specifically, Weight Watchers International, Jenny Craig, Nutri/System, and Diet Center Worldwide—to help them lose and keep off weight. Here, the scoop on each—plus pointers on making it work for you.

Weight Watchers International. The oldest and largest commercial diet program in this country, Weight Watchers emphasizes portion control and a healthy lifestyle that includes daily exercise and weekly weigh-ins. Eating supermarket food is encouraged, but prepackaged foods are available. With the center's 1-2-3 plan, foods are assigned a point value based on their calorie, fat, and fiber content. You're given a daily points limit based on your current weight. The cost is $30 to join, plus $12 weekly. Client counselors are trained former clients.

Be sure the program teaches you how to shop for and prepare food. You need to learn how to get the right types of food in the right proportions for maximum health, says Arthur Frank, M.D., medical director of the obesity management program at George Washington University Hospital in Washington, D.C.

Jenny Craig. The second-largest program, Jenny Craig requires that clients eat prepackaged foods until they lose half the weight they intend to lose. At that point, they can switch to supermarket foods. Minimum calories are determined for each individual. It costs $148 to join, plus $72 a week for prepackaged foods. Nonprofessional client counselors work one-on-one. Group support is offered, as are classes on lifestyle changes.

Gadgets That Are Hype

No-sweat machines. Exercise equipment that requires no effort to use isn't worth the effort required to order the stuff from infomercial hucksters. "Any machine that's supposed to be really, really easy and little work isn't going to burn many calories," says Dr. Chenoweth.

If you're not sure whether a particular machine will help you slim down or simply shrink your bank account, give it a trial run. If a friend bought it, ask to borrow it. Or rent it from a store. Lots of sporting goods shops lease exercise machines, notes Dr. Steelman. If the machine doesn't have you breaking a sweat after 5 to 10 minutes, don't break out your Visa card.

Spot reducers. Pitches for exercise equipment that "melts fat" from specified parts of your anatomy—your belly, your thighs, and so forth—regularly make the FTC's Operation Waistline list. The agency recently cited the makers of Abflex, for instance, for claiming that the gadget could help you "spot reduce."

Make sure the program offers psychological counseling or lessons in mental and emotional triggers for overeating. You need to know how stress affects your diet—specifically, whether you tend to reward or appease yourself with food—says Dr. Frank.

Nutri/System. This program emphasizes portion control and focuses on lifestyle modification. Prepackaged foods are required, but you are allowed fruits, vegetables, and skim milk. Costs range from $100 to $300 to join, plus $50 to $70 a week for food. Client counselors have some education in psychology, nutrition, and counseling.

Make sure the program offers a monitored exercise regimen and behavior-modification counseling. Don't rely only on a book as your behavior-modification component. While a book can suggest a specific strategy for changing an eating behavior, notes Dr. Frank, the strategy won't become an enduring habit unless you've had a chance to practice it, sort out your experiences with a counselor, modify your approach, and then try again.

Diet Center Worldwide. This program emphasizes losing body fat rather than pounds. Staffers encourage daily weigh-ins and also check body fat levels every 4 to 6 weeks. The center's Concept 1000 plan provides three diet shakes a day—for breakfast, lunch, and a snack—followed by a low-calorie dinner. Supermarket food is permitted, but prepackaged meals and shakes are available, and exclusive nutritional supplements are encouraged. Costs run about $75 a week for meals and shakes. Client counselors are trained nonprofessionals.

Make sure the staff is patient and committed for the long-term in helping you establish new, healthy habits.

Here's the real deal: There's absolutely no evidence that any exercise, machine, or diet will help you lose weight in a single spot on your body, says Dr. Steelman. Specific toning exercises, however, will help you firm certain areas—crunches, for instance, will tone your abdominal muscles but won't melt an ounce of fat from your belly, he says.

The Moves That Work

Walk, don't run. Here's some of the most encouraging weight-loss news in the last few years: Studies show that striding along at a good clip burns nearly as many calories as jogging at a moderate pace does. Plus, walking is easier on your knees and other joints than running. "When you walk at 5 miles an hour, you get the same fitness benefits you would if you were jogging but with a significantly lower risk of injury," explains John Duncan, clinical researcher at

Texas Woman's University in Denton and author of several studies on walking.

If you're walking already but not losing weight, walk more. Also, try gradually increasing your speed. "While cutting way back on calories will trigger a metabolic slowdown that thwarts your weight-loss plans, burning extra calories by adding exercise will speed up your metabolism and lower your set point (the point at which your calorie intake and calorie burn reach equilibrium)," says Dr. Chenoweth. For maximum weight loss, walk (or run, swim, or cycle) for 30 to 45 minutes a pop, six or seven times a week, he suggests.

What's more, keep moving between workouts. Park your car far from the mall entrance, and walk to the mailbox instead of driving. "In other words, don't work out for 30 minutes and then spend the rest of the day on the couch," Dr. Chenoweth warns.

Pump less iron. It's still smart to strength-train. As you no doubt know, strength training helps you lose weight because it helps build muscle, and muscle burns more calories than body fat. But the encouraging news here is that you don't have to strength-train as often as the experts once thought. New research suggests that training just twice a week is enough to garner the majority of the muscle-building/weight-shedding benefits. Experts used to think you had to train three times a week to do that. Studies also show that one set of strength-training exercises—say, 10 to 12 biceps curls—is almost as beneficial as three sets of 10 to 12 repetitions with the same amount of weight.

Don't forget to schedule your twice-a-week strength-training sessions for nonconsecutive days, which gives your muscles time to rest, says Wade Lillegard, M.D., co-director of the sports medicine division of the department of orthopedics at St. Mary's Duluth Clinic in Minnesota.

Trendy Moves That Work

Rock climbing. This activity burns an impressive 12 calories a minute. No wonder people are scrambling to sign up for lessons at climbing gyms—cavernous indoor spaces with steep walls studded with hand and foot grips (and ropes, pulleys, and harnesses to keep you from falling). If you have high blood pressure or are very overweight, check with your doctor before you make your first assault on the rock. Otherwise, get a good grip on the Yellow Pages and look under "health clubs" for gyms equipped for climbing. Introductory packages usually cost $25 and typically include a lesson and climbing-shoe rental.

Aerobic boxing. You feint, you swing, you jab—at no one in particular. While you can't knock anybody's block off, you can knock off some pounds with "noncontact" aerobic boxing (what Rocky Marciano would have called shadow boxing). South African scientists estimate that a typical noncontact boxing session burns as many calories as running 5.5 miles an hour.

The Lowdown on Drugs

Meridia. At the height of the diet-pill craze, people with a mere 5 to 10 pounds to lose were taking Phen-fen, a combination of the weight-loss drugs phentermine and fenfluramine. They were taking it at considerable risk, it turned out. On the heels of reports linking fenfluramine to heart-valve damage, the manufacturer pulled it from the shelves.

Now that the FDA has approved Meridia (the first new post–Phen-fen prescription diet drug), physicians are taking great pains to explain that it's not for small-time losers. The right candidate? Someone who's significantly overweight and hasn't been able to lose weight by changing her diet and exercising more, says Dr. Chenoweth. Studies show that Meridia, also known as sibutramine, boosts blood pressure in about 10 percent of the people who take it. Further, no one knows the long-term effects of the drug yet. So unless your doctor recommends it and persuades you otherwise, pass up this diet pill until more is known.

Phen-Pro. Recently divorced from fenfluramine, phentermine has hooked up with Prozac. Though fenfluramine was yanked from the shelves, phentermine (which wasn't implicated in heart-valve damage) remains on the market. Recently, doctors have been pairing it with the ever-popular antidepressant Prozac. Like fenfluramine, Prozac affects levels of serotonin, a neurotransmitter that influences both mood and appetite. But unlike fenfluramine, Prozac doesn't seem to hurt your heart. Bottom line: While there's no evidence that Phen-Pro is dangerous, there's no solid scientific evidence that this new combo can help you lose weight.

Herbs to Avoid

Brindall berry. Extracted and concentrated from brindall berry fruit, hydroxycitric acid (HCA) is the active ingredient in herbal weight-loss concoctions like CitriMax and CitraLean. Studies find that HCA helps laboratory animals eat less and slim down. But no one has adequately tested the stuff on humans. So whether it does the same for us—or is safe for humans—remains to be seen. Hold out for now.

Ephedra. Capitalizing on the popularity of St. John's wort, manufacturers have lately teamed the herbal antidepressant with ephedra, an herb long marketed as an appetite suppressant and metabolism booster. Years of trial and error, however, show that ephedra, a potent stimulant, can be potentially dangerous. "The FDA has reviewed numerous complaints about over-the-counter products containing ephedra, some linked to deaths," says Dr. Chenoweth. For starters, it can send your blood pressure sky-high as well as trigger heart palpitations in some people. The addition of St. John's wort doesn't make it any safer.

The FDA proposed limiting doses of ephedra to 24 milligrams per day for no more than 7 days. At that dose, the herb is useless as a diet aid, says Varro E. Tyler, Sc.D., Ph.D., dean emeritus of the Purdue University School of Pharmacy and Pharmacal Sciences in West Lafayette, Indiana. Moreover, there's no evidence that St. John's wort promotes weight loss.

Supplements to Shy Away From

Creatine monohydrate. Much lauded as a muscle builder, this supplement was implicated in the deaths of four wrestlers. But not fairly, it seems. Later reports raised questions as to whether creatine was to blame at all in the incidents.

Recent studies suggest the supplement can, in fact, help you build muscle, which can help you lose weight—since, pound for pound, muscle burns more calories than fat. Still, there have been no long-term safety studies to date, so the questions about side effects remain unanswered.

Chromium. Products containing chromium picolinate, a mineral, are also regulars on the FTC's hit list. There's simply no substantiating evidence that the reputed muscle builder works for weight loss. After sifting through the available data, researchers at several major universities were unable to find sufficient proof of its efficacy.

HMB. Its scientific name is beta-hydroxy beta-methylbutyrate. Supplement manufacturers claim that extra doses of this amino acid by-product can spur muscle growth. But experts say your body produces all the HMB you need. Adding more won't add more muscle to your physique but will subtract cash from your wallet.

A Feel-Good Plan to Lose 10, 20, or 30 Pounds

Y ou walk every day. You watch what you eat. So why are you still struggling to lose weight? The answer may be all in your head: Hating your body—a common reason for wanting to lose weight in the first place—can actually sabotage your weight-loss attempts.

The good news: You can learn to like your body and more than double your chances of getting slimmer.

Researchers at Stanford University School of Medicine found that people who started a weight-loss program feeling happiest with their bodies were more than twice as likely to lose weight as their counterparts who were least satisfied with their bodies.

But how do you get happy with your body before you lose weight? With advice from top body-image professionals, weight-loss experts, and women just like you who found that feeling good about their bodies made losing weight easier. In three simple steps, you can boost your body appreciation, shed pounds with ease, and get your best shape ever.

Step 1: Respect Your Body

"People who worry about how their bodies look often avoid the very things that can help them look and feel better, such as exercising and developing better coping skills," explains Elena Ramirez, Ph.D., clinical research associate in the department of nutrition and food sciences at the University of Vermont in Burlington. "Once women improve the way they feel about their bodies, they take better care of themselves, which helps them lose weight." Here's how to befriend your body.

Look in the mirror. Instead of cringing every time you see yourself, start accepting yourself, advises Dr. Ramirez. Slowly acclimate yourself to the image in the mirror by spending a few seconds a day looking at your body clothed. Slowly wear less and less, working up to viewing yourself unclothed for a few minutes.

"In a few weeks, you'll become comfortable with your reflection and realize that you have some positive physical qualities," says Kimberly Lavoi, 30, of Massachusetts, who has lost 22 pounds since beginning these body-image exercises. "You also begin to realize that you got yourself into the shape you're in, so you can also get yourself out of it."

Face your fears. It's common to avoid situations that make you feel worse about yourself, such as shopping for clothes or going to parties, says Dr. Ramirez. Feeling better about yourself requires facing those situations. "Pick one thing you avoid, such as wearing a bathing suit, and take small steps to conquer that fear," she says. "First, just buy the suit. The next day, wear it

Take Off 10 Years and 10 Pounds—Now!

You don't have to lose weight to start looking great. Try these simple tips from fashion pros.

Buy a good bra. "Too often, overweight women wear bras that let their breasts fall too low, making them look older, heavier, and short-waisted," says Jan Larkey, a Pittsburgh-based image consultant and author of *Flatter Your Figure.* "Get fitted for and invest in a good support bra."

Use color strategically. "Wear bright colors on your good features and dark colors on problem areas," advises Harriette Cole, president and creative director of Profundities, an image development company in New York City. "This lets you show off your best features while camouflaging trouble spots."

Sidestep sizes. "Squeezing into clothes that are too small can actually make you look larger," says Cole. If you can't stand to wear larger sizes, cut out the tags when you get home!

Try the boot cut. To slim your hips, try the new boot-cut pants, suggests Cole. "Instead of being tight at the ankles, these pants flare slightly from the knee, making you look more balanced and slimmer in the hips."

Pump up accessories. "It's hard to focus on any figure problems when a woman is wearing unusual, dangling earrings," says Larkey. "Pick up some eye-catching accessories—scarves, pins, handbags, shoes. They'll help you look great before, while, and after you lose weight."

Real-Life Success Story

Kimberly Lavoi, 30
Fall River, Massachusetts
Pounds lost: 22
Biggest obstacle: "I'd go to health clubs where everyone was super-skinny, and I'd lose my confidence. I felt fat and lazy."
Major accomplishment: "I have enough confidence to get in the pool for aqua aerobics."
How she did it: "I did mirror exercises to get used to the way I looked and to find positive attributes. I also stopped putting myself down. Now when I go shopping and something looks bad on me, I don't think, 'I'm stupid and fat.' I think, 'I tried on the wrong thing.'"

around the house for 10 minutes. Later, wear it in front of a friend. Soon, you'll feel comfortable enough to swim laps or take part in an aqua aerobics class."

Be polite! "If you had a friend who said, 'What a big butt you have!' every time you saw her, you wouldn't remain her friend," says Thomas F. Cash, Ph.D., professor of psychology at Old Dominion University in Norfolk, Virginia, and author of *The Body Image Workbook*. "Don't tolerate that treatment from yourself, either. Every time you start putting yourself down, stop cold. Instead, encourage yourself as you would a friend. Say, 'Yeah, my shape isn't what I would like, but I'm taking steps to change it. And that's a positive thing.'"

Ditch the magic number. Some women have their whole body image wrapped up in a number on the scale, says Joni E. Johnston, Psy.D., a clinical psychologist in Del Mar, California, and author of *Appearance Obsession*. "If they're just a couple of pounds off, they feel horrible about themselves. Give yourself an acceptable weight range between 5 and 10 pounds, so you can have healthy, normal weight fluctuations and still feel good about your body."

Hold your head high. When you're busy thinking that your thighs are too big, you assume everyone else is thinking that, too, so you feel self-conscious, says Dr. Cash. "People never judge us as harshly as we judge ourselves. If you hold your head up, smile, and project yourself as a healthy, confident person, that's what they'll see—and that's how you'll feel."

Step 2: Accept Your Power

Poor body image often comes with a little sound track in your head that repeats this tune: "My weight-loss efforts have never worked before, and they won't work now. I'm a failure," says Dr. Ramirez.

If you keep that negative sound track playing, you probably *will* fail.

Consider this: In one study, beginning tennis players who were told that they could improve their game by trying hard and practicing scored consistently better than those who were told that poor performance meant they lacked the innate ability. "If you believe you have bad genes, you're less likely to succeed than if you believe you have the power to control your actions, your attitude, and, consequently, your weight," says study leader Robert Singer, Ph.D., chairman of the exercise and sport science department at the University of Florida in Gainesville. It's all about developing what psychologists call self-efficacy—a big word for believing in yourself and your power to do what needs to be done. Here's how to boost yours.

Talk back. One quick way to stop the negative voices in your head is to simply tell them to quiet down, says Dr. Johnston. "Most people walk around putting themselves down without even realizing it. Pay attention when those self-defeating thoughts pop up. Every time your internal voice starts saying, 'I'm too fat,' 'I'm too uncoordinated,' or 'I can't do it,' answer back: 'That's enough. I can do whatever I put my mind to.'"

Write your résumé. Confidence changes from situation to situation, says Edward McAuley, Ph.D., professor of kinesiology at the University of Illinois at Urbana-Champaign. "It might be high in the office, yet low at the gym. You want to transfer all the assurance you can from one situation to the other." Think of it as writing your résumé. You don't always have the experience a job calls for, but you do have the skills. "Write down the skills you have to succeed at a fitness plan," he says. "List attributes such as 'I'm a hard worker,' 'I manage my time well,' and 'I'm a fast learner.' Then use these skills to succeed at your fitness program."

Recognize success. Think of developing confidence like building a house with a strong foundation brick by brick. "Each little success is a brick," says Joyce Nash, Ph.D., clinical psychologist in Menlo Park and San Francisco,

Real-Life Success Story

Carla Linder-Mayer, 39
Naperville, Illinois
Pounds lost: 120

Biggest obstacle: "Lack of self-confidence. I felt so bad about myself that all I would do was eat. I didn't believe I could do anything else."

Major accomplishment: "I completed the Chicago Marathon in 4 hours and 31 minutes."

How she did it: "I set small goals that wouldn't be overwhelming. My first goal was to walk ½ hour a week and lose 10 pounds. When I lost that 10, I thought, 'I can do that again.' As I lost more weight, I exercised more, and my confidence rose. It's all positive momentum. Anyone can do it."

No-Sweat Workouts

Feeling clumsy in aerobics class or the weight room can be devastating to your body image. Particularly at first, choose an activity that makes you simply enjoy moving. Here are some suggestions.

Take a stroll. "Feel your arms swing and your legs move," says Thomas F. Cash, Ph.D., professor of psychology at Old Dominion University in Norfolk, Virginia. "Enjoy the fresh air and how good it feels to be alive."

Seek the hills. "Hiking is wonderful for your body, mind, and spirit," says Rebecca Gorrell, director of fitness and movement therapy at Canyon Ranch Health Resort in Tucson. "No woman gets to the top of a mountain and still hates her thighs."

Find focus. "It's hard to dwell on how your body looks when you're concentrating on breathing and moving in yoga," says Joni E. Johnston, Psy.D., a clinical psychologist in Del Mar, California. "Plus, you can do yoga no matter what your size."

Unwind. Consider tai chi. Its gentle, fluid movements ease you from worrying about your body to moving with it, says Dr. Johnston. "It's relaxing and beautiful."

Dance, dance, dance! Pop in your favorite CD and boogie through the house. "When you move with music for fun, you forget about dance steps and how you look," says Dr. Cash.

California, and author of *The New Maximize Your Body Potential.* "Calling a gym that interests you is one brick. Going to observe an aerobics class is another. Don't disregard all these little steps: Applaud yourself for making progress."

Find new friends. A weight-loss buddy can go a long way toward building self-confidence, says Dr. Singer. "The more like-minded people you have to support you, the more confident you'll feel, and the more likely you are to succeed." Take advantage of the bulletin boards at the gym. Or look for a fitness buddy online at *Prevention* magazine's Healthy Ideas Web site (www.healthyideas.com). Click into the "weight-loss and fitness" area, then register under "finding support" in the "weight-loss program" section.

Step 3: Get Moving!

In order to boost your body image, build your confidence, and get a better body, you need to be active, says Dr. Nash. "It's essential for both looking and feeling your best."

When a group of middle-aged men and women started walking three times a week, they improved not only their heart health but also their self-esteem,

Real-Life Success Story

Diana Vertuccio, 50
Douglaston, New York
Pounds lost: 78
Biggest obstacle: "I felt so self-conscious that I hated to get undressed in front of my husband."
Major accomplishment: "Taking time for myself and finding a way to fit exercise into my daily schedule."
How she did it: "I dressed to accentuate my best features during the process. I found people who gave me positive support and looked at the treadmill as my buddy."

confidence, and body image. "It's positive momentum," says Dr. McAuley. Here are some tips to get you started.

Begin at home. Community gyms aren't for everyone, says Michaela Kiernan, Ph.D., research associate at Stanford University School of Medicine.

"Some overweight women may want to start with a home-based fitness program such as walking," Dr. Kiernan says. That way you don't have to face the stress or embarrassment of a group setting.

Start in first gear. A common mistake when starting a fitness program is setting your expectations too high, says Dr. Singer. You then become discouraged and quit when you don't reach those goals.

"Instead, picture a ladder, with your big goal at the top," Dr. Singer advises. "Develop short-term goals for each rung on that ladder."

If your ultimate goal, for instance, is to walk a 5-K race, make the first rung a 10-minute walk and then work your way up. Each small success you realize builds your confidence about reaching the big one.

Focus on bonuses. Exercise's benefits go way beyond the cosmetic, says Dr. Nash. "When you establish a goal to lower your blood pressure or your cholesterol, for example, you have something besides your clothing size to measure your progress—and you'll feel better about your body on another level."

Support a cause. "Getting involved in runs, walks, or bike rides for a cause that's important to you—whether it's breast cancer, AIDS, or multiple sclerosis—makes you feel good," says Ann Marie Miller, an exercise physiologist and fitness training manager at New York Sports Clubs in New York City.

"It also makes you grateful that you have a healthy body that can exercise," says Miller.

Seize those seconds. Just because you don't have 45 minutes to work out doesn't mean you should skip exercising entirely, says Dr. Johnston. "Doing something is always better than nothing. It all adds up in the long run." Even if you exercise for only 10 minutes, mark it on your calendar as a day you worked out. Being consistent will make you feel better about yourself and help you lose weight.

Slim Down in 30 Days— By Walking

D r. Suzanne Levine tried everything from ballet class to a home stair-climber to slim down her 178-pound figure. Then she discovered walking and lost more than 50 pounds—and has kept it off for 15 years.

As with Suzanne, walking could be the answer to your weight-loss prayers. Walking is easy, cheap, convenient, and not likely to result in an injury.

What's even better, if you're overweight, losing just 10 percent of your body weight can have tremendous health benefits by cutting your risk for cardiovascular disease, diabetes, cancer, and arthritis.

So get started today. You'll be surprised how easily you can walk off weight!

To get you going, Rebecca Gorrell, director of fitness and movement therapy at Canyon Ranch Health Resort in Tucson, developed four walking workouts guaranteed to have you dropping pounds in 30 days. Whether you're a beginner, stuck in a rut, looking for a new challenge, or an avid walker, you'll find the perfect program for you right here. So get moving—and start losing!

The Get-Started Plan

This plan is for you if you:

❖ Spend your days sitting at a desk or in a car and your evenings on the couch
❖ Walk less than 60 to 90 minutes a day doing your job or everyday activi-

ties such as walking to the bus stop, walking the dog, and chasing after kids

❖ Are severely overweight
❖ Are recovering from an illness or surgery
❖ Have a chronic disease or injury that limits activity

Even though you walk around every day, walking for weight loss is something that you need to build up to. When Suzanne, a New York City podiatrist, started walking, the extra pounds she carried made even short workouts feel intense.

"I walked at about 20 to 25 minutes per mile and was huffing and puffing," Suzanne remembers. "Now I do less than a 14-minute mile and walk 4 miles a day."

This program is designed to ease you into a regular walking routine. By starting out slowly, you'll enjoy exercising more, build your confidence, and reduce your risk of injury. Even at a slow pace, you'll still reap many benefits from your walking routine. From the beginning, you'll feel more energetic and flexible, and you'll be in a better mood. After about 2 weeks, your walks will feel easier because your heart will be getting fitter and your legs will be getting stronger.

Congratulations on starting a walking program! The next step: Stick with it. Here are some tips to keep you on track.

Notice the little things. Losing weight is a great motivator, but don't overlook the other benefits: stress reduction, improved mood, better-fitting clothes, performing daily activities with ease, leftover energy in the evening, and more.

Get-Started Workout

Duration	Frequency	Intensity	Speed
Week 1	10 min. for 3 days	Moderate*	Whatever is comfortable
Week 2	15 min. for 4 days	Moderate*	As if you're in a bit of a hurry; after walking for 10 min., you should have covered more distance than you did last week
Week 3	20 min. for 5 days	Moderate*	As if you're in a bit of a hurry
Week 4	30 min. for 5 days	Moderate*	As if you're in a bit of a hurry

Enough to get your heart pumping, but not enough to leave you out of breath

Easy Steps to a Slimmer, Stronger, Healthier Body

Walking does more than just whittle your waistline. Here's what you can expect from a good walking program.

❖ Lower blood pressure
❖ Decreased cholesterol levels
❖ Stronger bones
❖ Firmer muscles
❖ More energy
❖ Better mood
❖ More restful sleep
❖ Reduced stress
❖ Improved sex life
❖ Reduced risk of diabetes, heart disease, and cancer

Enjoy the great outdoors. While you're walking, breathe in the fresh air. Watch the sunrise. Check out the changing leaves or emerging flowers. Watch birds and animals.

Schedule it. Pick a specific time to walk and stick to it. That way, it becomes a regular part of your day—just like eating breakfast or reading the paper.

The Plateau-Busting Plan

This plan is for you if you:

❖ Have been walking regularly for at least 6 weeks
❖ Haven't seen the scale go down in the past month
❖ Are bored with walking and find yourself making excuses to justify skipping your workouts
❖ Don't do formal exercise, but your daily routine is somewhat active. For example, you are on your feet all day at your hospital job and then cook, clean, and try to keep up with a 3-year-old at night.

If you have been walking for a while and the weight has stopped coming off, you may have hit a plateau. Plateaus are practically a given when you're trying to lose weight. They might happen because you're bored or unchallenged, or you've stopped monitoring or setting goals for yourself. Fortunately, a simple change in your workout—such as intervals—can send those stubborn pounds packing.

That's what happened when Constance Costas traded in her aerobic classes for a treadmill and a weight program. "I got frustrated with the schedules, and

I wasn't able to work out consistently," says the 36-year-old freelance writer from Richmond, Virginia. So last year, she started walking on a treadmill or outdoors with her kids. "It liberated my workouts," she says. "It's no longer a struggle to exercise. When I tried on my summer clothes the next year, I could spin my skirts around my hips. I lost 13 pounds and went down two sizes—without dieting."

This interval walking program is guaranteed to help you take off those stubborn pounds, too.

It can be really difficult to stick with any exercise program when you're not seeing immediate results. But hang in there; the scale will start to inch its way down.

In the meantime, here are several ways that you can keep yourself motivated.

Take an alternate route. A change of scenery can inspire you. "Walk somewhere beautiful such as a hiking trail, along a river, or in a park," suggests Gorrell.

Savor your mileage. As you pick up speed, you'll go farther. Keep a log to

Rate Your Workout to Burn More Calories

The higher the intensity of your walk, the more calories you'll burn. But how do you know what intensity you're at? An easy, low-tech method to use is the Borg Scale for Rate of Perceived Exertion (RPE)—no arithmetic or heart rate monitors needed. This method is particularly helpful when you're doing the interval or pyramid workouts.

To use it, simply scan your body and consider how hard you're working. Is your breathing heavy? Are you sweating? Do your muscles feel warm? Are they burning? Now, rate how you feel.

Borg Scale for Rate of Perceived Exertion

6	
7	very, very light (lounging on the couch)
8	
9	very light (puttering around the house)
10	
11	fairly light (leisurely stroll)
12	
13	somewhat hard (normal walk)
14	
15	hard (walk as if in a hurry)
16	
17	very hard (jogging/running)
18	
19	very, very hard (sprinting)
20	

Plateau-Busting Workout

Duration	Frequency	Program	Rate of Perceived Exertion (RPE)
Week 1	35 min. for 5 days	Warmup (5 min.)	10–11
		Normal walk (5 min.)	13
		Speedup (5 min.)	15
		Recovery (10 min.)	13
		Speedup (5 min.)	15
		Cooldown (5 min.)	10–11
Week 2	35 min. for 5 days	Warmup (5 min.)	10–11
		Normal walk (5 min.)	13
		Speedup (5 min.)	16
		Recovery (10 min.)	13
		Speedup (5 min.)	16
		Cooldown (5 min.)	10–11
Week 3	45 min. for 5 days	Warmup (5 min.)	10–11
		Normal walk (5 min.)	13
		Speedup (5 min.)	16
		Recovery (8 min.)	13
		Speedup (5 min.)	16
		Recovery (7 min.)	13
		Speedup (5 min.)	16
		Cooldown (5 min.)	10–11
Week 4	45 min. for 5 days	Warmup (5 min.)	10–11
		Speedup (5 min.)	16
		Recovery (5 min.)	13
		Speedup (5 min.)	16
		Recovery (5 min.)	13
		Speedup (5 min.)	16
		Recovery (5 min.)	13
		Speedup (5 min.)	16
		Cooldown (5 min.)	10–11

track your improvements. Then reward yourself when you top last week's mileage entry.

Sign up for a walking trip. Plan a walking vacation to a gorgeous place like the lush, green New England countryside or the sunny California coast. The anticipation will keep you walking.

Be self-indulgent. Walks are your very own time. Relax, take deep breaths, dream, even problem-solve. There are no piles of laundry or ringing phones to distract you.

The Maximum Calorie-Burn Plan

This plan is for you if you:

❖ Think walking is too easy
❖ Want to lose weight fast
❖ Have been doing interval walking (or other exercise at a moderately high intensity) for at least 6 weeks
❖ Don't have time to take longer walks but want to burn more calories

This plan is designed to maximize calorie burn so you lose weight fast. It consists of "power pyramids," in which you do mini-intervals, working your way up to a brief but very high intensity walk or jog. Then you notch your way back down. That's how Rita Rover, a trim, 56-year-old nutritionist in private practice in Northport, New York, makes walking a challenging workout. Compared with her 30-mile bike rides and hour-plus tennis matches, walking might seem wimpy—but not with these high-intensity intervals.

"I combine walking short distances with running," Rita says. "It's more fun because of the challenge and variety—and I've lost weight without trying. In fact, I find that I have to eat more just to maintain my present weight!"

To do power pyramids, change your walking pace every 30 or 60 seconds based on your specific rates of perceived exertion (RPE).

Here are some ways to keep your workouts on schedule.

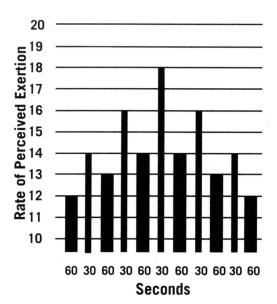

Power pyramid. Read the graph from left to right for time intervals. Then read up to find out what Rate of Perceived Exertion (RPE) you should be working at. After the first 60 seconds, move to the next time interval and continue.

Maximum Calorie-Burn Workout

Duration	Frequency	Program	Rate of Perceived Exertion (RPE)
Week 1	40 min. for 5 days	Warmup (5 min.)	10–11
		Pyramid (see figure)	
		Normal walk (7 min.)	13
		Pyramid	
		Normal walk (6 min.)	13
		Cooldown (5 min.)	10–11
Week 2	45 min. for 5 days	Warmup (5 min.)	10–11
		Pyramid	
		Normal walk (5 min.)	13
		Pyramid	
		Normal walk (5 min.)	13
		Pyramid	
		Cooldown (5 min.)	10–11
Week 3	50 min. for 5 days	Warmup (5 min.)	10–11
		Pyramid	
		Normal walk (5 min.)	13
		Pyramid	
		Normal walk (5 min.)	13
		Pyramid	
		Normal walk (5 min.)	13
		Cooldown (5 min.)	10–11
Week 4	60 min. for 5 days	Warmup (5 min.)	10–11
		Pyramid	
		Normal walk (5 min.)	13
		Pyramid	
		Normal walk (5 min.)	13
		Pyramid	
		Normal walk (5 min.)	13
		Pyramid	
		Cooldown (5 min.)	10–11

Train for a race. Pick a distance that's longer than you're used to. That way, you'll have to be consistent about training in order to do well.

Reward yourself. Buy a new walking outfit for not missing a workout in the past month. Or get a massage when you up your mileage.

Make intervals easier. Instead of constantly checking your watch, record upbeat music and then add a voice cue to mark your 30- and 60-second intervals.

The Toning Circuit Plan

This plan is for you if you:

❖ Want to firm up your butt, legs, abs, and more
❖ Want stronger legs
❖ Need some variety
❖ Have been walking regularly for at least 6 weeks

Walking not only sheds pounds but also can shape up your muscles. Mary Evans, a 40-something information systems expert from Emmaus, Pennsylvania, discovered that when she started hill walking. "My husband and I go up and down a steep hill for 2 to 3 miles almost every day," she says. And it shows: Mary has lost about 15 pounds and firmed her legs.

To shape more than just your legs, here's a toning circuit workout that uses different walking techniques to firm muscles.

Hill walking or stairclimbing. These exercises shape the fronts and backs of your thighs and calves.

Racewalking. This will firm your abs and upper back muscles. To do it, take shorter, quicker steps. Try to place each foot along a straight imaginary line in front of you, one foot in front of the other. Get your hips into the action by

Toning Circuit Workout

Duration	Frequency	Program	Rate of Perceived Exertion (RPE)
Week 1	30 min. for 5 days	Warmup (5 min.)	10–11
		Toning circuit (see figure; do each segment for 2 min.)	13–15
		Cooldown (5 min.)	10–11
Week 2	40 min. for 5 days	Warmup (5 min.)	10–11
		Toning circuit (do each segment for 3 min.)	13–15
		Cooldown (5 min.)	10–11
Week 3	50 min. for 5 days	Warmup (5 min.)	10–11
		Toning circuit (do each segment for 4 min.)	13–15
		Cooldown (5 min.)	10–11
Week 4	60 min. for 5 days	Warmup (5 min.)	10–11
		Toning circuit (do each segment for 5 min.)	13–15
		Cooldown (5 min.)	10–11

Perfect Walking Posture

Good walking posture helps boost your calorie burn and prevent injuries. To check your technique, have a friend watch you walk or walk on a treadmill in front of a mirror. According to Suki Munsell, Ph.D., founder of the Dynamic Health and Fitness Institute in Corte Madera, California, these are the key points of good posture.

❖ Look 6 feet in front of you.
❖ Drop your shoulders.
❖ Relax your arms and swing them forward as if each were a pendulum.
❖ Don't let your hands come across your body.
❖ Keep your abs firm but not so tight that you can't breathe.
❖ Tuck your pelvis slightly by bringing your belly button back toward your spine.
❖ Point your knees and toes forward, keeping your feet parallel.
❖ Roll from heel to toe; avoid falling to the inside or outside of your foot.
❖ Keep your head level; your ears should be over your shoulders.
❖ Bend your elbows to an 85° to 90° angle.
❖ Lift up and out of your hips to allow more swivel.
❖ Push off with your back foot.

swiveling them forward and back with each step. Think of them as an extension of your thighs. Bend your arms at 85° to 90° angles and let them swing from your shoulders like pendulums. Don't bounce.

The butt squeeze. This squeeze tightens your glutes. Use your normal walking form, but as you press off the toes of your back leg, squeeze your buttocks firmly, says Gorrell. "Be careful not to tense your lower back."

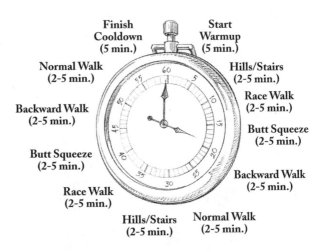

Toning circuit. Start at the top and walk your way around (clockwise), switching techniques as indicated.

Finish Cooldown (5 min.)
Start Warmup (5 min.)
Normal Walk (2-5 min.)
Hills/Stairs (2-5 min.)
Race Walk (2-5 min.)
Backward Walk (2-5 min.)
Butt Squeeze (2-5 min.)
Butt Squeeze (2-5 min.)
Backward Walk (2-5 min.)
Race Walk (2-5 min.)
Hills/Stairs (2-5 min.)
Normal Walk (2-5 min.)

Backward walking. This type of walking strengthens your back and abs because your balance is different. Reach back with the ball and toes of one foot without leaning forward, says Gorrell. Tuck your belly and put your hands on your hips. That makes your abs and back do all the work. For safety, limit backward walking to a level track or path.

Begin by doing each technique for 2 minutes, eventually working up to 5 minutes.

With the variety of techniques in this workout, you shouldn't get bored. But just in case, here are additional tips to inspire you.

Measure up. Record your waist, hip, thigh, or other measurements before you start the program. Then watch them shrink and firm up.

Get an incentive. Find a short, slim skirt or a form-fitting dress that you love. Then start walking toward the goal of buying it.

Find a walking partner. Take turns walking backward so you can look out for each other.

How Real Women Lose Weight

Add one set of situps every evening. Subtract one blueberry muffin every morning. Sometimes all it takes is just one new habit, one shift in perspective to push your body to the next level. Here, 10 women from around the country share the single simple-but-critical change that brought big fitness results. Read what worked for them and steal the moves that make sense for you.

"I Gave Up Mashed Potatoes"

One morning, Caroline Hwang, 29, noticed what she described as "this permanent ring around my waist." The editor and writer had always been a regular at the gym, and as a vegetarian, she watched what she ate. Her suddenly bulging middle mystified her until she thought hard about her diet—specifically, her passion for mashed potatoes.

In addition to ordering them at restaurants, she'd been having them nearly every day for lunch: "I was so busy that I didn't have time to go out, and there was nothing else edible at the company cafeteria," she says. "They weren't even real potatoes—just powdered. Really embarrassing." She resolved to give up her favorite comfort food, though she still allows herself a baked potato with salt, pepper, and broccoli. ("Occasionally, I add butter," she says. "But at least now I know how much is in there.") At restaurants, she requests a dollop, not a dish, of mashed potatoes. As a result, she lost 5 pounds without making any other changes in her diet, and the ring around her waist disappeared.

Steal her move: A big yen for one favorite food—whether it's Snickers bars or sunflower seeds—can hold your entire diet hostage. "It's not just the extra calories," says Vicki Ellis, a nutritionist with the Florida Institute of Nutrition and Dietetics in Miami Beach. "It's also a control issue. If you can give up that one comfort food, you gain a sense of control over other aspects of your diet as well."

"I Got a Dog"

Kerri-Lee Halkett, 27, credits her current 10-mile-a-week running regimen to her Dalmatian, Tully. As an on-air TV reporter in Washington, D.C., she's up at 3:30 every morning and understandably low on workout motivation in the evening. "It sounds awful, but that's the main reason I got my dog. Dalmatians are known for being hyper and desperate for exercise," says Halkett. "I figured Tully would force me to run regularly, and she's definitely living up to her end of the bargain."

Steal her move: Any creature that counts on you for exercise is a good thing, be it a dog, horse, sparring partner, or jogging buddy. She'll get you out of bed in the morning and make your workout feel speedy, social, and safe. If you're in the market for a dog you can run with, Robin Kovary of the American Dog Trainers Network in New York City recommends breeds with long legs and athletic bodies, such as Labrador retrievers, greyhounds, Doberman pinschers, or Halkett's favorite breed, Dalmatians.

"I Made My Job More Physical"

Three years ago, Kerensa Mabwa was a supervisor at a program for substance abusers in Chicago. Now she is a member of an African storytelling trio that blends narrative and dance. "It has been an amazing transformation for me," says the 31-year-old. "Plus, the dancing has really whipped my butt into shape." The change was motivated in part by Mabwa's desire to bring more movement into her clients' lives as well as her own. She created a series of seminars to spark the confidence of recovering addicts. Now other social service groups are clamoring for her courses, so Mabwa splits her time between teaching seminars and dancing. "Life is not just about using your mind," she says. "It's about making the connection between mind and body."

Steal her move: Dancing on the job won't win points with most employers, but adding just one element of movement to a sedentary routine can kick you off your plateau. According to the American Council on Exercise (ACE) in San Diego, three 10-minute stints of exercise each day are just as good as working out for 30 minutes straight. So try taking a brisk 10- or 15-minute walk during your lunch break and use the stairs instead of the elevator in your office building whenever possible, suggests Monica Schrader, ACE spokesperson.

You can also do wall pushups, squats, and lunges in your office (if you have one) as well as triceps dips: Sit on a sturdy chair, hands palms down on either side of your buttocks. Slide forward until your butt is off the seat and a few inches away from the chair; keep your thighs parallel to the floor and your elbows slightly bent. Slowly bend your arms, lowering your butt until your upper arms are parallel to the floor, then straighten your arms to return to the starting position. Do 15 repetitions. "These short bouts of exercise throughout the day give your mind and your body a break," Schrader says. After work, walk instead of driving to your favorite restaurant, if possible, or take a quick stroll after dinner.

"I Got a Great Mix Tape"

It's cheaper than a health-club membership, more motivating than a workout video. And the mix tape that Wendy Livingston listens to when she jogs has changed her attitude about cardio training. "I used to spend my whole run looking at my watch and thinking, 'It's only been 2 miles and I'm going to die,'" says the 31-year-old Durham, North Carolina, mother of one. Then her husband started mixing tapes for her to listen to during runs, and suddenly Livingston was logging 4 to 5 miles. "The music helps me sort of meditate through the workout and forget the pain," she says. "My husband keeps me guessing; he throws in some embarrassingly old stuff, like ZZ Top, but there's also lots of Spin Doctors and R.E.M." Hey, whatever gets you going.

Steal her move: Haven't made a mix tape since high school? Well, it's easier now. All you have to do is log on to one of the many custom CD Web sites, like www.musicmaker.com and www.customdisc.com, where you can scroll through a list of artists and song titles, then select a personalized mix for your CD. When you're done, type in your mailing address and credit card number (most custom CDs cost $15 to $25), and you'll get your CD in a few weeks. Copy onto a blank tape and you're ready to run—or blade or walk.

Once you've hit a music mix that really gets you going, listen to it only during exercise time: It will be part of your reward for working out. The same rule applies to your favorite TV fix; try permitting yourself *NYPD Blue* only when you're on the ski machine or treadmill.

"I Started Biking to Work"

Her mother was once known as the Bicycle Lady of Metuchen, New Jersey, which may explain why Elisabeth Ernish, 30, chooses to pedal to work across the Brooklyn Bridge into Manhattan every day—a hilly, traffic-packed, 14-mile round-trip commute—rather than hop on the subway like everyone else. "Mom didn't even bother getting a driver's license until she was well into her fifties," says Ernish. "I guess I got the biking bug from her."

When Ernish started grad school in New York City, she found that biking was the fastest way to shuttle between home, school, and two jobs. But what began as simple transportation soon became a cardio religion. "People go to such great lengths to work out—joining expensive gyms and hiring personal

A New Spin on Fitness

If regular workouts leave you cold, check out Spinning. It's indoor group cycling, also called Power Pacing, Cycle Reebok, or studio cycling. These bikes feel like the real thing. They're equipped with a weighted flywheel in the front that picks up speed as you pedal. They have toe clips and adjustable seats. There's a knob below the handlebars that allows you to adjust the tension, making pedaling easier or harder.

There are no group workout activities quite like Spinning. Above all, everyone in studio cycling is equal. No one knows at what level you have your tension adjusted, so you can ride at your personal workload. There are no choreographed moves, and unlike real cycling, you're never lagging behind the pack. Everyone finishes together. And everyone gets a great workout.

To find a Spinning class, call the health clubs in your area. You may need to reserve a spot, since class size is limited. Here's some other information you'll want to know before you go.

What it will cost: About $6 to $15 a class. A gym membership may include the cost of Spinning classes.

What you'll burn: Spinning burns 7 to 14 calories per minute, or up to 800 calories during a 1-hour class.

What to wear: To prevent saddle soreness, wear padded bike shorts or padded undies.

What to do first: Although cycling is especially good for people who have joint problems or trouble with weight-bearing exercise, you should check with your doctor first if you're new to exercise.

If you'd rather exercise at home, studio cycles retail at about $500 to $700. Schwinn and Reebok make two of the most popular models.

trainers. My bike commute builds in fitness. You should see my quads. They're as hard as a linebacker's."

Steal her move: Ernish finds she doesn't have to shower after her ride "because I'm not a real speedster," but sprinkling on some baby powder will help you freshen up before work. Also invest in waterproof gear for drizzly days. Ernish says she wears a jacket and pants that completely protect her work clothes, so she only misses 5 or 6 days of biking a year due to inclement weather.

Susan Boyle, bike program coordinator at Transportation Alternatives, a biking and walking advocacy group in New York City, suggests doing a practice run of your planned route on a weekend first. She also recommends wearing light-colored outerwear and a reflective vest for safety. Make sure your bike has a red back light and a white front light, which some states require by law. Ask your office building manager if bike access and storage are provided. If not, Boyle suggests that you lobby for them and that you try to line up support from co-workers. "You'd be surprised at the number of people who would ride to work if it were made easier," she says, "and you might even find a potential partner."

"I Swore Off Stairclimbing"

Getting stuck on one machine for too many months can zone out your mind and body. Dominique Saint-Louis, 32, says cutting herself loose from the thigh-punishing stairclimbing machine was her best gym decision ever. A TV producer in New York City, Saint-Louis switched from the StairMaster to the Versa Climber machine, a device that works both the arms and the legs. Within 3 months, she'd developed a stronger upper body without bulking up down below. "I've always wanted nicely defined muscles in my back, but I wasn't sure how to get them," she says. "Now I know."

Janet Israel, vice president of a Philadelphia catering company, kicked her stairclimbing addiction when her gym got its first elliptical fitness crosstrainer (Precor EFX) machines last year. "With EFX, there's no impact on my shins, and my legs aren't just going straight up and down," says Israel, age 37. "I can see a whole new set of muscles in my thighs and shoulders."

Steal her move: "People are such creatures of habit, especially when it comes to exercise," says Joan Hanscom, exercise program manager for the Washington Sports Clubs in Washington, D.C. "But if you do the same thing over and over, your body eventually adapts to the movement, and it won't be as effective." Instead, she says, try something new at your gym once in a while. "The StairMaster is great. Aerobics classes are great. But nothing is great every day."

"I Gave Up Drinking"

As a financially strapped law school student, Ann Kneeland decided to give up a lot of little extras—including alcohol. "Buying even the occasional beer just suddenly seemed like a big waste of money to me," she says. Her cost-cutting measure, however, came with a health bonus; when she skipped the campus bar, she was more motivated to exercise and eat right the next day. This translated into more energy for her studies and new Levi's a size smaller than her old ones. Kneeland, 32, now practices law with a Berkeley, California, public-interest group and still shuns alcohol for fitness reasons. "I haven't given up caffeine," she confesses. "But I have to keep some vices."

Steal her move: Drinking and eating go hand in hand, says Ellis of the Florida Institute of Nutrition and Dietetics. "If you have a cocktail in one hand, the other is probably reaching for the hors d'oeuvre plate." Cut down on drinks, and you'll nibble less; plus, you'll save the liquid calories (a vodka tonic has around 165 calories; a beer around 145).

"I Got a Babysitter"

When her first child was born, Lisa Goodman got back in shape by packing her baby in a jog stroller and going for power walks. But 3 years later, she had a second child, and suddenly exercise seemed impossible. "I have an exercise bike at home," says Goodman, a 37-year-old professor of psychology at the University of Maryland. "But now that my kids are no longer lulled into submission by *Lion King* videos, it's impossible to keep them distracted. After 10 minutes, they're at my feet screaming, 'My turn! My turn! My turn!'"

For a while, Goodman tried using her health club's day care facility. That was a flop: "My kids knew I was in the next room, and it drove them—and me—crazy." So she and her husband, Bill, bit the financial bullet and hired a sitter. "We gave up weekend babysitting so I could finally exercise," she says. "When it's the only thing that maintains my sanity, it's not a luxury," she says. "It's a necessity."

Steal her move: If day care or babysitting strains your budget, team up with a friend to swap sitting services. On alternate days, one of you exercises while the other watches the kids. If all goes well, you could each nab up to three fitness sessions a week—for free.

"I Found the Perfect Pushup"

They feel every bit as brutal as they sound, but Monica Ammann, 25, credits triceps hinge pushups with chiseling new cuts into her formerly undefined arms. "My upper body feels so much more powerful now, without being bulky," she says. "I never had a problem with my lower body because I play soccer and ski. But I had no upper-body definition before. Now my shoulders, biceps, and triceps are strong and stand out. And I can still only do four of these pushups in a row!"

Steal her move: Start in the usual "up" position, but place your hands in line with your waist instead of your shoulders, with your fingers forward, hands body-width apart. Keeping your abs tight, your elbows close to your sides, and your torso straight, slowly lower yourself to within a few inches of the floor. Now for the "hinge": Lower yourself those last 2 inches so your nose touches the floor, then come back up until your arms are straight but not locked. Repeat.

Too tough? Try these versions instead: Do the whole pushup with your weight on your knees, not your toes. Or place one hand in a traditional pushup position, about chest level, and place the other at waist level. Start with two sets of four, working up to two sets of eight.

"I Started Charting My Workouts"

For Jennifer Cadoff, it's all about creating a paper trail. Four years ago, the freelance writer began keeping track of each day she exercised—mostly to remind herself that a few missed days at the gym were nothing compared with all the days that she hadn't missed. Her system: One piece of paper, pinned up in the kitchen, lets her see a year at a glance. Each day she exercises, she marks down a tiny letter: T for tennis, B for bowling, W for walking, G for gym, and R for rowing machine. ("I haven't rowed in ages," she confides, but if her arms ache after raking the yard, she'll sneak in an R anyway.)

Cadoff's system keeps her focused on the importance of doing something every day—even if it's not exactly a biathlon. "My chart helps me remember the big picture," she says, "and the fact that fitness is a project for the rest of my life, not just for the duration of the tai chi class."

Steal her move: Start charting with a modest goal of, say, 3 workout days each week, then gradually add to it. ("I'm always trying to beat my record," says Cadoff. "It has become a private little game.") Since many gyms now monitor member attendance, ask for your record; you may be surprised at how often you're really going—and how knowing the numbers will help you keep the faith.

Flatten Your Stomach— Without Situps

Among fitness trends, Pilates (pronounced puh-LAH-tees) is one of the hottest because it helps build a long, lean, flexible body with killer abs.

Like yoga or ballet, Pilates is a series of controlled, balanced movements that create long, limber muscles by working them through a wide range of motion.

Until recently, however, most people had to go to a designated Pilates studio for classes because many of the exercises require special equipment. Now gyms across the country are offering "mat Pilates" classes that adapt the traditional moves so that you can do them with no more equipment than a floor mat.

The following exercises were designed by Laurie Hennessy, fitness coordinator of the Encino, California, branch of Bodies in Motion. These at-home moves, which can tone your abs and firm up your thighs and arms, are meant to be an introduction to the Pilates technique.

If you like the workout, look for a mat class where you can learn more. Nationwide gyms plan to feature group classes using portable Pilates machines.

Note: Every Pilates exercise targets the midsection, so keeping abs tight is key.

The Hundred

Targets: abdominals

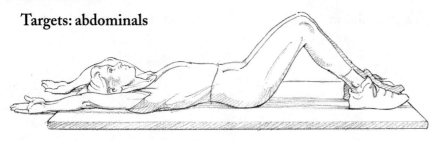

Lie on your back on an exercise mat, feet flat on the floor, with your arms on the floor above your head and your palms toward the ceiling.

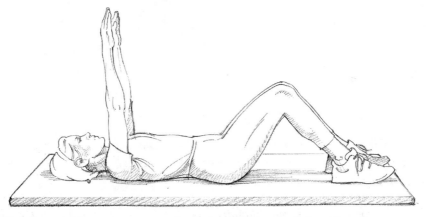

Inhale and raise your arms overhead, fingertips toward the ceiling.

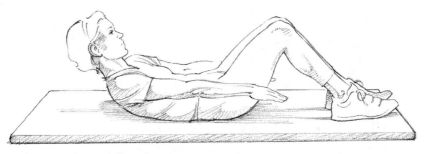

Exhale while you lower your arms, contract your abdominal muscles, and curl forward so your head, neck, and shoulders come off the floor. Stop lowering your arms when your hands are about 2 to 3 inches above the floor, palms down.

Hold this position and "pulse" your arms 10 times—reaching forward while inhaling and exhaling for five counts each. Then lower yourself back down. Rest and repeat. Start with 3 sets and build up to 10, for a total of 100.

Leg Circle

Targets: abdominals, quadriceps (front of thighs), and hamstrings

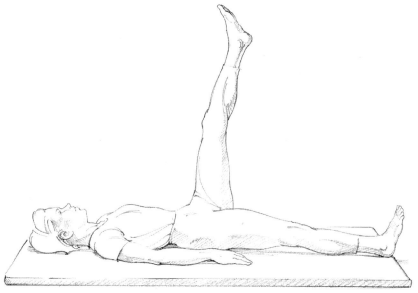

Lie flat on your back on the floor. (If you're a beginner, bend your knees.) Keep your hands at your sides, palms down, your abdominals tight, and your legs extended in front of you. Raise your extended left leg directly above your hip or as high as you can, with your toes gently pointed. Now draw four to six circles in the air with your entire leg while keeping your hips stable, then switch direction and circle the other way four to six times. Lower your left leg and switch to your right. Repeat.

Front Support
Targets: chest, arms, and abdominals

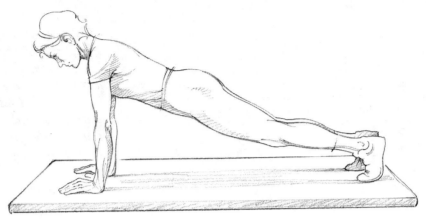

Lie facedown on the mat. Place your hands underneath your shoulders, or farther apart if that's more comfortable. Keeping your head, neck, back, and hips in a straight line, push up to straighten your arms.

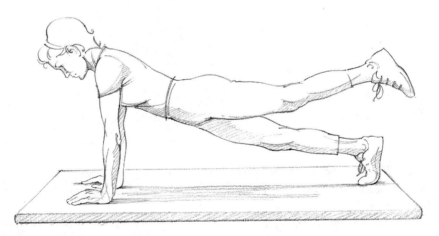

Lift your left heel toward the ceiling and hold for two or three counts, making sure that your head, neck, back, and hips are still in line. Don't move your hips.

Lower your left leg, and lift your right heel toward the ceiling. Hold for two or three counts. Repeat this entire sequence three or four times. At first, you may not be able to lift your toes more than an inch above the floor. As you develop more abdominal strength, you will be able to lift your foot higher.

Rolling

Don't do this unless your abs are already strong.
Targets: abdominals

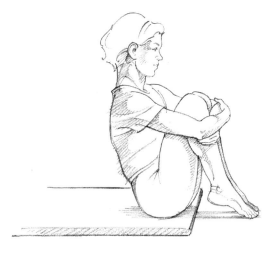

Sit close to the edge of your mat, hug your knees to your chest, and press your heels into your butt. Raise your feet an inch or two off the floor, point your toes gently, and tuck your chin to your chest.

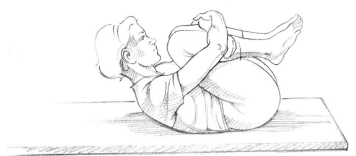

Keeping your shoulders pulled down and back and your abs tight, inhale and slowly rock back until your shoulders touch the floor. Avoid rolling onto your neck or head.

Exhale while you contract your abs to pull yourself forward and back to the starting position. Repeat five to eight times.

Beyond Menopause: Your Stay-in-Shape Guide

Ruth Steckelman Popkin never worried about her weight during her twenties and thirties. With the exception of three pregnancies, her 5'6" body never ventured past 125 pounds. "I'd exercise 4 or 5 days a week so I could eat whatever I wanted. I ate sensibly and was never on a diet," says Popkin, now 54, an attorney and owner of a title agency in Livingston, New Jersey.

She seemed cleared for takeoff—a symptom-free menopause. Then, at age 49, unwanted pounds piled around her midsection almost overnight. Clothes stopped fitting. She went from size 6 to 10 and stayed there, regardless of what or how little she ate.

Popkin's plight is one shared by millions of American women on the brink of menopause. It seems that healthy eating habits and exercise are suddenly no match for this life transition.

But with the help of Cristina Matera, M.D., assistant professor of clinical obstetrics and gynecology at Columbia University College of Physicians and Surgeons in New York City, Popkin made adjustments. She now eats a midafternoon snack, has salads without dressing, and begs off seconds at dinnertime. She lifts weights twice a week in addition to her four aerobic workouts. Now postmenopausal, she's happy with the way she looks, and she feels more fit and energetic than ever.

The Formula

Although each woman's situation is different, medical experts offer a formula that counters stubborn weight gain pegged to menopause. To breeze through your menopausal years fit and happy, they suggest you adopt this three-step approach.

❖ Eat less but more often.
❖ Enjoy a variety of exercise, including strength training.
❖ Adopt a healthy, self-promoting attitude.

What's the payoff? By embracing these easy-to-implement strategies, you may find that "the change" is the best time of your life. "Menopause is an incredible opportunity to take responsibility for your health and well-being," says Debra Waterhouse, R.D., author of *Outsmarting the Midlife Fat Cell*. "If you do something good for your body, when you exit this transition around age 55, you'll feel fit, strong, and the best you've ever been."

Eat Smarter

You've heard the old adage "You are what you eat." Well, that seems especially true during our forties. We look at a thick slab of chocolate cake, and it seems to gravitate instinctively to our thighs. But it doesn't have to be that way. With this eating game plan, food cravings won't get the best of you.

Eat small meals. Wave goodbye to meal skipping. Your body's metabolism slows by as much as 30 percent during menopause, so you need to eat smaller portions more often to help burn more for energy and store less as fat. This approach also helps minimize your mood swings and maximizes the efficient conversion of food into energy.

Make lunch your main meal. It seems that energy levels peak at high noon and dip at dinnertime for women. "Metabolism dips in the evening," says Waterhouse. "We're lucky if our bodies need 300 to 400 calories at night, but the typical woman eats a dinner containing 1,000 calories. That's 700 extra calories that will be converted and stored as fat while you sleep."

Go for variety. Choose from the different food groups, making sure you eat 5 servings of fruits and vegetables, 2 or 3 servings of protein and dairy products, and 6 to 11 servings of grains and pastas each day. If you're uncertain what's best for you, consult your doctor or a registered dietitian to get you on the right track.

Never surrender your favorite foods. Love pecan pie? Can't say no to ice cream sundaes? Enjoy them—in moderation. Diets that command you to stay away from specific foods are certain to fail, say nutrition experts. You only end up craving the banned food, abandoning the restrictive diet, and going on an eating binge.

Limit your salt and caffeine intake. Too much salt and caffeine can zap your bones of needed calcium and place you at greater risk for osteoporosis and hot flashes. Just 1 teaspoon of salt contains 2,300 milligrams of sodium—nearly double your daily quota. You should also limit your coffee to two cups a day.

Drink more water. Water is critical for maintaining your body's functions during your forties and fifties. Drink at least six to eight 8-ounce glasses every day.

Exercise Smarter

No one's asking you to spend all your waking hours sweating inside a gym. Instead, learn how to exercise smarter, not harder, says Miriam Nelson, Ph.D., associate chief of the physiology lab at Tufts University in Boston and author of *Strong Women Stay Slim*.

It's never too late to incorporate exercise into your life. Need some motivation? Regular exercisers report 39 percent fewer fat cravings and 22 percent fewer sugar cravings than inactive people, says Waterhouse, according to a survey she conducted. Exercisers also report that they experience half as many hot flashes.

Extend your aerobic workout. The 30-minute mall walk you've faithfully trekked three times a week just doesn't cut it anymore. As you approach menopause, you need to do 45 to 60 minutes of aerobic activity four or five

Climb Those Hills

At 5 feet tall and 120 pounds, Lynette Van Vlack of Newberg, Oregon, is 17 pounds heavier—but fitter and stronger—than when she was a 103-pound bride 28 years ago. She and her husband, Bob, recently moved into a three-story home on a mountain hillside with a challenging rocky slope. Lynette uses the hillside to add to her workout. "The gardening has been very challenging, and I've tripled the amount of exercise I get by running up and down the three flights of stairs all the time," she says.

No hillside house in your future? No problem. Try these tips instead.

❖ Climb hills in your neighborhood.
❖ Crank up the elevation on your electronic treadmill.
❖ Take the stairs often.

times a week to reduce your body fat. Why? Because your metabolic rate has slowed down, explains Dr. Nelson.

Introduce strength training. Aim for two muscle-building workouts lasting 30 to 40 minutes each week.

In her research, Dr. Nelson has discovered that strengthening exercises not only prevent muscle and bone loss but also help people lose weight. In fact, adding muscle can boost your calorie-burning potential by as much as 15 percent—about 300 calories a day for the average woman.

Vary your routines. If you love to walk, just vary how, when, and where you stride. Try scaling hills one day, walking mall laps the next. With your doctor's permission, try blending jogging with walking, or walking with a backpack filled with 5 to 10 pounds of newspaper. A variety of activity works all your muscles and prevents boredom.

Practice patience. Let your mind and body slowly adjust to your more active lifestyle. Don't expect to lose inches immediately. Experts say it takes at least 6 weeks for new workouts to become habit-forming and for your body to respond with weight loss.

Think Smarter

To ensure a healthy and happy voyage into menopause, your mind needs to be on your side. Be your own best friend by treating yourself with kindness, support, and compassion. Experts also suggest that you keep these thoughts in mind.

Stop trying to be 20. You never will—and never should attempt to—fit into jeans belonging to your slender 20-year-old daughter. Or look like a pencil-thin model from a fashion magazine. The average 40-year-old's body is shaped differently: fuller at the hips, waist, and chest than a younger woman's.

Strive to be fit, not thin. Possessing toned muscles is much healthier than being stick-thin as you approach menopause. The more lean muscle tissue you develop, the more energy you'll have and the quicker your body's metabolism will be. You'll also improve your mood, sleeping habits, balance, and flexibility while reducing your risk for heart disease, diabetes, cancer, and arthritis, adds Dr. Nelson. Not a bad deal.

Ditch the scale. Read your waistline for your best gauge of whether you're gaining or losing weight. "The scale is just a mechanical device and not an evaluation of our health or self-worth," notes Waterhouse. "Women need to take ownership of their bodies and judge how they feel, how their clothes fit, and how they look in the mirror."

Accept a modest weight gain of 3 to 10 pounds between ages 35 and 55 as real, necessary, and inevitable. (That is, as long as you eat a variety of healthy foods and exercise regularly.) This reserve helps fend off osteoporosis and

Your Ally in Menopause

As you enter your forties, your hormone levels begin to shift. Your ovaries—the biggest estrogen producers—start slacking a bit. As your estrogen dips, menopausal symptoms such as hot flashes and migraines may surface. You can minimize these symptoms by using an ally that's ready and willing to help produce estrogen: your fat cells.

Nutritional experts are discovering that if you work with—not against—your "midlife" fat cells, the transition into your menopausal years can be smoother.

When estrogen levels dip, the brain sends a message to activate fat cells. Instead of their usual function as fat-storage facilities, those fat cells have a biological role to produce estrogen. "Fat cells are our menopausal helpers," says Debra Waterhouse, R.D., author of *Outsmarting the Midlife Fat Cell*.

Recruit your 30 billion fat cells to your best advantage by avoiding any quick-loss or starvation diets. Regular exercise and sensible eating are the best ways to make your fat cells "work" for you. "The worst thing you can do during this transitional time is to try a restrictive diet in desperation," cautions Waterhouse. "Yo-yo dieting only gives your fat cells more strength and power. It makes them more stubborn. You only end up gaining more weight."

menopausal symptoms. (Don't forget that weight training can help turn those extra pounds from fat to muscle, which also gives you added energy and strength!)

Focus on accomplishments. Name a perfect person who always does the right thing at the right time. Impossible, yes? So why apply the same sky-high standards to yourself? Set realistic goals for weight management. Celebrate your minor victories and recognize, but don't dwell on, your setbacks as you steadily take steps to eat better and exercise more, says Dr. Nelson.

Empower yourself. Welcome menopause as a time to cater to your needs. Remind yourself that you have the power to affect these transitional years—as well as your weight—positively.

part six

True
Intimacy

6

His and Her
Health

Skyrocketing sales of Viagra have brought out from under the covers the topic of sex in the later years. "Both men and women experience changes related to sexual desire and response as they age," says Judith Seifer, R.N., Ph.D., certified sex therapist in Lewisburg, West Virginia, and past president of the American Association of Sex Educators. "These changes occur not only in their bodies but in their minds as well."

After menopause, a woman's estrogen level plummets, triggering a cascade of events. "One of the first things that happens to women as they make the transition from their forties to their fifties is that they don't lubricate as easily, or as well, when they become sexually aroused," says Dr. Seifer. "This drier, thinner vaginal tissue can make sex uncomfortable.

"The second thing that women notice is that they begin to have difficulty achieving orgasm. I've had women tell me they lose interest in sex because it's too much work. And when they do finally have an orgasm, it's not as intense," Dr. Seifer says.

Another problem is that a lack of estrogen can cause the vagina to shorten and tighten, making intercourse painful. In some women, the pain lasts for days. "A woman may start to complain that after orgasm, her uterus—and sometimes her bladder—goes into spasm. It doesn't take more than a few painful sexual encounters for a woman to start thinking, 'Is a man really worth this? Do I need this?'"

Besides physical changes, some women also notice a decrease in sexual desire. This can also have a biological basis, however. "Some women don't even want to be touched by their partners anymore," explains Dr. Seifer. "What used to feel good feels repulsive now. And many women don't know what's causing this." According to Dr. Seifer, post-menopausal women have less epinephrine and norepinephrine, two hormones that affect the skin's sense of touch. "This has a profound impact on an intimate sexual encounter. The woman doesn't know why she doesn't want her partner of 25 years to keep away from her, and the man thinks she doesn't love him anymore. It can be pretty terrifying for both of them."

By contrast, most men don't lose their sex drives after 50. "Their testosterone levels may go down over time, but it doesn't affect their interest in sex. Their biggest complaint is finding an interested partner," says Dr. Seifer.

How can a woman past menopause enjoy a healthy sex life? Dr. Seifer's advice is pretty simple.

❖ Pay attention to your body and take very good care of it. Consult your health care provider with any questions or concerns. If she doesn't ask you about your sex life, bring up the topic for discussion.
❖ Talk to your doctor about hormone-replacement therapy, including alternative forms of estrogen.
❖ Keep the lines of communication open with your partner. Sit down and talk about your grievances. Try to do everything you can to keep a healthy sex life. The old adage is true—if you don't use it, you'll lose it.

36

Eight Ways to Stress-Proof Your Relationship

Ever start out trying to have a simple chat with your man about rinsing the dishes before putting them in the dishwasher only to find World War III suddenly raging in your breakfast nook? Worse, are you hearing the voice of Psycho Woman from Hell coming out of your mouth?

Unfortunately, it's all too easy for conflicts about who does what in the house to escalate into full-fledged fights. Why? "If there's a major issue, you talk it out," explains professor Catherine Chambliss, Ph.D., an expert on stress and dual-career couples at Ursinus College in Collegeville, Pennsylvania. "But with minor issues, you think, 'Well, it doesn't matter.' Yet over time, resentment about these things builds up." This is why meltdowns happen.

Here are some typical stressful domestic issues and ways to defuse the frustration before you find yourself going nuclear.

Scenario #1: Dinner Daze

You both arrive home after work wiped out and realize the cupboards are bare. You're not in the mood to eat out or to order in the usual greasy fast food. To top it off, he asks, "So, honey, what's for dinner?"

Nuke-him response: Throw briefcase on floor. Roll eyes. Pull trigger. "I am beginning to think this relationship is sponsored by Pizza Hut. Since I know you won't volunteer to make a quick trip to Food Mart, tonight we'll be dining on a lovely condiments-only casserole."

On second thought, try: "Well, there's no food in the house, so let's order in. You choose, just not pizza, okay? And then we should figure out how to deal with this whole dinner thing to make it easier on both of us."

Why? Since no magic grocery fairy is going to swoop down bearing dinner, you have to deal with the current issue—eating—first. (The more famished you get, the nastier the fight.) Over takeout, you can discuss what to do about the lifetime of dinners ahead of you.

Create a fair system to handle grocery shopping, advises Dr. Chambliss. Take turns doing the weekly shopping. Put a list on the fridge with the designated shopper's name on it. The list is sacred. "Each person is responsible for writing down what he or she wants. If something doesn't make it to the list, it's no one's fault and you don't have to feel guilty about it," she adds. If you know it's going to be a bad week at work, plan on going out a few times or agree to forage separately on certain nights.

There may, however, be a larger issue at stake in a dinnertime war—something that has nothing to do with your stomach and everything to do with a tense day at work. "You need 'transition time,'" says Mary Sotile, coauthor with her husband of *Supercouple Syndrome: How Overworked Couples Can Beat Stress Together.* "You probably walk in the door and have kids attached to your jugular." She suggests trying 10 to 20 minutes of something that makes you

Bridge the Language Gap

Does it often seem like you and your man speak different languages? It's sort of true. "Men and women speak the same language—but differently," says Anthony Mulac, Ph.D., communications professor at the University of California, Santa Barbara. Men are more direct, he says, while women tend to favor "uncertainty verbs" ("It seems to be") and other hedges ("It's kind of nice"). So if you want a man to listen, try talking his way.

Men like to: Make references to quantity.
So you say: "It's 50 percent finished."

Men like to: Denote specific locations.
So you say: "The keys are on the left side of the desk."

Men like to: Use directives.
So you say: "Help me clean."

Men like to: Make "I" references.
So you say: "I have a lot of work."

feel good once you get home—try lighting a candle, putting on comfortable clothes, and popping in a favorite CD you haven't listened to in a while.

Scenario #2: Wasted Weekend

You're both so worn out from the week that when the weekend comes, you don't have anything planned; you end up piddling the time away at home or doing errands separately.

Nuke-him response: "Gosh, I remember when you thought I was more interesting than ESPN. Would it help if I wore a jersey and spit a lot?"

On second thought, try: "Let's spend this afternoon [insert one: sitting in the backyard, taking a walk, going for a drive], because I feel like I only get to see you when we're eating or watching *ER*."

Why? Most women suffer from "vital exhaustion," according to Sotile. You've had to organize so many things at work and home that you're sick of making plans. "Decide to meander together, which can mean even just going to the mall," she says. "And don't go anywhere near the washing machine."

Alternately, you could take turns playing social director, advises Lillian Glass, Ph.D., author of *Toxic People*. "I counseled one couple who took turns planning their weekends. He went along to her dog shows, and she went to boxing matches with him. He hated the dog shows, she started enjoying the fights. But the point was they were spending time together instead of fighting about their free time together."

Scenario #3: Bathroom Battle

One bathroom. Two people. One of you is always pounding on the door to push the other one along, and somebody's always late to the office.

Nuke-him response: "What are you doing, shaving one hair at a time? If I wanted to live like this, I'd still share a room with my sister!"

On second thought, try: "I need to get in there in 5 minutes so I'm not late to work. I'll put the coffee on and check the weather and then knock again in 5, okay?"

Why? No matter how good sarcasm feels, it's a no-no, reminds Dr. Glass. The better response highlights the issue of getting to work rather than the competition for sink time. (The coffee offer is just a nice touch that makes the prodding seem, well, less bitchy.)

Why is the bathroom issue such a stressor? Morning is another one of those transitional times of day that create frazzled feelings. But if you have a shower schedule, it can take away some of the blaming. You can say, "I'm counting on the schedule, and I get really frustrated when you don't follow it," instead of the oh-so-tempting, "Late again, nozzlehead!"

Scenario #4: Resident Slob

The house looks like Bruce Willis filmed a chase scene in it. And your man hasn't done any of his negotiated tasks—including cleaning the tub.

Nuke-him response: "Am I to conclude you actually like living in a pig sty? You must, because you never pitch in."

On second thought, try: "Have you noticed what a state our house is in? I thought you were going to tackle the bathroom—or do you want to renegotiate the duty list?"

Why? It's no wonder this issue is stressful. A University of Wisconsin study found that working wives spend an average of 14 hours a week more than their husbands on household tasks—and that's not including child care.

Moreover, universal terms like "always" and "never" take attention away from the cleaning issue and make him feel like his mother is scolding him—not exactly the role you want to appear in. One of the major reasons couples fight about housework, Dr. Chambliss says, is because a woman will complain about the way a man does his household duties. "He'll work less hard if he feels like he's your employee in the housework business." So if the bathroom is his job, let him do it the way he wants to. Maybe he's using the wrong kind of sponge, but don't correct him—it sends the message that the house is your territory, not his.

Also, consider cutting some corners. If you're both spending so much time keeping the house neat that it's causing friction, decide whether having clean windows—or fighting about who was supposed to clean them—is really more important than talking about your next vacation. Better yet, sit down and figure out if you can afford $50 a month for a cleaning service.

Scenario #5: Workaholic's Widow

He's working late—again. You're home wondering whether to eat without him. By the time he does trudge across the threshold, you're wondering what the point is of being married to a workaholic.

Nuke-him response: "If you loved me as much as your damn job . . ." or "I see the meter-reader more often than I see you . . ." or "Are you having an affair with your secretary?"

On second thought, try: "I miss you."

Why? These three little words are infinitely more effective than berating an

Bedtime Battle

While most people (nearly 7 out of 10) prefer to sleep in the same bed with their partners, a study found that a surprising number (32 percent) don't. In fact, women are slightly less likely to want to sleep in tandem than men. Those who prefer to sleep alone are annoyed by irritating nighttime behaviors that keep them awake. Here are the biggest bedtime gripes.

❖ Snoring
❖ Taking up too much room in the bed
❖ Hogging the covers or pillows
❖ Preferring the bedroom too hot or too cold
❖ Tossing and turning too much
❖ Watching TV, listening to the radio, or reading when you want to sleep

already exhausted mate, says Sotile, who admits she used to scream at her husband when he'd call to say he was working late again. "I'd be so mad I'd make his day ten times worse. That's when we agreed I wouldn't blow him out on the phone; we would wait and discuss it when I'd calmed down."

But how do you calm down? Instead of bottling up your rage so you can break it over his head when he gets home, do one of Sotile's transition exercises, such as getting a pair of binoculars and watching the birds outside for 20 minutes or renting a movie on your way home from work. Think of it as "me" time rather than "watching the clock and thinking of heaving it at him" time.

Scenario #6: In-Law Hell

You're having a rare relaxing evening, chatting about your respective days and drinking wine, when his mother calls and you hear him say, "Sure, c'mon over!"

Nuke-him response: "Did you have to invite her over? Now I have to clean the windows so your mother won't give me that Cruella de Vil look again. Oh, no I don't. I forgot: They're still clean—she was here yesterday."

On second thought, try: "Next time, could you tell her to wait an hour? I was really enjoying our quiet time."

Why? It's not a good move to make an issue of his mother's invading your privacy right before she arrives. He'll get offended, she'll sense the stress, and you're sure to wind up in a shouting match within a minute of her departure. Instead, focus on the positive—time with him—and bring up the subject during a less highly charged moment.

"Say, 'We need to figure out a plan for how often your parents are going to come around,'" says Sotile. It probably hasn't occurred to him to make clear boundaries between his relationship with you and his relationship with his family. Only he can establish this, but you can make sure it happens.

Scenario #7: Libido Feud

You had a rough day at work; the kids tried to stay up until midnight; there's a pile of laundry still waiting to be done in the hallway; he nods toward the bedroom, winks, and says, "Hey, honey, wanna . . ."

Nuke-him response: "Why are you blinking? A bit of lint from the dryer? Oh, sorry, it couldn't be that—you didn't have time to help with the laundry while you were listening to me wrangle with the kids, did you?"

On second thought, try: "You know, it's really hard to get in the mood when it's nearly midnight, I'm worn out, and there is a pile of laundry that's not getting any younger. Does that make sense?"

Why? You need to explain that you're not rejecting him because you don't find him attractive; it's just that you can't even think about whether he's attractive when you have so much else stressing you out. But he still may not get it, as Sotile explains: "Many men compartmentalize better than women, so when a man is tired, stressed, angry, or depressed, he can use sex to relax or feel better. Women usually want to have sex only when they're already relaxed or feeling good."

Reach Him with a Love Letter

Instead of simply counting the ways you love him, put them down on paper. A heartfelt note to your man can "strengthen your bond by creating a sense of connectedness," says Sandra Whitefield, a Chicago-based relationship therapist. "Mood-lifting endorphins are released when you receive compliments. And it feels good to give them, too." For a make-him-melt message, Whitefield recommends:

Open up. Begin with an appreciative statement, such as "I love you so much I need to tell you what's in my heart."

Shower him with praise. Write down everything you adore about him. Imagine your partner sitting in front of you. Write down what you love about his physical appearance, character, and actions.

Be true. If you aren't a mushy person, don't be mushy. Simple language and statements will still get your message across and will seem more genuine.

Present unqualified compliments. "I love when you hug me" shouldn't be followed by a negative statement such as "but you do it so seldom."

Add a personal touch. Include a photo of the two of you or a lipstick kiss.

You can try saying, "Let's just cuddle," but you've probably found that to him this is a quaint term for foreplay, so design your strategy to fit what you know about your guy. Why is this a stressful issue for you? Do you put pressure on yourself to do everything, including being a supersexpot? Since saying no can make you feel like a failure, explain to him what turns you on, when it turns you on, and how he can approach the issue in a way that makes you feel aroused—not annoyed.

Scenario #8: Dad Lite

When the kids are acting up, he always waits for you to play bad cop, and then he looks like Super Dad.

Nuke-him response: "You know, you're the father here, not an innocent bystander. I carried the Little Leaguer around for 9 months. Why don't you do a little of the heavy lifting once in a while?"

On second thought, try: "I really think you're a great dad to our kids, but there's one part of the process that really bothers me; I think we need to talk about it."

Why? Many men still have the view that their job is to "help out" with the kids instead of being an equal partner in their care. But in spite of themselves, women often don't want to share this territory with men and send the wrong signals about parenting duties. We want to be Super Mom, so we dub him Deputy Dad, explains Dr. Chambliss. Make sure you're sending him the signal that he's a full partner in the child-rearing enterprise: Keep him informed about things like the kids' schedules, lessons, and car pools—so that he's bringing the cookies for the school play instead of just showing up when you tell him to. By asking his opinion, you engage him in a discussion that's a "we" issue instead of "me versus you." Then when you talk about sharing the discipline duties, he may feel more open to taking on responsibility.

Is Your Sex Life Good Enough?

37

Sarah, happily coupled for several years, is idly reading a magazine sex survey. Her eyes land on the "frequency of intercourse" section, where she learns that two-thirds of all couples surveyed have intercourse twice as often as she and Robert do.

Reading the "frequency of multiple orgasms" section, she's horrified to discover that many women actually have multiple orgasms, never mind how often. Next she uncovers that a healthy percentage of men truly enjoy giving oral sex, that many can wait a full hour before coming, and that some are able to guarantee simultaneous orgasms.

Since everyone seems to be having more, better, kinkier, funkier, longer-lasting sex than she has with Robert, she wonders about the future of their twice-a-month so-called sex life. If the super-lovers in this survey are "normal," she and Robert are in a sexual coma. Will they ever awaken?

What Is "Normal" Sexual Activity?

Sarah is not alone. Most women in long-term relationships inevitably reach a point where they ask, "Is our sex life normal?" (Or the variations, "Am I normal?" or "Is he normal?") The question usually arises just as the passion they started out with mellows sweetly into something more comfortable and pre-

How to Boost Intimacy

The most soulful thing you can do during sex is to look at your husband. If making love in broad daylight is not your thing, at least try to leave on enough light so you can actually see each other.

According to David Schnarch, Ph.D., author of *Passionate Marriage*, "eyes-open sex" is the key to increasing intimacy. The aim isn't to check out each other's bodies, but rather to look deep into your partner's eyes—and soul. If you're not at this point yet, you're not alone. Only about 30 percent of couples have sex with their eyes open, and even fewer have eyes-open orgasms.

dictable. No matter that their mothers, aunts, best friends, and every expert in town warned of passion's fragility. When it actually goes into hiding (sometimes for months), all the consolation in the world cannot make up for the lack of earth-shattering sex.

When Shelley, 32, first noticed a slight decrease in desire for her husband, Bill, she chalked it up to their busy work schedules. "Most nights we have Chinese food in bed and look over our mutual funds and play with our puppy," she says. "And then we go to sleep." It was only when she awoke one morning and wondered idly if she could still flex her Kegel muscles that she gave her sex life a second thought.

Actually, that's not quite true. She had given it a thought a few weeks before, when she and Bill were at a party and suddenly this couple—let's call them Fred and Ginger—arrived looking tousled, flushed, and gorgeous in a clearly postcoital way. "While we were all standing around the kitchen checking the doneness of the roast beef," Shelley says, "they were eyeing each other with that 'let's get outta here and back into the sack' look. Dinner was clearly the last thing on their minds."

"I Want What She's Having"

For Shelley, couple envy had reared its little green-eyed head. Like survey reading, couple envy is usually an unpleasant but short-lived experience, one that leaves you a little agitated or just humbled but rarely so upset you can't get a grip. If the envy leaves you feeling nauseated, though, something is up, and you should ask yourself a few questions.

What, specifically, do you find yourself jealously comparing—how tender another man is? How wild or spontaneous he appears? How close that couple seems? What needs are not being met that make you feel so wistful, so wishful? Do you only occasionally feel this way—or always? Do you sometimes have good sex—or never? What has eluded you that you sense another couple possesses? What's your fantasy about the two of them? (After all, you're the writer, director, and producer of the fantasy; they're the actors.)

That couple you're envious of is interesting, not for what they have (since we'll never truly know what goes on behind their tousled facade) but for the needs they expose in you. Take Fred and Ginger, for instance: What was so awesome?

For Shelley it was their wildness, their obvious chemistry—a chemistry she'd never had with anyone in her whole life. But another woman at the same party might have envied their ease, the sense of openness between them. Another might have been struck by the sweet and constant attention they paid to each other. We all project onto couples like Fred and Ginger precisely what we feel our own personalities, lovers, or relationships lack.

Is the Perfect Sex Life Possible?

Once you figure out what's missing, decide if it's something truly crucial to your happiness, without which you'll feel increasingly deprived, or a more idle longing. We all, at some points in our lives, yearn for more than what we have— the road not taken, the love we lost, the personality that is just not his or ours.

If what you crave turns out to be an idealized, perfect sex life, maybe you're looking for something that doesn't exist. ("If sex is such a natural phenomenon, how come there are so many books on how-to?" Bette Midler once wisely observed.) The very qualities that assure the success of tender, long-term love are those that offset passion. Sociologist Pepper Schwartz, Ph.D., has found that lust requires both imbalance and tension to stay at the peak level. In her study of the way love works in deeply satisfying, egalitarian partnerships, Dr. Schwartz found a consistent lessening of passion over time. Why? Because, she says, "Peers operate under conditions of equity and equality, and because

Will Your Happiness Last?

To tell if you've found true, long-lasting love, answer the following questions, says Peggy Penn, a senior faculty member at the Ackerman Institute for the Family in New York City.

Do you know truly intimate things about each other? You and your partner should be able to express your secret hopes and dreams without fear of being judged.

Do you have shared life goals? True compatibility arises when you have a shared commitment to long-term goals.

Do you problem-solve and fight fair? If so, you discuss differences and understand the importance of compromise.

this reduces anger and insecurity, some passion is sacrificed as well." The couples she studied were more than willing, however, to give up fleeting bedroom highs for long-lasting, everyday happiness.

Getting Real

Shell-shocked after reading her sex survey, Sarah submitted to some brutal self-examination and remembered that she'd felt this same dissatisfaction, this same sense that wild passion had eluded her, in all of her serious, long-term relationships. "After about a year, I'd get tired of the day-to-day maintenance and start craving that emotional high that only comes at the beginning. I realized it's normal to want that, but it's not normal to keep leaving solid relationships, as I'd done several times, just for lust." She figured out the truth about what she wanted and the likelihood of getting it elsewhere (for very long)—and she stayed where she was.

Beware of "Intimacy Enhancer" Surgery

H E A L T H F L A S H

Lasers are being put to use in a controversial below-the-belt laser procedure purported to improve a woman's sex life. To decrease the vaginal diameter, practitioners use a laser to make incisions in the top and bottom of the vaginal canal. They overlap the muscles and remove excess surface tissue before stitching it all into place. (This is similar to an operation designed to relieve the leaking of urine from the bladders of elderly women.)

Neither the American College of Obstetricians and Gynecologists nor the Society of Gynecologic Surgeons endorses this procedure. Women concerned about sagging vaginal muscles after pregnancy can often get excellent results by performing Kegels, simple "clench and release" exercises targeting the pubococcygeus muscle that lies at the base of the pelvis.

"There's a considerable risk associated with surgery that tightens the vagina," says Christie Timmons, M.D., educational chairperson for the Society of Gynecologic Surgeons. "The tissue around the vagina can be scarred to the point where the woman may not be able to have sex or may even have extreme difficulty urinating."

In addition, the laser can burn the labia, causing a loss of sensation, warns Malcolm Lesavoy, M.D., chief of plastic surgery at Harbor-UCLA Medical Center.

We all judge ourselves against other people. But it's very hard to determine what's "normal" since the truth about all of our sex lives is so complicated, so deeply hidden. The people who are willing to talk about sex aren't necessarily reliable sources. Take Virginia. She rhapsodized about her joyous, over-the-moon sex life with Bob, the movie-producer boyfriend she adored. When her relationship ended abruptly, she explained it with a shrug and a thumbs-down gesture. "The sex just went," she said.

Went where? What could fuel such passion and then dissipate so quickly? We'll never get the real answers, of course. And that's the point. Others' sex lives may hold endless fascination, but we'll never know a thing about them.

The Pleasure of "Good-Enough" Sex

Like aiming for the perfect body or the perfect diet, aiming for the perfect sex life is just setting yourself up for disappointment. Better to wish for something you might actually get. British pediatrician and psychoanalyst D.W. Winnicott taught us all a thing or two when, more than 30 years ago, he introduced the idea of the "good-enough" mother, taking the pressure off anxious women who were trying to be perfect. If we follow his lead, we'll achieve something similar in our love lives: good-enough sex.

Such modified rapture may at first sound vaguely un-American. But it's not about settling for less; it's about appreciating what our bodies and psyches already deliver. If we relax and celebrate our flawed, prosaic, sometimes unspecial but often satisfying sex lives, we do two healthy things. One, we get real. And two, we make hotter sex optional, not mandatory, a mutual decision made when we're both ready to go for it, with none of the pressure and fear of disappointment that can so easily derail the pursuit of pleasure. All in all, the imperfect sex we most often have might be both normal and "good enough."

38

How Do You Define Infidelity?

I rene is a happily married 29-year-old woman who was having lunch with her old boyfriend Tom. As Tom was getting up to leave, he planted a kiss on Irene's lips that lasted an entire minute and left her not only stunned but electrified with pleasure. That was 2 weeks ago, and she still doesn't know whether to be horrified at her behavior ("Should I have been indignant?") or thrilled at the unexpected intensity of this blast from the past.

Is Our Definition of Infidelity Too Narrow?

Irene feels guilty—and also confused. "How do you define infidelity, really?" she wonders. She's finding that after 5 years of marriage, what used to be a clear-cut concept ("it meant sleeping with someone other than your mate—period") is increasingly open to debate. Perhaps it's not a single act but a whole series of them, she thinks; a bevy of behaviors rather than an isolated cataclysmic one. She's beginning to wonder whether, given longer life spans and increased sophistication, she should loosen her definition of infidelity a little. By the time she's in her early seventies, she argues, "I'll have been married half a century!"

On the other hand, Alison, a 31-year-old investment banker newly married to Pete, thinks we should tighten up, not loosen, the definition. "The real treachery occurs way before extramarital sex does," she says. "It starts not with the sex but the secrecy." She knows: She found out that Pete was having secret lunches with someone else at work. Even though the meetings were chaste and had begun long before Pete and Alison married, she considered the continuation of those lunches a serious betrayal. The fact that sex wasn't involved didn't help, since she felt Pete was nevertheless siphoning off an intensity that should have been reserved exclusively for her—and keeping it under wraps besides.

Debra, 30, not yet married but pledged to sexual exclusivity with her long-standing boyfriend, looks back wistfully on her dating-around days and admits to looking ahead with some trepidation to what she calls protracted, lifelong fidelity. She (along with the rest of the country) finds herself suddenly obsessed with definitions of faithlessness, of where to draw the line. Is secrecy part of the definition of adultery? Or is it the act of turning the twosome into a triangle? Is it when you confide in someone who knows you less well (and sympathizes with you more) than your partner? Is it okay to confide in a third party once? How about twice? And while we're at it, is it okay to flirt along the way?

What Matters More Than Sex

Trying to define infidelity according to the letter of the law is impossible, since laws themselves differ dramatically. In Jewish law, for instance, a married woman is guilty of adultery if she has sexual intercourse with any male other than her husband, while a married man is guilty of adultery only if he has intercourse with another man's wife. (The law considers the man's crime to be not an emotional one against his wife but a property crime against another man.) Other laws still allow, even demand, death for an unfaithful wife but assume a man's sexual wanderings to be simply what he's entitled to—married or not.

Even those of us who agree that infidelity is easy to define—it's sex with someone other than your partner, plain and simple—can go to town over the whole question of what, exactly, constitutes the act. Does petting while clothed count? Oral sex? Is sex, finally, even the point?

Some couples don't think so. At 31, Joanne, a travel agent married for 10 years, and her husband, Robert, a pilot, have devised unconventional marital rules for themselves. "We're more interested in our emotional well-being over the very long haul than in occasional lapses in sexual fidelity," she says. "We married young and traveled constantly. We decided then that a one-night stand on a business trip is permissible as long as it's neither discussed nor pursued beyond that one encounter," she says. Interestingly, while their pact began as a temporary, negotiable agreement, it remains intact today, "maybe because we don't travel all that much anymore," Joanne says dryly.

Some couples are even more unconventional, permitting their partners same-sex sexual involvements only or opposite-sex options with very precise

Infidelity: What the Numbers Say

- ❖ Percentage of men who think cheating is wrong: 91
- ❖ Of those men, percentage who have cheated: 20
- ❖ Percentage of men who think cheating is not wrong: 2
- ❖ Of those men, percentage who have cheated: 69
- ❖ Overall percentage of men who have cheated: 23
- ❖ Overall percentage of women who have cheated: 12
- ❖ Percentage of men who believe they'll have an affair in the coming year: 2
- ❖ Percentage of men who have had an affair in the past year: 4
- ❖ Percentage of women who believe they'll have an affair in the coming year: 4
- ❖ Percentage of women who have had an affair in the past year: 2
- ❖ Decade of life in which men are most likely to cheat: Thirties
- ❖ Decade of life in which women are most likely to cheat: Twenties
- ❖ Estimated number of women who say they would divorce their husbands if he flirted with another woman: 1 in 40
- ❖ Estimated number of women who say they would divorce their husbands if he kissed another woman: 1 in 4
- ❖ Estimated number of women who say they would divorce their husbands if he had a one-night stand with another woman: 1 in 2
- ❖ Estimated number of women who say they would divorce their husbands if he had a serious affair with another woman: 2 in 3
- ❖ Percentage of betrayed partners who knew about the affair at the time: 89
- ❖ Percentage of couples who divorce after an affair (even with counseling): 34
- ❖ Percentage of couples who preserve their marriage after an affair: 66
- ❖ Of those, percentage who later describe the marriage as unhappy or empty: 78
- ❖ Of men who cheated, percentage who were motivated by sexual excitement: 75
- ❖ Percentage of women who were motivated by sexual excitement: 53
- ❖ Percentage of men and women who were motivated by career advancement: 5
- ❖ Percentage of men who say they fell in love: 43
- ❖ Percentage of women who say they fell in love: 77

parameters. Marianne and Hal, for instance, both 37 and married 9 years, give each other "off" days once every 5 years. "This means," Marianne says, "that we go off on our own, overnight, no questions asked. It's a serious attempt to figure out a way of staying together forever and also having time apart. If an occasional lapse in sexual exclusivity is what we need to spend the next 30 or 40 years happily together, well, so be it."

Hal nods. "We know how weird our arrangement sounds to some people—like, 'Oh, they're the couple who take separate vacations . . . heh, heh, heh!' But we don't see it as a chance for promiscuity, and we certainly don't preach our views to anyone else. We've found that creating an actual ritual for an occasional indiscretion gives us some control over what happens."

On the other hand, some couples try to ensure relationship longevity by devising rules every bit as strict as Marianne and Hal's are flexible. "I was taught that lust itself, even in the imagination, is a sin," 38-year-old Sheila announces. "I kept fantasizing about my old boyfriend long after I married Alan, and I spent 2 years feeling guilty." It was Alan who finally talked her out of her misery, convincing her that fantasy had nothing to do with her love for him and that she had done nothing wrong.

A Blueprint for Fidelity

These couples are each struggling in their own ways to deal with a fact of life as old and as powerful as the institution of marriage itself: adultery. They're looking at the country's astronomical divorce rate—the highest on the planet—and devising interesting new ways to defy it. They're trying to draw their own sexual boundaries, alert to the spirit of fidelity's synonyms—allegiance, devotion, loyalty, faithfulness, honesty, integrity. They're aware that they must make their own rules and that no one else has the right to do that for them. "Hey, we all know what we should do, right?" Alison says. "We should be perfectly, undyingly sexually exclusive. But the history of the Western world, not to mention the body of Western literature, is filled with human beings who can't always do what they should do." So instead of looking at "shoulds," these couples are looking at reality and at what they think will give them the best chance for the long marriages they crave.

However you define it, fidelity is a choice made by both of you—and one of you is unfaithful when you renege on that choice without telling the other. The trick is to be with someone who makes the same choice, who views keeping the faith in the same way and with the same tenacity you do. To some, infidelity is less about a single indiscretion (like Irene's minute-long kiss) than a decision, conscious or not, to create a barrier between you and your partner;

it's a pattern of pulling away, of closing off channels of communication, be they sexual, verbal, emotional, or spiritual.

The motives behind the decision to be unfaithful are often psychologically complex and highly individual; they're rarely just a sign of faulty moral values. Anyone trying to come up with a single definition of infidelity will inevitably fail for the simple reason that, as novelist George Eliot put it long ago, we have no master key to fit all cases. Like love, which also eludes precise definition, fidelity is vaster than the customs governing it. Many couples are weary of probing the many ways trust can be eroded (for example, whether there was penetration, and if there wasn't, whether we can still call it adultery). Instead of dissecting the frailties that could or should lead to a breakup, they want to grasp the humanity that can keep them together. Most of all, couples feel that however unusual their sex lives, they're no one's business but their own.

Viagra One Year Later: Promise or Problem?

Viagra, the new oral medication for treating impotence, has raised more than the obvious. Many people have lots of questions—from how it's used and how it affects a couple's relationship to whether women can benefit from it. So here are the facts about what Viagra can do and what it can't.

Viagra (*sildenafil citrate*) was originally developed to treat angina, or chest pain, by increasing blood flow to the heart. While studies showed it wasn't very effective for angina, study participants noticed that blood flow to the penis improved. Men who had not been able to have an erection were suddenly able to.

Viagra increases the penis's response to sexual stimulation by enhancing the effect of certain chemical messengers that allow the smooth muscle of the penis to relax and stay relaxed, thereby increasing its blood flow. Viagra doesn't create sexual desire or produce an erection on its own, though. You and your partner need to do that the old-fashioned way: through sexual stimulation and arousal.

Who Can Benefit from Viagra

In clinical studies, Viagra was most effective in men with impotence due to physical or psychological reasons: hypertension, heart disease, diabetes,

How to Prevent Second-Honeymoon Cystitis

Although Viagra can reignite a dormant love life (if erectile dysfunction has been the cause), many older women are experiencing the kind of burning discomfort once considered a young woman's problem: "honeymoon cystitis," or urinary tract infections (UTIs) brought on by the friction of sexual intercourse.

The connection came to light when three doctors in Covington, Georgia, noticed a rise in UTI complaints among women patients between the ages of 55 and 75. "We checked our records and found that every one of their spouses had been given a prescription for Viagra," says Henry Patton, M.D., one of the physicians. "Out of 100 men who got Viagra, 15 of their wives came to us with cystitis." Since their observation was published in a medical journal, they've heard from other doctors—and women with UTIs—across the country who've also noted this side effect.

The symptoms. A frequent urge to urinate; burning pain and just a scant trickle when you do; passing blood with the urine.

The cause. Friction during lovemaking can nudge ever-present bacteria into the opening of a woman's urethra. From there, it's just a short distance to the bladder, where infection can easily develop.

Older women may be even more susceptible because they're likely to produce less vaginal lubrication.

What you can do. Drink six to eight 8-ounce glasses of water daily (even some just a few minutes before making love). Staying hydrated increases urine flow, which flushes harmful bacteria from your bladder. Also, be sure to empty your bladder immediately after sex.

If you do get a UTI. See your doctor—especially if you experience chills, nausea, vomiting, or lower-back pain. You may need an antibiotic to prevent kidney problems. Also, abstain from intercourse when UTI symptoms are present to prevent the infection from getting worse, Dr. Patton advises.

Cranberry or blueberry juice can help prevent the bacteria that cause urinary tract infections from sticking to the walls of the bladder. Since cranberry juice can be an irritant for some women, you may want to dilute it with a little water.

What your partner can do. A man should mention the sex-UTI connection to his partner, so she can take preventive steps. This is both partners' responsibility.

HEALTH FLASH

spinal cord injury, treatment of prostate cancer, depression, or anxiety. About 70 percent of men with these problems will benefit from the drug. Since some nerve function and blood flow to the penis are necessary for Viagra to work, men with no erectile function due to severe diabetes or vascular disease won't have as much success.

If a man takes Viagra hoping it will boost his already active sex life or prevent occasional performance anxiety, he'll be disappointed. There's no scientific evidence that it will improve the sexual performance of men who do not have erectile dysfunction. Nor should Viagra be taken in the hopes of preventing dysfunction in the future. Viagra is only indicated for men who consistently are unable to attain and/or maintain erections.

How to Use It

Stanton Honig, M.D., assistant clinical professor of urology at the University of Connecticut School of Medicine in Farmington and staff urologist at Yale University School of Medicine, advises his patients to take Viagra 1 hour before beginning sexual activity to allow time for it to be absorbed; its effects can last for up to 4 hours. He starts them on the standard dose of 50 milligrams. If a man doesn't respond on this dose, Dr. Honig increases it to 100 milligrams, which is the maximum dose recommended. If the patient experiences side effects, Dr. Honig reduces the dose to 25 milligrams. He adds that you should not exceed one pill a day regardless of the dose because that is the frequency used in studies of safety and effectiveness. The price is about $10 a pill, and some insurance companies either won't pay or limit pay to a certain number of pills a month. About 40 percent of prescriptions are covered by insurance.

Viagra's Side Effects

The most common side effects are headache (16 percent), flushing of the face (10 percent), indigestion (7 percent), and visual disturbances such as blurred vision or a blue halo effect (3 percent), reports Dr. Honig, who specializes in erectile dysfunction and male infertility. In general, the higher your dose, the more likely you are to experience side effects.

If you take nitroglycerin or other nitrates for angina or chest pain caused by heart disease, you should never take Viagra. Combining Viagra with these drugs can cause life-threatening low blood pressure. In fact, the American College of Cardiology and the American Heart Association have developed recommendations for physicians for prescribing Viagra to people with certain heart conditions.

What about Safety?

At least 69 men in the United States have died after having taken Viagra, according to the Food and Drug Administration (FDA). Both the FDA and Pfizer, the pharmaceutical company that makes the drug, said the men who died also had taken nitroglycerin or a nitrate medication or had serious cardiovascular problems that made the physical exertion of sexual activity dangerous. That's why it's so important for you to have a complete physical exam by your doctor before taking Viagra.

Viagra for Women?

Most experts say that for premenopausal women, using the drug even once is not a good idea. Since Viagra has never been studied in premenopausal women, there are concerns about its long-term effects. And no one knows the drug's impact on a woman's fertility or whether it causes birth defects. In fact, at this point there are no data to support its use by any woman. Yet the unknowns haven't stopped some doctors from prescribing Viagra for women, a practice that's legal once a drug is approved for any use by the FDA. Other women simply borrow their partners' medication, in hopes of steamier sexual experiences.

But Viagra isn't a guaranteed orgasm or even an aphrodisiac. It won't fire up a libido that has been dampened by oral contraceptives or antidepressants. "Viagra simply promotes blood flow to the genitals," says urologist John Mulhall, M.D., director of the Center for Male Sexual Health at Loyola University Medical Center in Maywood, Illinois. This means that it may help women who have difficulty with vaginal lubrication, clitoral swelling, or arousal problems.

At this point, some doctors, including Dr. Mulhall, prescribe Viagra only for women who have been through age- or surgery-induced menopause or who otherwise aren't able to have children. For now, younger women with sexual problems should seek out safer ways to increase their satisfaction. Some strategies:

❖ For vaginal dryness, lubricants such as Astroglide or Replens can help make intercourse more comfortable.

❖ If your libido has been quelled by the Pill, ask your doctor about switching to a different formulation.

❖ Antidepressants such as Prozac and Zoloft (the selective serotonin reuptake inhibitors, or SSRIs) can make orgasm elusive; if that's the case, consider the antidepressant Wellbutrin. Besides relieving the blues, it seems to jump-start the sex drive.

❖ Have your hormone levels checked. If low testosterone is behind dwindling desire, taking an oral form of the hormone can help. But keep in

No Safe Herbal Viagra Yet

Men continue to ask if there is a safe, effective, and inexpensive herbal remedy for impotence. "Probably not," says Varro E. Tyler, Sc.D., Ph.D., dean emeritus of the Purdue University School of Pharmacy and Pharmacal Sciences in West Lafayette, Indiana, "although one herb appears to be promising, and one is dangerous."

The promising herb for treating impotence is the multifaceted herb ginkgo. There has been evidence to suggest that ginkgo can put back the zing in the sex lives of men whose erections are affected by taking antidepressants. Though that preliminary study hasn't been followed up, you may want to try ginkgo for this troubling condition, says Dr. Tyler.

Yohimbe has some anti-impotence activity. Its active alkaloid, yohimbine, is currently available in this country as a prescription drug for erectile difficulties. The German Commission E (the world's leading authority on herbs) failed to approve yohimbe as a drug, however, because its use involves the risk of tremors, sleeplessness, high blood pressure, and rapid heartbeat, among other undesirable effects.

mind that the treatment can cause unpleasant side effects such as weight gain, hair growth, and deepening of the voice, so be sure you're monitored by a doctor.

❖ Stress, relationship ups and downs, or a deadline crunch at the office can all trigger a sexual slump, but if problems in the bedroom persist, some rest and a course of counseling (sexual or otherwise) can go a long way toward restoring the pleasure you've lost.

Viagra's Effect on Your Relationship

Most couples will find that being able to resume sexual intimacy strengthens their relationship, says Bonnie Saks, M.D., clinical associate professor of psychiatry at the University of South Florida in Tampa. Some, however, may find that it will force them to face deeper relationship issues that they were comfortably able to ignore when they weren't having sex.

A woman may not be very enthusiastic about the renewed sexual capabilities and interest of her partner. She may not want to reestablish sexual intimacy; it can be awkward or embarrassing. Further, she may be unprepared for any new sexual demands or may not be sexually attracted to her partner anymore.

Some couples may find that talking to a physician or counselor about their expectations will help avoid disappointment and frustration.

part seven

Inner Calm

7

His and Her
Health

Being a woman today means living in a pressure cooker, and a recent study proves it. Researchers in Canada had nearly 200 women wear blood pressure monitors for 24 hours. The women held white-collar, full-time positions, and about half had children. The researchers found that the combination of high job stress and many family responsibilities caused the women's blood pressures to rise as much as 11 points—and their elevated blood pressures remained high after they got home. This contrasts with other research that showed men's blood pressures went back down after work.

"The increase was present through work, evening, and night, suggesting a persistent effect beyond the work setting," says lead researcher Chantal Brisson, Ph.D., epidemiologist in the social and preventive medicine department at Laval University in Quebec. In other words, the women felt the sum total of both work and home stress, while the men felt the effects of work stress only.

"Stress is the pressure to produce," says Rosemary T. Bowes, Ph.D., a psychologist in Washington, D.C., who specializes in stress management, especially for dual-career couples. "Our earliest ancestors used stress, in the form of fight or flight, to survive. Today, we're not fighting tigers, we're fighting paper tigers."

Women can lessen their levels of stress by getting their husbands to help with household responsibilities, says Dr. Bowes, who's also a specialty advisor for the National Women's Health Resource Center in Washington, D.C. "Men can do all the things we can—wash dishes, help the kids with their homework. We learned how, so can they. What women need to realize is that men are going to do those tasks in their own ways. Women have to learn to accept that."

To lighten your load, follow these tips from Dr. Bowes.

❖ Sit down with your mate and tell him you're feeling stressed out. Ask him what he would be most comfortable doing regularly, then teach him how. Keep open the lines of communication and work together on solving the problem. Just make sure you end up delegating some of your responsibilities.

❖ Bring your husband into the housekeeping, child-rearing picture early on. For example, teach him how to give your baby a bath. Don't wait until your child is off to school and expect your mate to know how to take care of kids.

❖ For household chores, assign tasks and accept the way your husband or child takes care of them. For example, if you ask your husband to wash the dishes, don't be upset if he just places them in the rack and doesn't dry them right away.

40

No More Bad Days— Ever

We all have days when everything goes radically wrong. More elusive are those delicious days when everything goes right: Lights turn green, you finish your sales report early, and just before lunch your best friend calls to say there's a 50-percent-off sale at your favorite shoe store. Score! It all feels effortless—and so random.

Who knows what makes one day fall into place and another fall apart? Experts say they've solved the mystery. "Too often when we think, 'That was a fantastic day,' we assume it happened by chance," says psychologist Shane Murphy, Ph.D., president of Gold Medal Consultants in Monroe, Connecticut, and author of *The Achievement Zone: Eight Skills for Winning All the Time, from the Playing Field to the Boardroom*. But if you think that, you don't give yourself enough credit. "In fact, great days are often the result of good preparation," says Dr. Murphy.

A score of specialists on physical and mental health back him up: It's less that bad days are a cacophony of whatever you did wrong than that great days are a symphony of dozens of things you did right. The trick is figuring out those "right" things so you can do them regularly. This is life we're talking about; you can't control everything. But follow these steps and you'll up the ratio of good days to bad or turn around a morning that seems to be headed south.

Get More from Your Night's Sleep

Rest contributes enormously to our overall sense of well-being, optimism, and energy, says sleep expert Nigel Ball, Ph.D., director of the Sleep Disorders Center at the Virginia Mason Medical Center in Seattle. But most of us don't reap the maximum benefits, because a satisfying snooze isn't something you can pull off just by closing your eyes. Following are four keys suggested by Dr. Ball for high-quality shut-eye.

❖ Unwind in advance. Earlier in the evening, spend 5 to 10 minutes writing down everything you have to get done the next day. You'll exorcise all those gotta-remember demons that can make you toss and turn.

❖ Make your bedroom a no-stress zone. Remove anything distracting, like unpaid bills or the TV. "Your brain is like an engine; it needs to cool down before you can truly relax," explains Dr. Ball.

❖ Improve sleep conditions. Do you need water by the bed? A new pillow? "It's amazing how many people tell me they don't sleep well because there's light coming in through their windows—and yet they don't put up curtains," Dr. Ball says.

Simple Suggestions for Sounder Sleep

To get more quality Zzzs, try these suggestions.

Soothe yourself. If you're having trouble falling asleep, do what 111 patients did in a study conducted at Yale-New Haven Hospital in Connecticut. The group listened to relaxing tapes (classical music or nature sounds), drank a warm beverage (milk or herbal tea, no caffeine), or had a back rub (5 minutes of slow massage) prior to sleep. This approach reduced the use of sleep medications in that section of the hospital by more than 20 percent.

"Further, the more nondrug methods tried of the three offered, the better their quality of sleep," says Lorraine Mion, R.N., Ph.D., co-investigator of the study.

Stay cool. It's nice to be cozy, but one blanket too many or a thermostat set too high could rob you of deep sleep. "Your body temperature needs to drop at night, and too many covers can inhibit this," says John Herman, Ph.D., professor of psychiatry at the University of Texas Southwestern Medical Center in Dallas.

If you make it tough to cool down, your sleep won't be as deep or as restful. If you're getting plenty of sleep but don't feel rested, try making things a little less toasty. (Everyone is different, so it may take a few nights of experimenting to find a setup that's cooler, yet comfortable.)

❖ Shift your bedtime. Making it earlier or later could give you optimal rest. "Most people don't need a major sleep adjustment to feel more energetic," notes Dr. Ball. "They just need to tweak their total time by 30 minutes to an hour."

Slow Down Your Morning

If your typical morning goes by in a blur, you're getting off to a harried start. A calmer tempo and a few strategic morning pleasures will help you approach the day with confidence and self-possession.

Number one: Don't hit the snooze button! "If you set your whole schedule back 10 to 15 minutes, you wake up panicked and rushed—the exact opposite of the frame of mind you want," says Dr. Ball.

Kathy Cheun, a commercial producer in San Francisco, says she avoids the snooze temptation by placing her alarm clock out of arm's reach. "As long as I have to get up to turn it off, I'm halfway to the shower—and then I'm fine," she says.

Once you're up, think of your morning as time of your own, not just 2 hours you stumble through on your way to work. Tackle little tasks—like ironing a blouse or getting your briefcase packed and ready—the night before, suggests Dr. Ball. "The extra 10 minutes you don't have to spend on tasks starts your day with a sense of relaxation and freedom."

Then husband that sense of serenity: If reading the paper feels like a chore, put it off until later in the day. Cultivate pockets of pleasure, from a cup of lav-

Take a Few Deep Breaths

If you're going to do one positive thing for yourself during your day, says Christiane Northrup, M.D., author of *Women's Bodies, Women's Wisdom*, a round of several truly deep breaths is the way to go.

"Breathe fully, through your nose and down into your stomach, so you aerate the base of your lungs," says Dr. Northrup, who is also assistant clinical professor of obstetrics/gynecology at the University of Vermont College of Medicine in Burlington. "Most women only breathe into the upper third of their lungs." Those short breaths trigger the fight-or-flight response of the nervous system, while deep breathing sends soothing messages throughout your body.

Visualization can help. Think of a square and imagine each breath traveling up the left side, then over the top, down the right, and across the bottom. The goal is to make your inhalations and exhalations the same length.

Practice Saying No

Any perfect day will have to involve a few judicious nos—they enable you to turn down what you cannot reasonably handle. "Think of 'no' not as a rejection, which is how women often view it, but as a commitment," suggests Julia Smith, M.D., medical director of the personal health improvement program at the Virginia Mason Medical Center in Seattle. In essence, by not making promises you can't keep, you commit to keeping the promises you do make. "By saying no, you let the other person know you are taking his or her request seriously—it's not going straight to the bottom of your in box."

ishly scented tea to luxurious shower products made with herbs or essential oils. (Bergamot is the latest botanical to be touted for its energizing properties.) Kate Lipson, a Boston lawyer, keeps a space heater in her bathroom. "I step out of the shower and feel as if I'm in my own private sauna," she says.

Boost Your Emotional Immune System

On a good day, the same number of frustrations and irritations arise as on any other day—you just handle them differently. "If you wake up in a really good mood, and then your stocking rips, you just shrug it off and put on another pair," says Steven Stosny, Ph.D., a psychotherapist in Washington, D.C.

The key is to adopt that same no-sweat attitude the rest of the time, whether the problem is a ripped stocking, traffic jam, work deadline, or day care snafu.

Pay attention to your morning programming. "If you wake up feeling that the day will be a nightmare, your brain will access its 'horrible day' files," says Dr. Stosny. "As long as you are in that mindset, finding solutions to the problems that arise will be like looking for a summer dress in a closet full of sweaters."

Stop the downward spiral by reminding yourself that a bad mood doesn't make a bad day—just as a long line at the coffee shop when you're already running late is not a sign that your entire morning is fated to go badly. When you give yourself those negative messages, you put yourself into what Dr. Stosny calls a weak mode of self. No matter what happens, you focus on damages, defects, and failures.

Instead, Dr. Stosny says, respond to setbacks by concentrating on how you met similar challenges in the past. "Once you're engaged in finding a solution, you switch into a competent mode, and things go well because you are making them go well." (For extra insurance, keep a spare pair of hose in your desk drawer.)

Just Add Water

Drinking more water throughout the day is one of the easiest ways to boost both mood and motivation. "Most Americans are marginally dehydrated," says Felicia Busch, R.D., spokesperson for the American Dietetic Association. "Some of the symptoms include loss of concentration, irritation, fatigue—a lot of little things that can make your day go badly."

Unfortunately, water often loses out to coffee, tea, or soda because people don't like the taste, Busch says. She suggests making up a Thermos of decaffeinated herbal tea or adding slices of lemon, lime, orange, "or a splash of fruit juice to your water—anything that makes it more appealing."

Pace Yourself for Productivity

Even the best mood comes under fire the minute you set foot in the office. How do you maintain that I'm-on-top-of-it feeling? Put off the thousands of little things that are clamoring for attention—your expenses, that messy pile of correspondence—and tackle big projects first, so you hit the afternoon with a sense of accomplishment and momentum.

Dr. Murphy also stresses the importance of distinguishing between what's urgent and what's important. "Urgent things are external, like answering your

Write Off the Blues

Have you ever spent hours writing a letter you never sent—but just writing it seemed to make you feel better? That instinct to write is a healthy one, according to two recent studies. Researchers at Saint Joseph's University in Philadelphia showed that when students wrote in journals about stressful events, they felt they gained more control over them. As a result, they experienced fewer medical problems.

The participants who showed the greatest improvement engaged in what researchers call self-regulatory writing: Not only did they pour out their problems, but they also came up with a list of three ways to cope.

A separate study led by psychologist James Pennebaker, Ph.D., at the University of Texas at Dallas, yielded similar findings. Students who were instructed to write about past traumas reported fewer doctor visits than those who wrote about more frivolous affairs.

Grab a pen and paper (or your trusty laptop) and go to work. If you need help getting started, check out these books on writing: *The Artist's Way at Work: Riding the Dragon* by Julia Cameron with Mark Bryan and *Bird by Bird: Some Instructions on Writing and Life* by Anne Lamott.

boss's e-mail. What's important is something you decide is a priority based on personal goals."

The key is to give time to what's important without neglecting what's urgent. If you have a presentation due that could land you a promotion, spend 2 hours of your morning on that. But answer your boss's e-mail quickly before you get started and use the natural lulls of the day—say, the 30 minutes between working on your presentation and a lunchtime meeting—to catch up on other business.

Make Busywork Meaningful

What is it that makes work such a pleasure on certain days or some duties suddenly less of a chore? According to Mihaly Csikszentmihalyi, Ph.D., best-selling author of *Flow: The Psychology of Optimal Experience*, it's all about connection.

If you feel stuck at your job or bored by certain tasks, "you're probably doing everything you can to procrastinate—sharpening pencils, talking on the phone," says Dr. Csikszentmihalyi. "That doesn't work—it doesn't advance you or make you feel happy."

Instead of disconnecting and secretly bemoaning the data entry that awaits you at the end of every day, do everything you can to connect to your task. "Rather than do as little as possible, focus and try to cross every *t* and dot every *i*—you'll immediately feel a sense of confidence and competence," says Dr. Csikszentmihalyi.

"Entering various complaints and criminal offenses into the computer system is part of my job at the district attorney's office," says Ginny Perre-Dowd, a domestic violence outreach worker in Dutchess County, New York. "It's rote work, but I see it as my downtime. I block out all distractions, put some classical music on the radio, light a small vanilla-scented candle—it's very meditative."

Take a "Friend Break"

If you simply put your head down and keep going until quitting time, you won't have a perfect day. Social breaks are critical to keep your equilibrium and sense of humor. A quick call to a friend or a few e-mail sallies bring your personality to the surface.

A purely personal call is especially necessary when work demands leave you feeling overwhelmed or annoyed. Dial up your best friend/boyfriend/husband and let off steam, says Dr. Murphy. "In moments of stress, you need to connect with someone you can trust." Just don't let it turn into an extended, self-pitying

Making Life Better

A telephone poll commissioned by the Spiegel catalog cited the following as the top twentieth-century inventions that most improved women's lives.

1. Women's right to vote
2. Birth control
3. Mammograms
4. Tampons
5. Household conveniences (refrigerator, dishwasher, washing machine, microwave)
6. Maternity leave
7. Cosmetic surgery
8. Portable/cell phones
9. Prenatal health care
10. Sneakers

wallow. Vent briefly, he suggests, "then step back and say, 'Okay, now what do I really need to do to fix the problem?'"

Create an End-of-Day Oasis

"Every woman I talk to seems to have one resolution in her heart that she never acts on," says Joan Borysenko, Ph.D., author of *A Woman's Book of Life*. "That's to create a Sabbath of sorts within each day." Most of us think of the Sabbath as a time of rest, but it's also a time to take stock and reconnect with where you are, what you want, and all that's going right in your life. You might, for example, appreciate the ordinary magic of getting home from work half an hour early and having the time to experiment with a new recipe or sit down and write a letter. As Benjamin Franklin observed, happiness "is produced not so much by the great pieces of good fortune that seldom happen as by the little advantages that occur every day."

Whether you tend the garden for 30 minutes, have a nightly "let's catch up" conversation with your partner, or follow Oprah's example and give daily thanks (before you go to sleep, write down five things you're thankful for, however insignificant), make a point of ending your day by appreciating the quality of your life. Then commit to making it happen all over again tomorrow.

41

The Impulsive Woman's Guide to Willpower

Every New Year's Eve, as the ball drops in Times Square and the champagne bubbles up in our glasses, we promise ourselves we'll lose those 5 pounds or stick to our exercise schedule or sew all our own clothes or dump that cheating boyfriend. This year will be different. Oh, if only we had more willpower!

About 40 to 45 percent of adults make at least one New Year's resolution, according to John C. Norcross, Ph.D., clinical psychologist, professor of psychology at the University of Scranton in Pennsylvania, and coauthor of *Changing for Good*. Of those, 71 percent are successful after 2 weeks, and 46 percent are successful after 6 months. He explains that people who rely exclusively on willpower without doing any preparation are more likely to fail. "Wanting to change isn't enough," he says. "It's readiness that counts."

We think of willpower as a magic muscle to tone and flex, a well of discipline we can simply draw from. By relying on sheer willpower to reach a goal, however, we set ourselves up for failure and disappointment. Whether your weakness is as nominal as chewing your cuticles or as harmful as an abusive lover, it's important to know that bringing about change is a process that takes time and involves missteps. We hair-twirling, credit card–using, social-smoking fridge bingers need more than willpower to overcome our Ben and Jerry's trysts. According to the experts, successfully changing a behavior entails being realistic, planning ahead, learning our triggers, coming up with replacements for habits, and rewarding and forgiving ourselves.

"We think of willpower as 'just say no,'" explains Gary McClain, Ph.D., a psychologist and coauthor of *The Complete Idiot's Guide to Breaking Bad Habits*. "But I think it should be 'don't just say no.' Because after you say no, you wonder, 'What am I supposed to do with myself now? I'm at a party and everyone is drinking.' You have to go beyond saying no, retrain yourself, and come up with alternatives."

Think Fulfillment, Not Self-Denial

The term *pullpower*, rather than willpower, is preferred by Ronald G. Nathan, Ph.D., clinical professor of family practice at Albany Medical College and author of the audiotape *Relieving Your Holiday Stress and Achieving Your New Year's Resolutions*. By pullpower, he means that you're drawn to a goal and attracted by possible outcomes, rather than that you use iron will to do or not do something.

Experts say we need to accept that we may not get it right the first time. On average, people who are trying to quit smoking, for example, quit two or three times before they kick the habit for good. "Few people ever really fail; they just give up trying," explains Dr. Nathan. "The important thing is to keep going; don't let the first failure derail your efforts."

Some people seem to wallow in willpower. Lisa, for example, always eats teeny, well-balanced meals and never bloats out of her perfect-size-four sex goddess ensembles. Judy gets up at 5:00 A.M. to write for 2 hours before going to work. What's their secret? Sheer willpower with a penchant for being hard on themselves? No, it's more that they have a knack for being good to themselves. The rules they're enforcing aren't for denying pleasure but for feeling fulfilled. They're able to keep in perspective the fact that what feels good at the moment—two ice cream bars, sleeping late—often feels lousy in the long run.

Here are guidelines that will help you be good and, most important, good to yourself.

Take It One Step at a Time

To help keep those New Year's resolutions, set realistic, obtainable goals and break big, general goals into specific mini-goals.

"It's best to pick small things you can imagine doing for the rest of your life that will add up to your goal," advises Dr. Nathan. "Including a salad or soup at every meal except breakfast, for example, may decrease your overall calorie intake for the meal by about 50 calories. Over time, the cumulative effect may be healthy weight loss."

"Start with something easy to accomplish and accomplish it," advises Peter A. Wish, Ph.D., a psychologist in Long Boat Key, Florida, and author of *Don't Stop at Green Lights*. "Nothing builds on success like success. It makes you feel good, want to continue, and feel optimistic."

"You need to know what a realistic schedule is," Dr. McClain adds. "Sometimes this means seeking advice from a professional—a doctor for weight loss, a therapist for destructive relationships, a credit counselor for paying off credit cards. Ask: What's realistic for a year from now, and what schedule can I get on? People who have experience can help, because we're often not the best authority for ourselves."

Karen exercises for 20 minutes every day. Sometimes she's so busy that this means jumping up and down in her pj's in the kitchen. The bottom line, though, is that she gets her 20 minutes in. You, on the other hand, have the larger, less specific goal of "working out at the gym more often." The gym workouts you envision take nearly 2 hours once you add in changing, driving to the gym, cardio work, free weights, and loitering around the water fountain. As a result, you go for days without exercising at all, especially when deadlines loom.

Try this instead. Test-drive Karen's 20-minute rule. Grab your Walkman and walk briskly to the drugstore or use the patio steps to do 20 minutes of step aerobics. You'll get in some exercise and not be so inclined to slack off on busy days.

Forget Rigid Rules

We usually enforce willpower by setting up little rules for ourselves. But experts advise caution when creating rules: "I prefer goals to rules," says Dr. Nathan. "It's a matter of small, doable steps. A patient of mine decided she wouldn't eat anything she couldn't wash. That meant she stuck to eating fruits and vegetables, because you can't really wash Twinkies."

"Rules can be helpful if they're not an excuse to beat ourselves up, which is as destructive as bad habits," adds Dr. McClain. "Instead of rules, think of promises. A good promise would be: 'I promise to stand back and think about why I'm doing something before doing it and think of alternatives.'"

It's key to keep the reason for the rule in mind: Instead of saying, "I have to exercise," focus on the fact that studies suggest that 20 to 30 minutes of exercise promotes cardiovascular health. You'll increase your metabolism and blood flow, gain energy, and feel better. The only way you can be successful is if the rule is yours and not someone else's. If it's someone else's, then it's their fault that you can't have a snack or cigarette, and you become resentful.

Know What Sets You Off

Willpower begins with understanding your triggers, some of which are environmental and some of which are internal, says Dr. McClain. "Life is filled with triggers. Many habits, such as eating and drinking, are culturally based, so they're particularly hard to control. We celebrate with food, for example. It's important to recognize these environmental triggers and figure out what to do when they go off."

Then there are the internal triggers—the feelings—that make us do things like drink too much at parties. If we're aware of the trigger (we feel shy, for example), we can plan ahead, maybe bringing a friend along for support.

Ride Out Impulses

Once you learn your triggers, you're better prepared to get past impulses. Rehearse mentally what will happen when you face an impulse, recommends Dr. Nathan. What will you do or say? "If you imagine yourself doing something healthy ahead of time, you're more likely to do it."

Another way to ride out an impulse is to have a buddy you can call. Make a pact that you'll help each other when you're tempted and bolster each other when you have a setback.

When you're fighting the urge to call a guy, Dr. McClain says that it's important to break down that urge and ask yourself, "What am I looking for? What does it stem from? What do I get out of this? What are the consequences?" "It's not easy," he adds, "but sometimes you have to sit down, grit your teeth, and examine the urge."

Do you sometimes have to ride out the impulse to buy something, like yet another pair of absolutely perfect pumps? Do you find those "special gift for you" promotions at cosmetic counters especially enticing and convince yourself that you can't live without a teeny lipstick and mascara—and then buy stuff you don't really need to qualify for the freebies? Stop and examine the urge: Do you really need this stuff? More important, do you even want it? If you discover the answers are no and no, you can leave the store feeling liberated.

Look on the Bright Side

Instead of trying to deny ourselves, it's important to focus on the things we can have. "Building willpower doesn't have to be all negative," says Dr. McClain. "It's about finding positive alternatives for your behavior and making use of them." He adds that over time, by replacing habits with alternatives, we learn the alternative as a new behavior. "At first it's not easy. Maybe you need

Calm "Female Only" Cravings

A craving is a strong urge for a specific food or specific type of food—say, salty or sweet—that can strike at any time, including right after a meal, says Mindy Kurzer, Ph.D., associate professor of nutrition at the University of Minnesota's department of food science and nutrition in St. Paul. More women than men report having cravings, possibly because of hormonal changes. Still, you can keep cravings from getting out of control. Here's how.

Keep a cravings calendar. Experts recommend writing down what your cravings are, how you feel both before and after eating, and where you are in your menstrual cycle. If your cravings are in sync with your period, you can relax a little bit, knowing your body is compensating for a few of those extra calories. But if your cravings tend to strike when you're feeling lonely or anxious, you have to conquer the emotional triggers before you can control the cravings. Sometimes that's as simple as talking to a friend who's a good listener or heading to the gym for a mood-boosting workout.

Pick the forbidden fruit. Depriving yourself of something you want can only increase the desire. Instead, allow yourself to indulge occasionally—and in moderation. Savor every little bit. And tell yourself that you can have it again, that you're not being deprived.

Load up on carbs. Eating complex carbohydrates like pasta, bagels, and whole-wheat bread before the onset of your period will help curb cravings and can boost calm-inducing serotonin levels.

Find a substitute. Try to swap one food for another less fatty version, like low-fat frozen yogurt instead of ice cream.

Sweat it out. Exercise is one of the best ways to help manage cravings, for two reasons: It can decrease your appetite and therefore may kill your craving, and it helps lower anxiety, which may have triggered your snack attack.

Do the five Ds. If you really want to conquer a craving, remember the five Ds, suggests the iVillage's Better Health Web site (www.betterhealth.com).

❖ Delay at least 10 minutes before you eat so you don't act on impulse.
❖ Distract yourself by doing an activity that requires you to focus.
❖ Distance yourself from the food (take a walk to get away from the fridge, for example).
❖ Determine how important it is for you to eat the food you're craving.
❖ Decide on a reasonable amount (maybe four Hershey's Kisses—not the whole bag—are enough to satisfy you).

to set up some structure—signing up for a class so you don't eat out of boredom, for example—so you're not left to your own devices."

"Turn on something positive instead of trying to turn off something negative," adds Dr. Nathan. "When you have the urge to smoke, take a walk."

When your snacking trigger goes off, for instance, try this: Hit the living room, play one song on a CD, and dance, jog in place, or stretch. Just keep moving to one song. The neighbors might think you've turned into a party animal, but you'll ride out the urge to snack and be ready to resume whatever else you were doing. The upside might be that you get to listen to music that you might otherwise not get around to. Sometimes, when you look at what you can have instead of trying to pound into your head what you can't have, the answers are incredibly obvious and life doesn't seem so restrictive.

Monitor Yourself in Writing

For many people, keeping a diary of whatever it is they're trying to do or not do is helpful.

"Just monitoring food intake has been shown to have a positive effect on weight loss, because it promotes awareness," says Dr. Nathan. "Writing down what you eat helps because a diary shows you where you're vulnerable and what your specific responses are. By knowing this, you can prepare for triggers."

"Writing it down makes it real," says Karen, who jots her exercise activities down in her day planner. "And it's rewarding."

Your diary shouldn't be another restriction, however. "Don't use the diary as another rule for yourself," advises Dr. McClain. "Use it as a way of thinking through things. 'Why did I want to do this? How did I feel afterward?' Not: 'I have to write in this journal at seven o'clock every morning.'"

Don't Overdo It

It can take willpower not to overdo good behavior, such as working, exercising, or even brushing your teeth, explains Dr. McClain. "Of course it's good to go to the gym, but not if it's instead of meeting people or working on your career—if it interferes with the balance in your life. Essentially, anything that interferes with having a balanced life may be a negative habit."

Loosen the Reins

Sometimes it's okay to give in to cravings and go with your impulses, such as allowing yourself to sleep in or enjoy a cookie. Paradoxically, if we loosen the grip a little and go with our cravings and impulses, we're better able to exert willpower, because we're leading a more balanced life.

"Use letting go to help build structure and balance," advises Dr. McClain.

"You might tell yourself, 'I'm not going to have a big breakfast Monday through Friday, but on Saturday morning, I'm going to have Belgian waffles.' You need to schedule breaks with things you really enjoy."

This doesn't apply to physically destructive habits such as smoking or drinking, adds Dr. McClain. You can't schedule a cigarette or highball on Saturday morning. It doesn't work to do this with destructive relationships, either. You can't let your guard down and call once. Instead, come up with something else that's satisfying.

Treat Yourself

"Small rewards early in the process are important," advises Dr. Nathan. "Don't say, 'When I lose 20 pounds, I'll buy myself an outfit.' That's too late. Even if you haven't lost weight yet, you may have eaten less and exercised more." So focus on something fun. Go to the movies or buy a good book after a couple of days of dieting. For many people, those first few days are really the tough ones.

An important reward is feedback, which helps boost willpower, Dr. Wish adds. Positive feedback can be the good feeling that endorphins give you after exercising or the satisfaction of fitting into clothes after eating less. Identify and enjoy these reinforcers.

Rewards can also work as safety nets, says Dr. McClain. Instead of saving them for the end of a big project, schedule them in to help structure your day.

Give Yourself Permission to Be Human

We're all bound to have little setbacks along the way. What's the best way to handle them?

"Each time you screw up, realize that it's an opportunity to learn something about yourself and to restrategize," says Dr. McClain. "You might learn what doesn't work, what your triggers are, when you can't let your guard down. Forgive yourself and say, 'What else can I try?'"

We often fail because we didn't do enough preparation, Dr. Nathan explains. "Often, we make the decision to change, and we haven't prepared ourselves. Preparation helps us think ahead to who else to call instead of an old boyfriend, for example. Instead of saying, 'I'm a failure,' we need to realize that sometimes we just weren't prepared enough."

Maybe you didn't really get 20 minutes of exercise in on Sunday—unless you count shopping for a couch. Tell yourself it's okay: "I still exercised more than last week, and maybe I'll do even better next week." Sometimes it takes a little willpower to tell yourself these nice things.

Discover the Power of Forgiveness

It wasn't something Susan expected to hear: "I've done something very wrong."

Carefully closing the door behind her, Susan's friend Robin walked into her office and sat down. "I've come to apologize," she admitted, awkwardly smoothing her skirt.

Startled, Susan sat back in her chair. At 45, Robin was an ambitious woman who went after what she wanted. Apologies were not her style.

Susan looked over the top of her glasses at Robin. "You better tell me what you've done," she said. And for the next 5 minutes, she did. Robin told Susan how, from the day 3 years earlier when the two of them had been promoted to senior positions within the company, she had privately bad-mouthed Susan's work to their boss. Jealous of Susan's success, she'd even encouraged their childless-by-choice boss to think that, as a working mother, Susan wouldn't be able to give the job the kind of time it required.

Robin took a deep breath and looked out the window. "I don't like who I've become," she said quietly. "I'm trying to change."

She looked directly at Susan. "Can you ever forgive me?"

Forgive her? Why would anyone forgive someone who had deliberately and knowingly betrayed her?

Because, says forgiveness researcher Robert Enright, Ph.D., professor of educational psychology at the University of Wisconsin at Madison, unless you forgive someone who tried to ruin your life, you could end up ruining it yourself.

What's in It for You?

While anger and resentment are perfectly natural under the circumstances—it's the way humans respond to injustice, says Dr. Enright—you run the risk of letting such an experience darken your attitude. Your bitterness could become a negative view of life that would affect how you think about everyone. If you stop trusting people because you think they will always stab you in the back, you could miss out on some valuable and enriching friendships. And that would make you vulnerable to chronic anxiety, serious depression, general distrust, poor self-esteem, and a pervading sense of hopelessness.

What's more, those negative feelings can also trigger a cascade of stress hormones that accelerate the heart rate, shut down the immune system, and encourage blood clotting, which can lead to heart attacks and stroke, adds Richard Fitzgibbons, M.D., a psychiatrist in suburban Philadelphia. In fact, studies show that hanging on to anger and resentment increases your chance

Identify Hidden Sources of Anger

Sometimes we bury our anger so deeply that we no longer recognize its source. But it's easier to forgive when you can remember who did what to whom. For most people, the deepest disappointment in childhood and adolescence is with their fathers. "Their fathers simply haven't been there for them when they needed them. If you're in that particular boat, pay attention to the feelings you have for your dad," suggests Richard Fitzgibbons, M.D., a psychiatrist in suburban Philadelphia.

Here are other sources of hidden anger that Dr. Fitzgibbons says might be likely to affect you.

❖ Anger with your children for not being sensitive to your needs
❖ Anger with your spouse for ways in which he has disappointed you
❖ Anger with an employer or a spouse's employer—particularly if you or your spouse has recently been downsized

HEALTH FLASH

of a heart attack fivefold. It also increases your risk of cancer, high blood pressure, high cholesterol, and a host of chronic illnesses.

Forgiveness, on the other hand, short-circuits that process entirely, says Dr. Fitzgibbons. It fosters healthful changes in both your attitude and your body, boosting your self-esteem and feelings of hope as it lowers your blood pressure and heart rate. It can even help you sleep better.

What Forgiving Is—And Isn't

There are many benefits to forgiving, but that's not to say forgiveness is easy. If your spouse cheats on you or your best friend betrays a confidence, forgiving them may take time—and it probably won't come easily. For most of us, "forgiveness is an intellectual decision you make to give up your anger and feelings for revenge," says Dr. Fitzgibbons.

Knowing what forgiveness is, and isn't, may help ease you into it. For example, forgiving someone who has done you wrong is not condoning what she did or absolving her of guilt. It doesn't mean that you've gone all soft and fuzzy toward her or that you're going to trust her or make yourself vulnerable in any way.

If you decide to trust her at a later date, that's fine, says Dr. Fitzgibbons. But it's not necessary to trust, or even like, the other person again in order to heal or maintain a healthy life. Further, forgiving is not forgetting: It is letting go of anger and hurt and moving on.

What Doesn't Work

"There are three ways to handle anger when someone hurts you," explains Dr. Fitzgibbons. "Deny it, express it, or forgive the person who caused it."

Denial doesn't work. That's just burying your anger, and anger rarely stays buried. What's more, studies show that denial leads to all sorts of mental illnesses, such as depression, which in turn can increase your risk of physical illnesses such as heart disease.

Expressing anger, while it seems helpful, can actually be equally harmful, according to Dr. Fitzgibbons, who first proposed using forgiveness as a therapeutic technique more than a decade ago. The problem is that most of us have tried the denial tactic at some point in our lives. But with so much buried anger, when we do finally express it, we risk detonating a hidden arsenal of deadly explosives that could ruin friendships, wreck marriages, and even harm our children.

The most important thing is to decide whether your anger requires action or not, according to Redford B. Williams, M.D., the director of the Behav-

How Forgiving Are You?

The Enright Forgiveness Inventory is a scientific test that measures how much you've forgiven someone for a particular offense. It's too long to reproduce here, but forgiveness researcher Robert Enright, Ph.D., professor of educational psychology at the University of Wisconsin at Madison and the psychologist who developed it, has come up with this shortened form.

To see whether or not you've truly forgiven someone who has hurt you, think about a specific person and what he or she has done, says Dr. Enright. If there are a number of injustices, center on the most recent. Then respond to a, b, and c following each of the three statements below by circling the number next to the answer that represents how you feel about the person who has hurt you.

SD = strongly disagree

D = disagree

A = agree

SA = strongly agree

1. The best description of my feelings is that I
    a. resent him or her (SD–4, D–3, A–2, SA–1)
    b. dislike him or her (SD–4, D–3, A–2, SA–1)
    c. love him or her (SD–1, D–2, A–3, SA–4)
2. When I think about the person, I
    a. wish him or her well (SD–1, D–2, A–3, SA–4)
    b. think kindly about him or her (SD–1, D–2, A–3, SA–4)
    c. do not respect the person at all (SD–4, D–3, A–2, SA–1)
3. If given the opportunity, I would
    a. return his or her phone call (SD–1, D–2, A–3, SA–4)
    b. put the person down (SD–4, D–3, A–2, SA–1)
    c. try to be helpful (SD–1, D–2, A–3, SA–4)

Scoring

Total your points and compare them with the scoring below.

9–12 points: You're not forgiving the person and perhaps you're still angry.

13–20 points: You're not forgiving but are moving in the direction of forgiveness.

21–26 points: You're in transition to forgiveness.

27–36 points: You're forgiving.

ioral Medicine Research Center at Duke University Medical Center in Durham, North Carolina. "True anger is justifiable, and you'll need to act on it. Express it by assertion rather than blowing up." At other times, you may be angry about something small or something that can't be changed. Either way, he adds, you can practice forgiveness as a way of getting out from under the anger.

How Forgiveness Can Heal You

Forgiveness heals by removing certain amounts of excess anger within you each time you forgive someone. It also decreases the need for revenge and the need to make someone else change, explains Dr. Williams.

There's now scientific support: Dr. Enright measured study participants' emotional states before and after they forgave those who had hurt them. He discovered that those who forgave eliminated feelings of anxiety and depression and boosted their self-esteem and sense of hope. Other researchers have found that forgiving results in better sleep, increased feelings of love, an enhanced ability to trust, and an end to the physical symptoms and illness caused by anger. It even lessens the impact of mental illness such as depression.

Forget the Silent Treatment

Ever been tempted to give your spouse or friend the silent treatment? Don't. The mental effort you exert to consciously ignore him could drain your own brainpower.

Researchers at Case Western Reserve University in Cleveland discovered the brain-sapping effect of the silent treatment when they paired students with research team members and stuck them in a room alone together for 4 minutes. They told half the students to ignore their partners and half to strike up a conversation.

Later, the researchers gave each student 20 word puzzles to do. Those who had talked with their companions were more persistent in their efforts to solve the puzzles than those who had ignored their partners. "This suggests that consciously ignoring people requires a lot of mental energy," says study leader Kristin Sommer, Ph.D., now assistant professor of psychology at Baruch College in New York City.

Try these suggestions from Dr. Sommer the next time you're tempted to punish someone with silence.

❖ Remember that you're also punishing yourself: It saps mental energy.
❖ Empathize with the other person. "Recall an occasion when you were given the silent treatment," she says, "and how awful it felt to be ignored."

The bottom line: "Talking is almost always the best approach," says Dr. Sommer. "It's communication that solves problems, not silence."

How to Forgive Those Who Trespass against You

Now that we know that forgiveness heals, how do we use it? The process looks surprisingly simple—but it may be one of the toughest things you'll ever do. Here's what Drs. Fitzgibbons and Enright suggest.

Acknowledge your anger—all of it. Think about how you were hurt, your response, and how you feel right now, says Dr. Enright. Just because you're not boiling mad doesn't mean you're not angry. Anger frequently disguises itself as depleted energy, a preoccupation with what happened, impatience with other people, and a tendency to look at the world in a negative way. If you're not sure at whom your anger is directed or if you suspect that much of it has gotten buried under a veneer of "making nice," then every morning when you get up, just say, "I want to forgive the people who disappointed me and caused me to feel sad or lonely." After a while, the source of your anger will emerge. You may be angrier than ever when you realize who it is and what they've done, adds Dr. Fitzgibbons. But that's the time to follow the next recommendation.

Decide to forgive. Some people decide to forgive because their religious beliefs demand that they turn the other cheek, embrace their enemies, and go on. Others decide to forgive because their anger is causing them so much emotional pain that they'll try anything to relieve it. Still others simply recognize that if anger is dictating how they feel, then their entire lives are being controlled by the people who hurt them.

If none of those things are motivating you, you need to "go through the motions" in your head until you can truly feel forgiveness in your heart. Get up every morning and say to yourself, "I want to forgive so-and-so for what he or she has done," says Dr. Fitzgibbons. If it helps, stand in front of an empty chair, pretend the person who hurt you is sitting there, and say, "I forgive you."

Don't Get Mad, Get Distracted

When you feel your blood start to boil, try distracting yourself. You'll feel better—and maybe even live longer. In a study at the University of Michigan in Ann Arbor, researchers riled up 256 people to see how they handled it. They found that women tend to choose distraction to cope with anger, while men choose rumination and distraction equally.

The female response probably works better. Evidence suggests that dwelling on anger increases its intensity, whereas distraction reduces it, says study author Cheryl L. Rusting, Ph.D., now assistant professor at the State University of New York at Buffalo. Some experts believe that anger is as much of a risk factor for heart disease in both sexes as cholesterol, smoking, or high blood pressure.

Do no evil. Resolve not to act negatively against the person who hurt you, says Dr. Enright. You don't have to do anything good on her behalf—just don't do anything bad. For example, if the wrongdoer's name comes up in conversation, don't give in to the temptation to do some serious "dissing." That's the time to obey the old chestnut, "If you can't say something nice, don't say anything at all."

Consider the source. Is there anything in the background of the offender that could explain her behavior? If there is, don't let it sidetrack you into feeling sorry for her, says Dr. Enright. It's no excuse. But it will help you to forgive and move on if you can see some reason for her actions.

In the case of Robin and Susan, both of Robin's parents died when she was 16, and she was left on her own to raise a younger sister. They had no money and no relatives to look out for them. But Robin kept the family together, put food on the table, and even got both herself and her sister full scholarships to prestigious universities. Although knowing that didn't make what Robin did to Susan right, it did help Susan understand Robin's need to get all the marbles she can in any game she plays.

Put yourself in the other person's shoes. This is empathy. Think about what was going on in the life of the person who hurt you when she did it, suggests Dr. Enright. Maybe she hit a rough stretch and needed to strike out—and you got in the way. Robin, for example, had married a guy who couldn't seem to keep a job. Did that make her feel like she was all alone and responsible for her family's financial security again? Susan didn't know, but just thinking about it helped her anger toward Robin to soften.

Give yourself some time. Forgiving with both head and heart isn't something you can do overnight, says Dr. Fitzgibbons. "Some people think, 'Well, if I make the decision to forgive—bingo! There goes my anger and it's over.' Unfortunately, it takes weeks, months, sometimes years to get over being disappointed and angry," he explains. "It's like draining an abscess. When you decide to forgive, you can drain only a certain amount of anger from the heart and the unconscious at a time."

Consider reconciliation. Forgiveness doesn't always lead to reconciliation, says Dr. Fitzgibbons. In some cases, you need to keep hurtful people at arm's length so they can't continue hurting you. But if you know the person is clearly not going to hurt you again or if she seems truly sorry, then reconciliation becomes possible.

It's up to you.

part eight

Best Bets
in Beauty

8

His and Her Health

Closing the Gender Gap in Cosmetic Surgery

The wicked queen in *Snow White* asks, "Mirror, mirror on the wall—who's the fairest of them all?" These days, both women *and* men are asking that question. What's different between the sexes is deciding whether or not to opt for cosmetic surgery.

"Women still have more cosmetic surgery than men, but an increasing number of men are opting for it, too," says plastic surgeon Diane Gerber, M.D., who practices in Chicago and is a spokesperson for the American Society of Plastic and Reconstructive Surgeons. "Women tend to be more in touch with their bodies and are less embarrassed about plastic surgery. Men fear people will think they're vain if they schedule elective surgery. But that's changing now. Like women, men work in a competitive corporate environment, and they want to look as young and healthy as the next guy."

The most common cosmetic surgeries women get are liposuction, eyelid surgery, and breast augmentation. For men, it's nose reshaping, hair transplants, and liposuction. "Liposuction is one of the top three for both sexes because there has always been a demand for people to reduce the amount of fat on their bodies," says Dr. Gerber. "Fat is simply not beautiful on certain parts of the body."

The area where Dr. Gerber finds a distinct gender difference is making the decision to schedule the surgery. "Women are more sure of their decisions," she notices. "They are generally calmer going into it than men, especially if it's the first time they've had elective surgery. Men are more apprehensive, and sometimes they second-guess themselves. I don't think they fear the pain of injections or surgery. I suspect it's because they are not used to making these kinds of decisions, especially regarding elective, cosmetic surgery. Once men have made up their minds to have surgery, they are generally in a big hurry to schedule. In most households, even if both partners are working, it's the woman who schedules the doctor visits for the entire family. It's a part of women's daily lives."

If you're considering cosmetic surgery but are not sure if it's right for you, Dr. Gerber suggests asking yourself the following questions.

❖ Am I basically happy with my life but looking to improve or change a specific body part or region? "If you can answer yes to that question, you're a good candidate for cosmetic surgery because you want to make a physical change," says Dr. Gerber.

❖ Am I unhappy with my life and myself and think cosmetic surgery will make my life better? "If you answer yes to this question, cosmetic surgery may not be right for you because you want to change your life," says Dr. Gerber. "If your spouse left you or there was a death in the family or you don't like yourself, surgery won't fix the situation. That is not a realistic expectation. A realistic expectation is, 'My thighs are too fat, I'd like them thinner, and surgery can make them thinner.'"

Vitamins That Beautify Your Skin

Think how much easier our mothers' jobs would have been if they'd told us we could make mush of our peas and oranges and smear them over our faces to get the benefit of the vitamins they contain. Well, Mom, today we can slather ourselves with essential nutrients—and look lovely doing it.

Vitamins are big beauty news, turning up in every possible kind of elixir for skin, hair, and nails. It's hard to say what's more alluring—the promises they make for the future or the pretty, pampered way they make us feel right now. Still, the trend has become so huge that it's hard not to feel a little overwhelmed.

Are all vitamin products created equal, or do some work harder than others? How are you supposed to pick and choose? Here's how.

Vitamin A: The Strongest Wrinkle Fighter

When it comes to beauty, creams containing A are the only vitamin-enriched products that have been shown—in properly designed, scientific trials on people—to smooth skin, reduce fine lines, and fade age spots.

We're talking of course about Retin-A and Renova, which get their strength from the vitamin-A derivative tretinoin. This prescription chemical

Men's Products for Women

You don't need to stop at your half of the bathroom shelf to look your best. Here are products for men that you can use, too.

Polo Sport Scrub Face Wash. The cooling menthol lather softens up that craggy face of his after he gets out of bed in the morning.

What's in it for you: Jojoba microspheres that will work their exfoliating magic on your dead skin before you hop into bed at night.

Chanel Technique Pour Homme High Performance Moisture Formula. It pampers his razor-scraped flesh into something nice and nuzzle-worthy.

What's in it for you: Vitamin E and other ingredients that will hydrate your face while moisturizing your hands and cuticles at the same time.

Tend Skin. Prevents ingrown hairs on his delicate face and reduces irritation.

What's in it for you: Prevents ingrown hairs on your delicate bikini line and reduces irritation.

Gillette Mach3 razor. It has three extra-thin blades that are a triple threat for giving him a superclose shave.

What's in it for you: Great for mornings when you decide at the last minute to wear a sleeveless shell.

RazorGuard. The between-uses soaking solution keeps his razor sharp for a whole month.

What's in it for you: The same.

Orly Nails for Males. Its natural-looking and protective coat will hide his nail-biting habit.

What's in it for you: Its semigloss finish is perfect for those minimal makeup days.

seems to short-circuit the process by which ultraviolet light breaks down collagen and elastin, proteins that help keep skin plump and uncreased. Tretinoin also stimulates the production of new collagen.

What about over-the-counter vitamin A products? They use different, less well-studied forms of A, so it's hard to say how well they work. This much we know: They're generally weaker and thus kinder to skin than Renova, but this also means that their wrinkle-fading action isn't as powerful.

Of the vitamin A cousins, experts are most impressed by one called retinol, though it is less easily absorbed into skin than tretinoin. You'll find it in Avon's Anew Retinol Recovery Complex PM Treatment and Estée Lauder's Diminish. Both are skin treatments rather than moisturizers, so dab them on fine lines, crow's-feet, and other problem areas, then follow with your favorite lotion and sunscreen. Since retinol has the potential to irritate skin, start slowly. If you notice irritation, use it every other day for a couple of weeks.

Vitamin B: Conditioning for Your Hair and Nails

A quick survey of what could happen if you didn't get enough of the eight B vitamins illustrates their importance to physical appearance. You might end up with dark-pigmented nails; hair loss; or oily, crusty, scaly skin. People with brittle nail syndrome—chronic cracking and splitting—are sometimes treated with large oral doses of biotin, a B vitamin that used to be mislabeled vitamin H. (Doctors poached the remedy from veterinarians, who feed biotin to horses to strengthen their hooves.) Also treatable with biotin is a rare condition called uncombable hair syndrome (the name says it all).

In the world of cosmetics, pro-vitamin B_5, also known as panthenol, is the most common form of B, turning up frequently in shampoos and other hair care products. Will it tame your mane and nourish your hide?

Don't expect miracles. While a rat's fur goes gray and drops out if its food is lacking in vitamin B_5, your tresses won't noticeably thicken or regain their youthful brightness after you lather up with a panthenol-enriched shampoo. On the other hand, because it's oily, panthenol does have some moisturizing benefits.

Vitamin C: Your Skin's Best Defense

Vitamin C is vital to making collagen; that's why in olden days, sailors warded off the hideous skin and gum sores of scurvy by taking a barrel of limes to sea and snacking on their juicy pulp. Vitamin C is also an antioxidant, able to neutralize the dangerous molecules called free radicals that form when the body is exposed to sunlight, smog, and cigarette smoke—in fact, they're formed during the very process of living and breathing. If unchecked, the theory goes, free radicals may damage collagen, elastin, and DNA, leading to wrinkles and worse.

Because of this, vitamin C lotions and serums have become very appealing. When scientists rub the vitamin onto the backs of rats and pigs, their skin takes twice as long as normal to sunburn, suggesting that cosmetics or sunscreen imbued with C could add another line of defense against cancer- and wrinkle-causing ultraviolet (UV) rays. In petri dishes, C prompts skin cells to divide and produce fresh collagen. So far, though, studies haven't tested whether vitamin C potions can make humans grow new collagen. Still, some dermatologists swear that faces get rosier and less furrowed when vitamin C is applied, and this year scientists reported that a lotion containing C lessened fine lines after 18 months of use.

How do you choose among all the new C products? Your best bet is to select a version—such as Cellex-C, SkinCeuticals, or C-Esta—with plenty of the vitamin in it: 5 to 15 percent, in line with quantities used in animal studies.

As with the retinol products, these serums are meant to be used underneath your regular moisturizer. And while they do provide some sun protection, it's not so much that you can afford to skip sunscreen.

Once you buy that precious box or vial—top brands cost $45 and up—take good care of it. Vitamin C can break down rapidly. Some products are chemically stabilized, but to be on the safe side, store your C in a cool, dark place.

Vitamin E: A Little Extra Protection

As with C, there's good evidence that vitamin E guards against sun damage when smeared onto skin. Vitamin E has the additional benefit of being oily, so it softens the complexion and conditions hair a bit. (This soothing oiliness, rather than the vitamin itself, is probably behind the folk remedy of breaking a vitamin E capsule onto a cut or scrape to limit scarring.)

For these reasons, it makes sense to choose moisturizers with vitamin E whenever you have the option. But remember: Not all E's are the same. Many products contain a form of the vitamin—known as alpha-tocopherol acetate—that is more chemically stable but less effective (studies suggest it doesn't protect against UV damage). The more potent version is alpha-tocopherol, which you can find in L'Oréal's Futur-E or in gels containing aloe vera, a particularly rich source. If the vitamin E cream you've been using has the acetate version, don't fret: Experts say a small amount of this E does get converted to the more effective kind once it's on your skin—and this may be enough to offer some protection from those nasty free radicals.

Is it okay to use more than one vitamin cream at a time? Yes, but practice common sense. If you really want to boost the beauty benefits vitamins have to offer, you might try a retinol product in the morning, follow it with a dollop of vitamin E moisturizer, and then go for some C serum at night. If you notice any irritation, give your face a break.

Food Fixes for Beauty Woes

I f you're spending a lot of money at the hairdresser and cosmetic counter but neglecting what you eat, you may be sabotaging your elaborate beauty regimens—and all the lipstick and blush in the world won't help. (Good genes have a lot to do with it, too, of course, not to mention staying generally healthy and getting enough sleep and exercise.)

"Beauty begins with healthy eating," says Ann Louise Gittleman, a certified nutritionist and author of *Super Nutrition for Women*. "So many women focus on the outside, but without proper nutrition you won't look your best." Dry skin, lackluster hair, brittle nails—these are just a few red flags that may let you know you aren't eating right.

Happily, small diet changes can bring about big cosmetic benefits. Here are some strategies to nourish the inner and outer you.

You Have More Wrinkles Than a Shar-Pei

What you need: Vitamin A

What it does: Vitamin A maintains your outer layer of skin, thereby helping to prevent premature aging. "It's the same thing that's in Retin-A," says Robert Skidmore, M.D., medical director of dermatology at Shands Hospital, University of Florida College of Medicine, Gainesville, who warns against taking high doses (by taking vitamins that exceed the RDA, for instance), because A is stored in the body.

What you should eat: Carrots, sweet potatoes, leafy green vegetables, peaches, apricots

Your Body Is Black and Blue (You Bruise Easily)

What you need: Vitamin C

What it does: It forms collagen, which holds cells together (this helps prevent bruising) and may speed the healing of skin wounds. (Bruising can be a sign of vitamin C deficiency, or it may be hormonal.)

What you should eat: Citrus fruits, strawberries, tomatoes, broccoli, squash ("Drinking a glass of citrus juice every day should help," says Gittleman.)

Your Face Is as Puffy as Marlon Brando's

What you need: To avoid excess sodium

What it does: Sodium pulls water out of your body's cells and into the spaces between them.

What you should eat: Herbs and spices on your food rather than salt; also avoid processed foods, which tend to contain buckets of sodium

You Have Unsightly Spider Veins

What you need: Water

What it does: Water keeps your skin cool by allowing it to sweat; this prevents the eruption of tiny capillaries, which occurs when the face is overheated and flushed, says Dr. Skidmore.

What you should drink: Water (or plenty of caffeine-free beverages)

You're as Pale as a Plate of Tofu

What you need: Iron

What it does: Iron prevents anemia, which causes a pale, drawn complexion.

What you should eat: Red meat—the darker the color, the greater the iron content—liver, beans, eggs, spinach, and broccoli

Age-Defying Remedies You Can Make at Home

These four simple remedies—made with pure ingredients like papaya, olive oil, milk, and honey—can help renew your complexion, soothe your skin, and smooth out fine lines and wrinkles. Best of all, they're inexpensive and easy to make.

Tropical Fruit Masque

What it does: Smoothes wrinkles, refreshes your skin

What's in it: 1 cup fresh pineapple, ½ cup fresh papaya (slightly green), and 2 tablespoons honey

How it works: Pineapple and papaya are rich in alpha hydroxy acids (AHAs), which dissolve dead skin cells, increase hydration, and stimulate the production of collagen. AHAs also smooth the skin's surface, which can even out skin tone and make tiny lines appear less visible. Honey is a natural humectant that hydrates your skin.

How to make it: Puree the pineapple and papaya in a food processor or blender. Add the honey and mix thoroughly.

How to use it: Wash your face, then spread the mixture over your skin, avoiding the eye area. Leave it on for no more than 5 minutes; rinse with cool water. Follow with a moisturizer. Don't use the masque more than once a week. Store it in the refrigerator for 3 to 4 days, and use the leftovers for your hands, elbows, feet, or other areas.

Jojoba–Grapefruit Body Moisturizer

What it does: Smoothes dry skin

What's in it: 3 tablespoons jojoba oil, 3 drops grapefruit essential oil, and 1 grapefruit

How it works: The grapefruit is a source of AHAs, and the jojoba oil lubricates the skin and keeps it smooth.

How to make it: Combine the oils and set aside. Remove the yellow skin of the grapefruit with a vegetable peeler, avoiding the white pith underneath. Toss the peel in the oil mix until it's coated. Put the mixture aside to infuse for at least 24 hours. Remove the peel, squeezing it against a spoon to retain as much of the oil as possible; discard the peel. Pour the mixture into a storage container.

How to use it: Moisturize right after a bath or shower so your moisturizer can form a barrier to keep water from evaporating out of your skin. Store in a colored bottle in a cool, dark place for up to a month.

Buttery Night Cream

What it does: Softens neck lines

What's in it: 2 tablespoons cocoa butter, 2 teaspoons light olive oil, 1 tablespoon lanolin, and ½ teaspoon vitamin E oil

How it works: It moisturizes while you sleep. Cocoa butter is good for nighttime preparations because it can be too heavy for daytime use. Light olive oil is easily absorbed by the skin and seals in moisture. Lanolin also seals in moisture and is easily absorbed. Vitamin E oil naturally preserves the cream and adds its own moistness to the product.

Note: If your complexion is oily or blemish-prone, this recipe may be too rich for your skin.

How to make it: Mix the cocoa butter, light olive oil, lanolin, and vitamin E oil in a glass container, cover, and microwave on high for 45 seconds. Stir the mixture thoroughly and cool. Pour the cream into a jar with a tight-fitting lid.

How to use it: Massage an amount the size of a quarter into your neck every night before you go to bed. The lotion will last up to 4 months. Store in a cool, dry place.

Green Tea Soak

What it does: Soothes sensitive skin

What's in it: ½ cup loose green tea leaves and ½ cup rolled oats or instant oatmeal

How it works: Green tea is a marvelous and versatile remedy. A green tea bath is a terrific way to tone your skin and to unwind after a stressful day at home or in the office. Oatmeal is a wonderful soother, especially for sensitive skin. The starchy nature of oatmeal makes it naturally soothing.

How to make it: Combine the green tea leaves and oatmeal in a muslin or cheesecloth bag. Suspend the bag from your bathtub spout with string or ribbon. Let the mixture steep as you fill the tub with warm water.

How to use it: Soak for 10 to 15 minutes. Then rub your body gently with a loofah and rinse. Towel dry and apply moisturizer lavishly. Make a fresh bag each time.

Safety First

Just because a home remedy is natural and homemade doesn't mean you can't have a bad reaction to it.

Before you try any of the products mentioned above, test them by dabbing a dime-size drop on your inner arm. Leave it on for 20 minutes. Don't use the product if the area becomes red or itchy. Finally, don't use any product that contains an ingredient to which you already know you're allergic.

Your Skin Is as Scaly as Godzilla's

What you need: Zinc

What it does: Zinc helps dead skin cells slough off normally. (Think of it as a loofah you swallow.) "Dry, scaly skin can often be remedied by adding zinc to the diet," says Dr. Skidmore.

What you should eat: Oysters, red meat, crabmeat, turkey, whole grains, nuts, beans, pumpkin seeds

Also reach for: Water ("It's the forgotten beauty nutrient," says Jackie Newgent, a spokeswoman for the American Dietetic Association.)

What it does: It can help prevent dry skin by keeping your skin hydrated.

What you should drink: "Six to eight glasses daily will help skin stay moist," Newgent says.

Also reach for: Linoleic acid, or essential fats the body can't produce on its own ("They play an important role in sebum [oil] production, which keeps skin soft and supple," notes Dr. Skidmore.)

What it does: It maintains smooth, moist skin.

What you should eat: Safflower oil, olive oil, canola oil, nuts, seeds, whole grains

Your Lips Feel like Dried Paint

What you need: Water

What it does: It hydrates lip tissues. "Lips have no oil glands, which makes them prone to dryness. Keeping the body hydrated helps keep them moist," says Newgent.

What you should drink: Water!

Your Lips Have Cracks in the Corners

What you need: Vitamin B$_2$, otherwise known as riboflavin

What it does: It prevents deficiency, which can cause blisters and cracks.

What you should eat or drink: Milk, dark green vegetables, whole grains

Your Nails Are Brittle

What you need: Protein

What it does: It fortifies your nails, which get their strength from protein, says Newgent.

What you should eat or drink: Meat, fish, chicken, milk, eggs, beans

**H
E
A
L
T
H

F
L
A
S
H**

Top 10
Beauty
Foods

All fruits and vegetables have antioxidant power—a formidable weapon against aging. Here are the very best picks. Make sure you eat lots of them.

❖ Blueberries

❖ Blackberries

❖ Strawberries

❖ Kale, cooked

❖ Spinach, cooked

❖ Oranges

❖ Beets, cooked

❖ Brussels sprouts, cooked

❖ Plums

❖ Broccoli florets

Your Eyes Are Dry or Red

What you need: Vitamin A

What it does: It promotes healthy eye tissue and helps your eyes adjust to dim light. "Vitamin A is important for overall eye health," says Gittleman.

What you should eat: Carrots, sweet potatoes, leafy green vegetables, peaches, apricots

Your Teeth Are Dingy

What you need: Anything but coffee, tea, or brewed iced tea

What it does: Avoiding these dark-colored drinks protects your teeth (and tongue) from stains, says Douglas Berkey, D.M.D., professor and chairman of applied dentistry at the University of Colorado School of Dentistry in Denver.

What you should drink: Light-colored herbal teas, fruit juices, sparkling water

Your Hair Is as Dull as Dishwater

What you need: Linoleic acid (fat)

What it does: It aids sebum production, which lubricates hair. "Fats play an important part in maintaining lustrous hair," says Newgent. "Women who cut out too much fat from their diets may complain of dull, dry hair."

What you should eat: Safflower oil, olive oil, canola oil, nuts, seeds in moderation as well as whole grains

Also reach for: Silica, a trace mineral that helps create hair's protein structure and adds sheen

What it does: It keeps hair strong and shiny.

What you should eat: Whole grains

You've Gone Gray Prematurely (and It Doesn't Look Distinguished)

What you need: Trace minerals such as iron and copper

What they do: They help maintain hair pigment. "Some research suggests that a diet rich in minerals may combat premature gray," says Gittleman.

What you should eat or drink: Meats, whole grains, milk, yogurt, eggs, blackstrap molasses, and a variety of colorful fruits and vegetables

Your Hair Is Thinning

What you need: Zinc

What it does: It prevents hair loss. "Studies show that people who are zinc-deficient can start losing hair. Zinc also strengthens hair," says Gittleman.

What you should eat: Oysters, red meat, crabmeat, turkey, whole grains, nuts, beans, pumpkin seeds

45

Rescue Tactics for Skin-Care Emergencies

S till searching for the perfect skin solution? Let the experts show you the shortcuts to your softest skin—no matter what shape it's in.

Dry Skin

Doctor on call: Debra Wattenberg, M.D., a New York City dermatologist

Symptoms: Flakiness, particularly on the outer corners of the nose, mouth, and eyes

Daily regime: Wash with a nonsoap cleanser and moisturize, twice daily. (Using a heavy cream or one made for extremely dry skin is okay unless you're prone to breakouts.) Drink plenty of fluids and get regular exercise, which generates blood flow, hydrating the skin. Finally, wear sunblock every day—a sunburn will dry out your skin and cause excessive flaking.

Weekly regime: Avoid alpha hydroxy acid (AHA) as well as benzoyl peroxide, since they dry skin. Instead, use beta hydroxy acid twice a week to gently remove dead surface skin cells and hydrate the layer underneath. If your skin has a mild reaction to the acid, mix it with your regular moisturizer to weaken its effect. Once a week, use a mud mask to deep clean and moisturize.

Monthly regime: Get a facial specifically designed to hydrate the skin once a month.

The Ultimate Anti-Aging Ammo for Your Skin

Is overexposure to the elements wreaking havoc on your complexion? Here's how to fight back.

For the beginner: Your mission is to keep the skin you have and prevent future damage.

What you should do: Wear sunscreen every time you step outside. In addition to daily cleansing and moisturizing, use eye serums and night creams to care for your delicate facial skin while you get your Zzzs.

For the intermediate: You've had lots of days at the beach, and the laugh lines have landed.

What you should do: Perk up your existing routine with vitamins—topically! With a little vitamin C serum, you'll see results in days. The results last only as long as you continue to use the product, but that's where alpha hydroxy acid (AHA) and firming creams come in.

For the advanced: No more kidding around. You've tried it all and heard it all before.

What you should do: Facials will keep your skin toned and healthy. If chemical peels frighten you, try a kinder, gentler version: Ask your dermatologist about low-concentration AHA or beta hydroxy acid peels, which simply exfoliate the top layer of the epidermis.

Oily Skin

Doctor on call: Greg Jenkins, M.D., a Silicon Valley dermatologist

Symptoms: An all-over greasy feeling; occasional bouts of acne; oil in the T-zone, even after washing; oil shining through makeup; oily scalp, sometimes accompanied by dandruff

Daily regime: In the morning, wash with gel cleanser or bar soap specifically made for acne to remove oil from the surface of your skin. Follow with an oil-free, noncomedogenic moisturizer with sunscreen and oil-free makeup. In the evening, use a toner to clean skin and remove excess oil and makeup, then follow with a moisturizer. (Nix the night creams—they can be too heavy; your daytime moisturizer should do the trick.) Avoid stress and alcohol consumption as well as anything that rubs against your face (like your hands or the telephone).

Note: If you're already taking the Pill, the brand Ortho Tri-cyclen has been found to be more effective in treating oily skin and reducing acne.

Weekly regime: Use a seaweed or clay mask to deep clean pores once or twice a week.

Monthly regime: Consult a skin care expert at a spa or salon about steaming your face to remove blackheads.

Sensitive Skin

Doctor on call: Deborah S. Sarnoff, M.D., a New York City dermatologist

Symptoms: Reacts to changes in climate and treatment as well as to many cosmetics; prone to blemishes (which could be the result of oil buildup or a reaction to specific ingredients in makeup) and flakiness, burning, chafing, and cracking skin

Daily regime: Use a mild lotion cleanser (the kind you use tissues to remove) and an oil-free moisturizer for day and night. Make sure sunscreen is part of your morning routine. (Before using any new product, test it on your inner arm, where the skin is most similar to the face; no reaction means it's probably face-safe. If a slight irritation develops, use a low-dose hydrocortisone cream on the area.) Drink plenty of water, get lots of rest, and exercise regularly. Avoid washcloths, loofahs, toners, and bar soaps—all of them can cause mild irritation. Finally, if you must exfoliate, remember that beta hydroxy acid is gentler than alpha hydroxy acid.

Weekly regime: Keep a diary of what you react to. Try a mask of milk of magnesia once a week to hydrate your skin.

Monthly regime: Get a monthly facial, making sure to avoid steam treatments, since extreme temperatures can irritate the skin.

Winter Skin Care

Here's how to survive skin's harshest season.

Make a clean sweep. First, wash up. This ensures that you'll get the maximum effect from the products that follow. But because it's crucial in the winter to keep your skin hydrated, avoid soaps, which tend to strip away skin's natural oils. Instead, use a gentle body wash or gel.

Scrub and smooth. Items from your pantry, like salt and ground almonds, can be used to exfoliate dead skin cells, which accumulate to cause dull, flaky skin (especially where skin is thicker, like the knees and elbows). To make sure your hands don't get roughed up, use a mesh sponge, loofah, or pouf.

Lubricate. Smooth on lotion immediately after showering or bathing, when your skin is still wet, to lock in moisture. You don't have to see dry skin to have it—so start treating yourself to luxurious body lotions before the temperature drops. If you've already gone from flaky to freeze-dried, try a cream instead of a lotion for extra moisture.

Combination Skin

Doctor on call: Jim Baral, M.D., a New York City dermatologist

Symptoms: Dry cheeks one day, oily T-zone the next; constant changes in complexion; drier in the winter (since most rooms are overheated and very dry)

Daily regime: Use a gentle cleanser twice daily, patting your skin dry (because rubbing can irritate it). Use a light moisturizer in the morning and a heavier one at night. Keep a humidifier in your room, especially in the winter, so your skin doesn't dry out. And always wear a sunscreen with a sun protection factor (SPF) of at least 15 under your makeup, because you're exposed to harmful rays even when it's cloudy.

Weekly regime: Take vitamins (C and E in particular) a few times a week to reduce the signs of aging and boost your skin's natural glow. Eat a healthy diet of grains, fruits, and vegetables and get aerobic exercise a few days each week to improve your skin tone.

Monthly regime: Ask a dermatologist or a skin care expert about using a low-concentration AHA peel once every few months to improve the texture of your skin.

46

Nine New Age-Erasing Uses for Lasers

L asers are no longer just the province of surgeons on the front lines of medicine. They've now been drafted for duty against a host of common (but pesky) cosmetic problems: dull teeth, wrinkles, even stretch marks.

You have to tread with caution, however. "Laser surgery is a completely unregulated specialty. There's nothing to stop someone—be it an M.D. or someone with a degree in veterinary medicine—from buying a laser and aiming it at patients," warns Tina Alster, M.D., director of the Washington Institute of Dermatologic Laser Surgery and assistant clinical professor of dermatology at Georgetown University School of Medicine in Washington, D.C.

Because of this, it pays to do your homework. Here some of the country's leading laser specialists tell about the most exciting new techniques, so you can get the job done right.

The Smile Sweetener

The old way: Hydrogen peroxide home bleaching kits, which involved sleeping in a night guard for weeks.

The new way: A more powerful hydrogen peroxide bleaching solution is applied to your teeth and zapped with a laser in your dentist's office. "The laser energy makes the bleaching solution work faster," explains Robert Reyto, D.D.S., a dentist in Beverly Hills, California. The procedure takes about an hour. (Cost: about $1,000.)

It's best for: People whose teeth are stained as a result of years of smoking and coffee drinking. But beware: If you keep up your old habits, the stains will return.

Is it risky or painful? Some women notice tooth sensitivity during the procedure. "There's also a small chance that a dentist will apply an over-heated laser to the tooth and cause damage to the pulp (the soft tissue that holds a tooth's nerve and blood vessels)," explains Kenneth Burrell, D.D.S., senior director of the American Dental Association Council on Scientific Affairs.

Recovery time: Virtually none. You may need to take ibuprofen (Motrin or Advil) for a few days if your teeth feel tingly.

The Skin Smoother

The old way: Wrinkle-fighting injections, such as collagen or Botox.

The new way: Dermatologists use two types of lasers—the CO_2 laser (for deep wrinkles) and the Erbium-YAG laser (for smaller lines, like crow's-feet)—to strip away top layers of skin, leaving the surface baby smooth. (Cost: $3,500 to $10,000 for full facial resurfacing.)

It's best for: Light-skinned women. "Those with naturally dark or olive skin tones tend to experience prolonged redness and are more likely to show pigment changes," says Dr. Alster. You can get the procedure done at the first sign of wrinkles, but most patients are in their forties or fifties. Be sure to inform your doctor if you've ever had a cold sore, herpes infection, or shingles, since the procedure can reactivate the viruses that cause these conditions.

Is it risky or painful? Darker-skinned women should approach any laser with caution but should have fewer problems with the Erbium-YAG. With the CO_2 laser, they're more likely to experience delayed hypopigmentation, in which the lasered skin appears lighter than the surrounding tissue, says Laurie Polis, M.D., director of New York City's Soho Skin and Laser Center.

Recovery time: Your skin will look badly sunburned but will probably feel fine; painkillers are rarely needed. If you've gone under the CO_2 laser, you'll need to hide for about a week. "Initially, your eyes may be swollen and your face may be bright red. It won't hurt; you'll just look scary," says Dr. Polis. The redness will fade within a couple of months. The Erbium-YAG laser is much kinder: You'll be pink for a week or two, but you should be back in business within 10 days.

The Acne Eraser

The old way: Acne scars required dermabrasion, an abrasive and painful surgical procedure that left you looking like the Swamp Thing for weeks.

The new way: Doctors beam the CO_2 laser at the affected area and vaporize the top layers of your skin. Studies presented at the American Academy of Dermatology showed that one to two treatments improved scarring by more than 80 percent. "The laser promotes collagen growth, which fills in many remaining scar depressions after the procedure," explains Dr. Polis. If you have deep scarring, you may need a second resurfacing treatment about 9 months later. (Cost: approximately $200 to $500 per scar.)

It's best for: Anyone with residual acne scars. If you still have active acne, however, your doctor will want to get it under control first, since zapping pimples can increase your chances of pigment changes or scars. If you've been on Accutane, most doctors recommend waiting at least a year after you've stopped treatment (the drug dries your skin, making it more prone to scarring).

The risk factor: As with wrinkle removal, dark-skinned women are more prone to pigment changes.

Recovery time: Expect some tenderness and soreness for up to a week afterward. That first week also brings intense swelling, oozing, and blistering (so you'll want to hide out); an intensely sunburned look will linger for 6 weeks to 2 months.

The Vein Vanisher

The old way: Sclerotherapy—in which the blood vessel was injected with a salt solution, causing it to collapse and disappear.

The new way: "It's more effective to use a laser, which incinerates red blood cells and destroys veins from the inside out," says Bruce Katz, M.D., director of cosmetic and laser surgery at Columbia University College of Physicians and Surgeons in New York City. You'll usually require only one to two sessions; each can take 15 to 20 minutes. (Cost: $400 to $800, depending on the number of veins to be removed.)

It's best for: Anyone with broken spider veins on the face and legs. Sclerotherapy is still more effective for larger leg veins.

Is it risky or painful? Each pulse stings on impact, like the snap of a rubber band against your skin. Most people don't need anesthetic, but if you're squeamish, you can ask your doctor for a topical numbing cream. There's a very slight chance (less than 5 percent) that you'll blister.

Recovery time: Older lasers left patients black and blue for up to 10 days. "Today we use the Versapulse laser, which leaves you just slightly swollen and red for a day, as if you were sunburned," explains Dr. Katz. You can easily cover

Find a Qualified Laser Specialist

With doctors advertising their procedures in magazines, on subway cars, and on TV, it's hard to determine who's a quality M.D. and who's a quack. "Since laser surgery is a new and rapidly evolving specialty, there are relatively few doctors with extensive experience in the field," cautions Tina Alster, M.D., director of the Washington Institute of Dermatologic Laser Surgery and assistant clinical professor of dermatology at Georgetown University School of Medicine in Washington, D.C. Here are some tips for finding a doctor who can make you look sensational.

Check credentials. Membership in the American Society of Laser Medicine and Surgery is a must. Ideally, your doctor should also be affiliated with a respected university medical school. Since there's no board certification procedure for laser surgery, look for doctors who have completed academic courses. Training courses offered by laser companies offer only minimal preparation.

Ask about the laser. Make sure the doctor owns it. To keep costs down, some doctors rent a specific laser for a day or two and schedule all their procedures for those days. "This is a dead giveaway that a doctor lacks clinical experience with that laser," says Bruce Katz, M.D., director of cosmetic and laser surgery at Columbia University College of Physicians and Surgeons in New York City. "The doctor should be doing the procedure enough so that it's more cost-effective to own the laser than to rent it."

Ask to see the goods. Other people's goods, that is. Cosmetic laser specialists should have before-and-after photos of patients who have gone under the laser. "Be sure you see pictures of the doctor's own patients—some doctors will try to pass off photos obtained from laser companies as their own," warns Dr. Alster.

Be wary of guarantees. "Be very, very suspicious of someone who promises 100 percent improvement," says Laurie Polis, M.D., director of New York City's Soho Skin and Laser Center. "We can never fully predict results, but we can give a predictable range of improvement."

HEALTH FLASH

it up with makeup. The lasered areas may also feel slightly sore and itchy for a day or two.

The Spot Assassin

The old way: Dermabrasion—a deep chemical peeling or burning with acids, which produced pain and scarring—or surgery.

The new way: Lasers can vaporize brown spots, brown and red birthmarks, sun spots, red blood vessels, and age spots with minimal pain and virtually no scar risk. "The laser targets the spots on the skin, destroying blood vessels, pigment molecules, and pigment cells on contact," explains Arielle N.B. Kauvar, M.D., assistant professor of dermatology at New York University Medical Center. For red blood vessels and brown spots, one treatment is usually all you'll need. Brown and red birthmarks may require multiple sessions. (Cost: $200 to $1,000, depending on the number and size of spots.)

It's best for: Basically anybody. "Treatment options may be limited in darker-complexioned women because many lasers cannot differentiate between brown spots and normal pigment," says Dr. Kauvar, but even they may want to look into it.

Is it risky or painful? You may feel mild discomfort. Ask your doctor to apply a topical anesthetic cream beforehand.

Recovery time: Some lasers cause temporary pink blotches, while others form red spots and scabs that can last up to 2 weeks. Apply sunscreen with a sun protection factor (SPF) of 15 to treated areas, since sun exposure might cause permanent darkening of skin.

The Stretch Mark Shrinker

The old way: Retin-A, which had limited effects.

The new way: "We now can use a new laser called a pulsed dye laser to improve stretch marks; it causes your skin to generate increased amounts of elastic fiber, forming a new pattern of fibers that look like normal skin," explains Dr. Kauvar. You may need up to four treatments before you notice a significant improvement. (Cost: $250 to $650, depending on the size, number, and location of stretch marks.)

It's best for: Fair-skinned women. "If you have dark skin, the wrinkled appearance of the area will improve, but the color will not return to normal; you'll still have some white stripes," warns Dr. Kauvar. Attention new moms: Recently acquired stretch marks seem to improve more than older marks, so consider getting your marks zapped a few months after delivery.

Is it risky or painful? Hardly. Most women do not even need topical anesthetic.

Recovery time: The lasered area will turn slightly red for several days. Within 8 weeks you should see a significant improvement in the wrinkled texture of the stretch marks.

The Tattoo Remover

The old way: Dermabrasion, which produced pain and scarring (and inspired you to hang on to that youthful mistake).

The new way: A laser sends hundreds of rapid-fire pulses to the tattooed skin. "Each laser blast shatters the pigmented cells, which are then swept away by your body's immune system," explains Melanie Grossman, M.D., assistant clinical professor of dermatology at Weill Medical College of Cornell University in New York City. Depending on the size of the tattoo, a treatment session can last anywhere from 5 minutes to an hour. You'll usually require one to five sessions. (Cost: $200 to $1,000, depending on the tattoo's size.)

It's best for: People with black, red, and green tattoos, which are easier to remove than aqua and fluorescent ones.

Is it risky or painful? No. Your doctor will numb the affected area with anesthesia, so you'll feel minimal pain. If you're dark-skinned, you may notice your skin's natural tone lightening because its own pigment (melanin) is destroyed along with the tattoo; when the series of laser treatments is over, all should return to normal.

Recovery time: Three to 10 days. Don't be surprised if you have deep bruising and even bleeding. "It does look worse before it looks better," warns Dr. Grossman. You'll have to avoid sunbathing throughout the course of the treatments, because a tan fills the skin with excess melanin, which makes it harder for the laser to reach underlying tattoo pigments.

The Laser Razor

The old way: Electrolysis, a painful procedure in which a fine needle zapped electricity into a hair follicle to disable it.

The new way: A laser is used to disable the hair follicles. Expect a minimum of three sessions spaced a month apart. After that, you'll have to come in a couple of times a year for maintenance treatments. Studies presented to the American Academy of Laser Surgeons show that lasers can reduce hair growth significantly—from 50 to 80 percent—but don't offer a truly permanent solution. (Cost: around $1,250 for a package of three treatments for the bikini area; a smaller area, like your upper lip, is around $500.)

It's best for: Women with pale skin and dark hair, because the laser can specifically target the dark pigment in the hair follicle. "It's not as effective for dark-skinned women, because the laser has trouble differentiating between the skin and the hair follicle," explains Debra Luftman, M.D., clinical instructor of dermatology at UCLA School of Medicine.

Is it risky or painful? Always make sure the laser procedure is supervised by an M.D. "Never go to a hair removal place where there are no medical personnel on site, because technicians don't have nearly as much training and are much more likely to cause burning or scarring," warns Dr. Luftman. You'll feel some slight tingling during the procedure, but it's not as painful as waxing or electrolysis.

The Faster Facial

The old way: An esthetician massaged special lotions and masks on your face to remove the top layer of dead skin.

The new way: "We use a mild laser like the Erbium-YAG to vaporize the skin's top layer, which exfoliates the skin and stimulates skin growth," explains New York City dermatologist Steven Victor, M.D. "It's like a chemical peel, only the results are faster." (Cost: $200 to $300 per session.)

It's best for: Anyone seeking a traditional facial.

Is it risky or painful? There's virtually no pain, but you do take a risk that it won't work: Some doctors claim it's a pricey way to get minimal improvement. "Doctors are giving the impression that these laser facials are the same as laser skin resurfacing," says Dr. Alster. "But if you can get the same results from a chemical peel at half the cost, it just seems like a gimmick."

The recovery: There's no downtime; you leave your doctor's office with a pink, glowing face, similar to the look of a traditional facial.

Secrets of Sexy, Carefree Hair

H ere's hot news for healthy hair. A new group of conditioners (called heat-activated or heat-defense conditioners) claims to improve the condition of hair while you style with hair dryers and curling irons. According to cosmetic chemist and ingredients specialist David Steinberg, who is also president of Steinberg and Associates Consulting Firm in Plainsboro, New Jersey, heat helps these products penetrate better to condition and strengthen hair. In truth, their ingredients have been in conditioners for decades. But these new formulations allow them to be sprayed on and left in. This makes the protection stick around for the styling phase.

Although many people love the shine and softness conditioners produce, some women find that their hair becomes too soft to style. If you have fine hair, experiment with how much conditioner is needed for benefits without sacrificing body.

Here are more foolproof ways to keep your hair looking its best.

Easy-to-Make Homemade Conditioners

Kitchen-based treatments for shiny, healthy-looking hair are cheap, easy, and fun to make. These come from Leslie Baumann, M.D., director of cosmetic dermatology at the University of Miami. Find the right one for you and try it after shampooing (leave in for 5 minutes). Repeat every few weeks or as needed.

Lemon juice or vinegar removes buildup on dirty, oily, or frequently conditioned hair. To use, pour 1 cup through your hair, wait, then rinse and use your regular conditioner. Since overuse can strip natural oils, which will damage hair, do not use every day or on treated hair. Left on, lemon juice or vinegar will lighten hair in sun.

Beer adds body and shine to fine, limp hair, but it's good for all hair types. To use, pour one full can of beer onto your hair, wait, and then rinse. Condition if your hair is dry. Note that the beer must be fresh, not flat, and that the benefit washes out in the next shampoo. There's no harm in using it every day.

Egg yolks add shine to dry, dull hair and condition slightly. To use, massage two yolks into your hair, wait, then rinse. No additional conditioner is needed. Note that the benefits wash out in your next shampoo, and the yolks may make fine hair a bit oily.

Mayonnaise adds shine to very dry, dull hair and deep-moisturizes it. To use, massage 2 tablespoons into your hair. Wait, then rinse. No additional conditioner is needed. This is best for very dry hair only since it could leave normal hair looking greasy for days.

Revitalize Abused Hair

If your hair is showing signs of abuse from sun, chlorine, or salt water, you can undo an entire summer's worth of damage in less time than it takes to try on a bathing suit. Try these four easy tips.

Cut it out. A good cut is the only solution for split ends. With fewer sticking out, hair looks sleeker. (No product repairs split ends; so-called end-healers may glue ends together, but the effect is temporary.)

Go deep. To replace lost moisture, apply a deep conditioner—or make your own by adding 3 ounces each of softened butter and heavy cream to 3 ounces of regular conditioner. Cover with a warm, damp towel. (For shorter hair, store what's left over in the fridge for up to 10 days.) Wait 15 minutes, then shampoo and rinse thoroughly. Repeat the process several times a week at first, then every couple of weeks for maintenance.

Clean. Frequent shampooing doesn't dry out hair, but it removes dulling oil. In fact, with a remoisturizing shampoo, you can add moisture.

Gloss. Apply a protective serum before drying. These products contain silicone (or methicone or dimethicone) to add shine, protect against heat styling, and prevent frizz. One drawback: They can be difficult to wash out, leaving hair feeling brittle, says Philip Kingsley, of the Philip Kingsley Trichological Centre in New York City and author of *Hair: An Owner's Handbook*. Choose

Is Your Hair Dye Safe?

Hair dyes that slowly darken gray contain lead. Should you be worried?

Yes, says Howard Mielke, Ph.D., associate professor of environmental toxicology at Xavier University of Louisiana College of Pharmacy in New Orleans. Progressive hair dyes do pose a potential health threat. Unlike most dyes (permanent, semipermanent, and temporary), progressives usually contain lead acetate. They darken gray hair by forming a lead salt that binds with hair proteins. According to a study headed by Dr. Mielke, these dyes contain 2,300 to 6,000 micrograms of lead per gram. That's up to 10 times the limit allowed in house paint (a lead source that remains a major hazard).

Dr. Mielke's research team found that from 26 to 80 micrograms of lead remained on each hand after using the product, even after washing with soap and water. In fact, lead was found on everything subsequently touched—combs, hair dryers, and even phones.

While washing your hands or wearing gloves may help, it doesn't eliminate all risk. "The dye is clear and does not stain, so you can't know where it has dripped," says Dr. Mielke. That means you could contaminate clean hands and, if you touch your mouth, ingest the dye unknowingly.

Even passing a hand through dry, dyed hair picked up 286 micrograms of lead. Some studies say that children 6 years old and younger can safely ingest only 6 micrograms of lead per day; adults, 30 to 60 micrograms.

"The more we study lead, the more we find harmful effects at lower doses than previously suspected," adds Herbert Needleman, M.D., lead poisoning expert and professor of pediatrics at the University of Pittsburgh School of Medicine.

The FDA, currently reviewing the evidence, maintains that lead acetate–containing hair dye products can be used safely by carefully following label directions. Still, Dr. Mielke has stopped such tests on humans. "If it's too hazardous for my lab, I say it's too hazardous for your bathroom."

Quick tip: Check the label. If lead acetate is not listed, then your hair dye is okay.

HEALTH FLASH

creamy products, or serums, which have less silicone and more conditioners than "shine" sprays. Look for formulas that contain water.

Choose Hair Color Carefully

Whether it's a major switch or just a color lift, the key to getting what you want from your hair color is having a vision. Here are four steps you should take before making any change. (Note: It's a myth that you should always "go lighter with age." Going too blond, if it doesn't balance with your skin tone, can make you look older.)

Choose colors. Take pictures of colors you like to your colorist so she can tell you what's realistic for you.

Play with wigs. This is the best way to prepare yourself for a color change. A wig in your former color may surprise you if you're significantly gray now. Skin tone changes over time, and you've likely become accustomed to the flattering lightness around your face, explains colorist Anthony Rocanello, from Manhattan's chic Salon A.K.S.

Schedule a consultation. Good colorists welcome a preappointment visit (at no charge) to ensure that your new color will be harmonious with your skin tone and to decide which product is best for you.

Get patched. The initial consultation is also a good time to do a skin patch test for allergies to the hair colorants.

Safeguard Your Color

By depositing temporary pigment molecules onto hair, color-refresher shampoos can return depth and brilliance to fading color and tone down brassiness. But used incorrectly, they can damage hair by overdrying it, says Rocanello, maker of customized enhancing shampoos at Salon A.K.S. Here are four of his recommendations.

Wait 2 weeks. You should wait 2 weeks to use an enhancing shampoo after coloring your hair. Use it only when your color starts fading.

Count to 60. Massage it in like regular shampoo, then wait 1 minute before rinsing; waiting longer may dry hair.

Space it out. Wait another week or so before you reapply color-enhancing shampoo. Everyday use can actually change the shade of colored hair when the goal is to enhance it. (From the time you have one salon touch-up to the next, you should use it no more than three times.)

Baby your hair. To counteract the drying effect, finish with a moisturizing, detangling treatment.

Rescue a Disaster Perm

If you've ever been "fuzzed" with a bad perm, you know the sudden longing for straighter hair again. There is hope, though, says Susan MacCoy, hair artist and master colorist at the Elizabeth Adam Salon and Day Spa in Chicago. She offers this advice for dealing with a bad perm.

Tame it. Before styling, comb some leave-in conditioner through your hair to weigh down the curl. Then, several times a week, use a deep-moisturizing product for about 10 minutes. This restores curl and softens dry, chemically treated ends so hair is easier to style.

Trim it. A perm is tightest at the ends, so a trim can help loosen your look. If you want to walk out of the salon perm-free, however, you're talking about a buzz cut. Generally, you need at least 3 inches of virgin hair to successfully cut out a perm, and that can take 6 months to grow.

How to Survive That Awkward "Growing-Out" Stage

How is it that stars bounce from the Oscars to movie premieres sporting new hairstyles, when we never saw them grow out the ones they had before? Easy: by knowing the little tricks that make in-limbo locks look like the latest in haute coiffure. Here's how you can do the same.

Bangs

The wait: Ten months to a year before bangs reach your shoulders.

The strategy: If you have angled bangs (shorter in the center), wait until you can pull them below your lashes, then get a trim (1/8 inch). Ask your stylist to angle the sides into your hair and not touch the center. With straight-across bangs, just let them grow, trimming only if you get split ends.

Styling tips: Part bangs in the middle, pull back two sections (twisting them once or twice if desired), and secure with mini-barrettes 2 to 3 inches behind your hairline. To hide longer bangs, hold them to one side with a bobby pin and let the bulk of your hair hang over. You can also work bangs into your hair as you blow-dry, pulling them straight back with a round brush.

Shag Cut

The wait: It'll take a year to grow all your layers out to shoulder-length.

The strategy: Let your hair grow until the longest parts in the back touch your shoulders, then have it blunt-cut at the shoulders once every 3 to 4 months.

Warning: If the back is cut any shorter than shoulder-length, the effect might be more matronly than you had in mind.

Styling tips: You can twist a chunk off your face and hold it with a mini-barrette (or you can do this in two or three places). Not in an accessory

Loosen it. If your hair's elasticity hasn't been damaged (if it's not brittle or breaking), you could be a candidate for the following solutions.

❖ Have your hairstylist hide an old perm with a new one by giving your hair a no-visible-curl body perm, using super-large rollers and a low-pH, no-test-curl perm. (These perms have a built-in "stopwatch.")

❖ Turn unruly curls into waves by combing a nonalkaline, delicate waving lotion through your hair for 10 to 12 minutes. Rinse well and comb neutralizer through your hair. Leave on for 5 minutes. You can also undo your perm completely by using a mild formula straightener designed for naturally curly hair. Apply it gently with a wide-tooth comb. Since the hair is already chemically processed, it takes only 2 to 5 minutes to do the job.

Let an expert fix it. If your "disaster" perm was the result of a do-it-yourselfer effort, turn to a salon for solutions.

mood? Work in a nickel-size blob of styling cream and shake hair as you blow-dry. When it's half-dry, add more cream; the layers will look tousled, not droopy.

Layers

The wait: It depends on how short the shorter sections of your hair are, but probably 5 to 7 months to hit your shoulders.

The strategy: Option one: Take the plunge and have all your hair cut to the length of one of the shortest chunks. Option two: Have shorter sections angled into the body of your hair. Option three: Have long sections trimmed every three months as you let your shorter sections play catch-up.

Styling tips: An accordion-style headband can be placed anywhere on the head to scoop up errant strands. You can also gather hair into a high ponytail, chignon, or braids, letting shorter pieces hang out.

Angled Bob

The wait: If your shorter-in-back bob is shaved at the neck, it'll take about 10 months to get to shoulder-length; if not, 6 to 8 months.

The strategy: Lucky you—you can let this style grow out without a lot of maintenance. Since the basic shape remains, you'll still appear to have a real haircut. When the shorter part in the back reaches your collar, head to the salon and ask your stylist to start blunting the angled sides.

Styling tips: Stick in a barrette, pinning a section so that it falls toward your face. (A variation: Take a ½- to 1-inch section of hair at the front, twist it three times, and fasten it with a barrette at eye level.) Also, try slipping in a jeweled bobby pin or two anywhere along your hairline.

New Rx for Hair Loss

When Propecia hit pharmacy shelves in 1999, it brought to the balding population a huge promise—and plenty of questions. Here are the facts about the first and only hair-regrowth pill.

Does it work? Propecia (the generic name is finasteride) shows great promise for men. In clinical trials of 1,879 balding men, more than 80 percent of those taking Propecia experienced no hair loss during the 2-year period— even better, 66 percent showed hair regrowth. In some men, results were seen in 3 months, but it may take longer.

Unlike minoxidil (Rogaine), whose mechanism has never been understood, Propecia's success makes sense, says Ivan Cohen, M.D., assistant professor of dermatology at Yale University School of Medicine. Propecia works by blocking the conversion of testosterone into DHT (dihydrotes-tosterone), a hormone that shrinks hair follicles—a key factor in male hair loss.

By reducing DHT levels 60 percent, Propecia can stop hair loss and in many cases trigger hair growth, explains Keith Kaufman, M.D., of Merck Research Laboratories, Propecia's makers in Rahway, New Jersey.

Can women use it? Not if they're of childbearing age, says Dr. Kaufman. Propecia can cause birth defects when taken during pregnancy. In fact, pregnant women are discouraged from handling broken pills because the drug may be absorbed through the skin.

As for other women, the jury's still out. Propecia works by acting on hormones such as testosterone. Since women tend to have lower levels of this hormone, the results may be different.

For women whose hair loss is due to high testosterone or low estrogen after menopause, there's a chance Propecia may work, says Dr. Cohen. A more definitive answer is on the way: Results of a study on postmenopausal women with thinning hair are expected soon.

Are there side effects? The only reported side effects are decreased libido and impotence, but they're extremely rare. Only 1.8 percent of the men taking Propecia experienced decreased libido, while 1.3 percent of those taking the placebo (dummy pill) did. Of the men taking Propecia, 1.3 percent experienced impotence; 0.7 percent of those taking the placebo did. Better news: When they stopped taking the drug, these side effects went away. And in roughly 60 percent of the men who continued taking it, side effects disappeared.

How much does it cost? A month's prescription costs $45 to $49, or about $550 a year. It's a lifelong investment. If you stop taking it, you'll start losing your hair again.

Other options for female hair loss. Rogaine, the topical over-the-counter treatment, has been successful for some women. So have estrogen supplements. "Sometimes women on hormone replacement therapy find that their hair loss slows down," explains Dr. Cohen.

Credits

"Why We Need Gender-Specific Medicine" on page 4 and the box on page 5 are adapted from "Diagnosing the Gender Gap," an article by Sue Landry that originally appeared in the St. Petersburg (Florida) *Times*. Copyright © 1997 by St. Petersburg *Times*. Reprinted with permission.

"Don't Take Your Medicine like a Man" on page 10 is an article by Robert Lipsyte that originally appeared in *The New York Times*. Copyright © 1999 by the New York Times Co. Reprinted by permission.

"Six Medical Tests You Really Need" on page 24 is adapted from "Which Tests Do You Need?" an article by Karen Cicero that originally appeared in *American Health for Women*. Copyright © 1998 by *American Health for Women*. Reprinted with permission.

"Amazing Facts about the Pill" on page 47 and the boxes on pages 48, 50, and 52–53 are adapted from "The Power of the Pill," an article by Jennifer Cadoff that originally appeared in *New Woman*. Copyright © 1998 by Jennifer Cadoff. Reprinted with permission.

"Survival Tactics for the Female Heart" on page 89 is adapted from "Heart of a Woman," an article by Marion Asnes that originally appeared in *New Woman*. Copyright © 1998 by Marion Asnes. Reprinted with permission.

"Power over Pain: The Female Advantage" on page 127 and the box on page 128 are adapted from "The Painful Truth," an article by Alice Lesch Kelly that originally appeared in the April 1999 issue of *Walking* magazine. Copyright © 1999 by Alice Lesch Kelly. Reprinted with permission.

"What Men Eat: A Woman's Guide" on page 138 is adapted from "He Eats, She Eats," an article by Dana Silbiger that originally appeared in *Marie Claire*. Copyright © 1998 by *Marie Claire*. Reprinted with permission.

"Is Your Sex Life Good Enough?" on page 239 is adapted from an article of the same name by Dalma Heyn that originally appeared in *New Woman*. Copyright © 1999 by Dalma Heyn. Reprinted with permission of the author.

"How Do You Define Infidelity?" on page 244 is adapted from an article of the same name by Dalma Heyn that originally appeared in *New Woman*. Copyright © 1999 by Dalma Heyn. Reprinted with permission of the author.

Part of "Viagra One Year Later: Promise or Problem?" on page 249 is adapted from "Viagra For Women?," an article by Stacey Colino that originally appeared in *New Woman*. Copyright © 1999 by Stacey Colino. Reprinted with permission of the author.

"Discover the Power of Forgiveness" on page 272 and the boxes on pages 273 and 275 are adapted from an article of the same name by Ellen Michaud that originally appeared in *Prevention*. Copyright © 1999 by Ellen Michaud. Reprinted with permission.

"Vitamins That Beautify Your Skin" on page 282 is adapted from "Beautiful Skin from A to E," an article by Rosie Mestel that originally appeared in *Health*. Reprinted with permission from HEALTH, © 1998.

"How to Survive That Awkward 'Growing-Out' Stage" on pages 308–309 are adapted from the article "Growing-Out Pains" by Brooke Eastburn that originally appeared in *Mademoiselle*. Courtesy *Mademoiselle*. Copyright © 1998 by Condé Nast Publications, Inc.

Index

<u>Underscored</u> page references indicate boxed text. *Italicized* references indicate illustrations.

A

ABCD checklist, for skin cancer, 80
Abdominals, exercise for, *219–22*
Acceptance, of your body, weight loss
    and, 195–97
Accessories, for appearing slimmer, <u>196</u>
ACE inhibitors, to lower blood pressure,
    111
Acne
    oral contraceptives for, <u>52</u>
    scars due to, treatment of, 299
Activity. *See also* Exercise(s)
    at work, for weight loss, 212–13
Acupuncture, 55–56
Adultery. *See* Infidelity
Aerobic boxing, for weight loss, 192
African-American women, heart disease
    among, 95
Age spots, laser treatment of, 301
Air conditioners, to prevent allergic reac-
    tions, 123
ALA, 167
Alcohol
    gender difference in handling of, 9
    interaction with oral contraceptives, 39
    limiting intake of, 69, 216
    menopausal symptoms and, 69
Aleve, for breast pain, <u>37</u>

Allergies, 121–26
    avoiding reactions and, 122–24
    colds vs., <u>124</u>
    menstrual cycle and, <u>125</u>
    during pregnancy, <u>125</u>
    relief of, <u>122</u>, 125–26
Aloe vera, 285
Alpha-linolenic acid (ALA), 167
Alpha-lipoic acid, to prevent heart
    disease, <u>91</u>
Alpha-tocopherol, 285
Alpha-tocopherol acetate, 285
Alternative therapies, 55–62. *See also*
    Herbal products
    acceptance of, <u>57</u>
    acupuncture, 55–56
    ayurveda, 56–58
    chiropractic, 58
    homeopathy, 58–60
    insurance coverage for, <u>59</u>
    naturopathy, 60
    osteopathy, 60
    for pain, <u>128</u>
    traditional Chinese medicine, 61–62
American Board of Medical Specialties, 36
Amitriptyline, for interstitial cystitis, 20
Anemia, 287
Angelica sinensis, for menopausal symp-
    toms, <u>69</u>

Anger
acknowledging, 277
forgiveness and (*see* Forgiveness)
hanging on to, 273–74
identifying sources of, 273
ways to handle, 274–76
Angina, 92
medications for, as contraindication to
Viagra, 251
Angiography, 96
Angioplasty, gender differences in effectiveness of, 16
Anthocyanins, in blueberries, 147
Antibiotics
interaction with oral contraceptives,
39, 53
side effects of, 9
Anticoagulants, interaction with herbs, 181
Anticonvulsants, interaction with oral
contraceptives, 39
Antidepressants
interactions of
with herbs, 179
with oral contraceptives, 39
for interstitial cystitis, 20
side effects of, 9
Anti-estrogens. *See* Raloxifene; Tamoxifen
Antihistamines, for allergies, 125–26
Antioxidants
antiaging action of, 291
to prevent heart disease, 91
in whole grains, 153
Antiseizure medications, interaction with
oral contraceptives, 39, 53
Anxiety, perimenopausal, 70–71
Appetite
exercise vs. skipping meals and, 187
indulging, weight loss and, 187–88
Arms, exercise for, *221*
Arrhythmias
drugs triggering, 9
PSVT, 22–23
Arthritis, devil's claw for, 180
Artichoke, health benefits of, 180
Aspirin
interaction with herbs, 181
to prevent colon cancer, 111
Association of State Medical Board Executive Directors' Web site, 36
Astelin, 126
Asthma, 125
Atherosclerosis
smoking and, 101
stroke and, 92, 99, 101

Attitude. *See also* Outlook
toward body, weight loss and, 195
toward pain, 128
for staying in shape after menopause,
226–27
AutoPap, 26
Avon's Anew Retinol Recovery Complex
PM Treatment, 283
Ayurveda, 56–58

B

Back pain
chiropractic for, 58
osteoporosis and, 115
Backward walking, 210
Bacterial vaginosis (BV), 33–34
Bad breath, home remedies for, 172–73
Bad days, avoiding, 258–64
deep breathing for, 260
drinking water and, 262
end-of-day oasis for, 264
"friend breaks" for, 263–64
improving sleep for, 259–60, 259
making work meaningful and, 263
outlook and, 261
pacing yourself and, 262–63
saying no and, 261
slowing morning pace for, 260–61
writing down feelings for, 262
Baikal skullcap, melatonin in, 182
Basil tea, 175
Bathroom, conflict in morning over
using, 234–35
Beans, health benefits of, 145
Beauty, 279–310
cosmetic surgery and, 280–81
diet and, 286–92
hair and, 304–5, 306, 307–10, 308–9
home remedies for, 288–89
lasers for, 297–99, 300, 301–3
men's products to use for, 283
skin care and, 293–96
vitamins for, 282–85
Beer, as hair conditioner, 305
Berries, health benefits of, 146, 147
Beta-carotene, to prevent cancer, 86
Beta-hydroxy beta-methylbutyrate
(HMB), caution regarding, 194
Biking, for weight loss, 214–15
Biotin, for hair and nails, 284
Birth control, emergency, 50

Birth control pills. *See* Oral
    contraceptives
Birthmarks, laser treatment of, 301
Black cohosh, for menopausal symptoms,
    68
Bleaching teeth, 297–98
Blood cholesterol, lowering, <u>94</u>, <u>108</u>
Blood clots
    anti-estrogen drugs and, 75
    oral contraceptives and, 51, 67
    stroke and, 99
Blood pressure, lowering, 99–100, <u>99</u>,
    103–4
Blood pressure checks, 30, <u>90</u>
Blood vessels, laser treatment of, 301
Blueberries, health benefits of, <u>147</u>
Body, respecting, weight loss and, 195–97
Body composition, measuring, 189
Body fat. *See also* Weight loss
    burning, <u>188</u>
    visceral, gender difference in, <u>184</u>
Body weight. *See also* Weight loss
    gain of, oral contraceptives and, <u>53</u>
    low, osteoporosis related to, 114–15
Bone-density scans, 28–29, <u>28</u>, <u>116</u>
Borg Scale for Rate of Perceived Exertion
    (RPE), <u>204</u>
Borrelia burgdorferi. *See* Lyme disease
Boxing, aerobic, for weight loss, 192
Bras, <u>37</u>, <u>196</u>
Breast cancer
    gene mutations causing, <u>106</u>
    hormone-replacement therapy and, <u>45</u>
    mammography to detect, 26–28, <u>27</u>, <u>28</u>
    medications for treating, 73–77, <u>74</u>, <u>76</u>
    omega-3 fatty acids for, 168
    oral contraceptives and, 54, 67
    prevention of, <u>106</u>, 111
        diet and, 153, <u>159</u>
        medications for, 73–77, <u>74</u>, <u>76</u>
        natural products for, 83–84, 85, <u>86</u>
    risk factors for, <u>76</u>
    risk of, calculating, <u>74</u>
    screening for, 26–28, <u>27</u>
Breast Cancer Risk Assessment Tool, <u>74</u>
Breast pain, <u>37</u>
    around period, stopping, <u>37</u>
    oral contraceptives and, <u>52</u>
Breathing, deep, <u>260</u>
    for menopausal symptoms, <u>68</u>
Breathing techniques, for pain manage-
    ment, <u>128</u>
Brindall berry, caution regarding, 193
Broccoli, health benefits of, 146

Brown spots, laser treatment of, 301
Bruising, vitamin C for, 287
Buttocks, squeezing, 209
BV, 33–34
Bypass surgery, gender differences in
    effectiveness of, 16

C

Caffeine, avoiding
    for menopausal symptoms, 69
    to stop breast pain, <u>37</u>
Calcium, osteoporosis and, <u>114</u>, <u>117</u>,
    119–20
Calcium D-glucarate, to prevent cancer,
    83–85
Calming down, 236
Cancer
    of breast (*see* Breast cancer)
    cervical, Pap test to detect, 24–26, <u>25</u>,
        34–35
    of colon (*see* Colon cancer)
    dietary prevention of, 157–61
    endometrial, 67, 75
    gastric, prevention of, 83
    gender differences in, 17
    inherited mutations causing, 105–6,
        107–9, <u>110</u>, 111
    of liver, prevention of, 85
    of lung (*see* Lung cancer)
    medications to prevent, 73–77, <u>74</u>, <u>76</u>,
        <u>106</u>, 111
    natural products to prevent, 81–88, <u>82</u>,
        <u>84</u>, <u>86</u>
    oral contraceptives and risk of, 54
    ovarian (*see* Ovarian cancer)
    prostate, 82, <u>84</u>
    rectal, prevention of, <u>84</u>
    of skin (*see* Skin cancer)
    surgery to prevent, <u>106</u>, 111
Candy, low-fat, 164
Canola oil, 168
CAP, 34
Carbohydrates, 152–56
    labeling and, <u>155</u>
    refined, 152–53
    requirements for, 154–55
    whole grains and, 153–54, 155–56,
        <u>155</u>, <u>156</u>
Cardamom, for bad breath, 172–73
Cardiac arrhythmias. *See* Arrhythmias
Caregiving role, gender and, 11, 12–13

Diet *(continued)*
    gender differences in, 138–44
    giving up single favorite food and,
        211–12
    high-protein, 189
    for interstitial cystitis, 19
    low-fat snacks for, 162–65
    for staying in shape after menopause,
        224–25
    to lower blood pressure, 100–101
    to lower risk of genetic diseases, 108–9
Dietary fats
    avoiding trans fats, 169
    beneficial, 166–71, 166, 167, 171
    monounsaturated, 169–70
    omega-3 *(see* Omega-3 fatty acids)
    omega-6, 170–71
    saturated, reducing to prevent genetic
        disease, 109
Diet Center Worldwide, 191
Diet programs, 190–91
Digital mammography, 26–27
Dilantin, interaction with oral contracep-
    tives, 53
Dimethyl sulfoxide (DMSO), for inter-
    stitial cystitis, 20
Distraction, for coping with anger, 277
Diuretics, interaction with herbs, 181
Diuril, interaction with herbs, 181
DMSO, for interstitial cystitis, 20
Docosahexaenoic acid (DHA), 167
Dogs, walking, weight loss and, 212
Dong quai, for menopausal symptoms, 69
Douching, 34
Dressing. *See* Clothing
Dry skin, 293
Dual energy x-ray absorptiometry
    (DEXA), 28–29, 116

E

Egg yolks, as hair conditioner, 305
Eicosapentaenoic acid (EPA), 167
Elavil
    interactions with
        herbs, 179
        oral contraceptives, 39
    side effect of, 9
Electrocardiogram, 23, 95
Electrolysis, lasers for, 302–3
Electrophysiologic study and ablation, for
    PSVT, 23

Elliptical exercise machines, 189
Elmiron, for interstitial cystitis, 19
Emergency contraception, 50
Emotional symptoms, perimenopausal,
    70–71
Emotional well-being, infidelity and,
    245–46
Empathy, 278
Endometrial cancer
    oral contraceptives and, 67
    tamoxifen and, 75
Endometriosis, treatment of, osteoporosis
    and, 118
Endovaginal ultrasound, 25
Energy, sagging, home remedy for,
    178
Enright Forgiveness Inventory, 275
Envy, of other couples, 240–41
EPA, 167
Ephedra
    caution regarding, 193–94
    interaction with drugs, 179
Erectile dysfunction
    heart disease related to, 96
    herbal remedies for, 253
    Viagra and *(see* Viagra)
Erythromycin, side effect of, 9
Estée Lauder's Diminish, 283
Estratab, 45
Estrogen
    menopausal decline in, 230
    in oral contraceptives, 49, 51
    osteoporosis and, in men, 119
    produced by fat cells, 227
    protection against heart disease by, 6
Ethinyl estradiol, 49
Evening primrose oil, for breast pain,
    37
Evista. *See* Raloxifene
Exercise(s)
    appetite and, 187
    charting workouts and, 217
    Kegel, 38–39, 242
    for lowering blood pressure, 99, 100
    making time for, 216
    for managing cravings, 269
    for menopausal symptoms, 69, 70, 72
    after menopause, 225–26, 225
    Pilates, 218, *219–22*
    to prevent genetic diseases, 109
    to prevent osteoporosis, 114
    to prevent stroke, 99, 100, 103
    triceps hinge pushups, 216–17
    for weight loss, 199–200

Exercise machines
elliptical, 189
requiring no effort, 191
spot reducers, 191–92
varying use of, 215
Exercise stress testing, 95
Extramarital sex. *See* Infidelity
Eyes, diet and, 291

F

Facials, lasers for, 303
Failures
accepting, 271
at smoking cessation, 266
Fasting plasma glucose test, 28, 29–30
Fat cells, estrogen produced by, 227
Fatigue, home remedy for, 178
Feedback, building willpower and, 271
Fenfluramine, 193
Fertility, oral contraceptives and, 49
Feverfew
interaction with anticoagulants, 181
melatonin in, 182
Fiber
need for, 149
sources of, 150, 153, 154
Fibroids, removal of, 35
Fidelity, achieving, 247–48
Finasteride, 310
Fish
health benefits of, 146
omega-3 fatty acids from, 167, 167, 168
Flaxseed
for menopausal symptoms, 70
omega-3 fatty acids in, 168
Flu, home remedy for, 177
Food(s). *See also* Diet; *specific foods*
healing, 145–48
Food cravings
curbing, 137
gender differences in, 136–37
giving in to, 270–71
managing, 269
Forgetfulness, perimenopausal, 71–72
Forgiveness, 272–78
alternatives to, 274–76
benefits of, 273–74
healing provided by, 276
identifying sources of anger and, 273
inventory of, 275

Fractures, osteoporosis and, 115, 116
Frozen treats, low-fat, 165
Fruits
for beauty, 291
health benefits of, 157–61
as low-fat snacks, 165

G

Garlic
for allergies, 124
for heart disease, 94
interaction with anticoagulants, 181
to prevent cancer, 82, 82–83
Gas, home remedy for, 174
Gastric cancer, prevention of, 83
Gender differences
alcohol tolerance and, 9
cosmetic surgery use and, 280–81
diet and, 138–44
disease effects and, 16–17
drug metabolism and, 9
effects of medical treatments and, 16, 17
food cravings and, 136–37
gender-based medicine and, 6–7
heart disease and, 6, 16–17, 91–92, 93
improving health of both sexes and, 7
language and, 233
longevity and, 64–65
pain experience and, 127–29
physiological, 5
sex after 50 and, 230–31
smoking consequences and, 9
stress and, 256–57
stroke and, 102
unrecognized, 5–6
vulnerability to sexual disease and, 8
weight loss and, 184–85
women's health centers and, 2–3
Genetic counselors, 108
Genetic diseases, 105–11
cancer as, 105–6, 107–9, 110, 111
heart disease as, 105, 106–9, 108, 110
lowering risk of, 107–9
German chamomile tea, 175
Germander, caution regarding, 177
Gillette Mach3 razor, 283
Ginger
for headache, 175
for indigestion, 174
interaction with anticoagulants, 181
for motion sickness, 176–77

interaction with drugs, 179, 181–82
for menopausal symptoms, <u>43</u>, 68, 69, <u>69</u>, 71, 72
to prevent cancer, 81–88
to regulate periods, <u>39</u>
Herbal teas
brewing, <u>175</u>
as home remedies, 173, 174–77, 178
Herpes virus infections, lemon balm for, <u>180</u>
High blood pressure. *See* Blood pressure, lowering; Blood pressure checks
High-density lipoprotein (HDL) level, 32, <u>90</u>, <u>94</u>
High-protein diets, 189
High-tech scales, 189
Hill walking, 208, <u>225</u>
Hismanal, side effect of, 9
HMB, caution regarding, 194
HMG-CoA reductase inhibitors, to reduce blood cholesterol, <u>94</u>, 103, <u>108</u>, 111
HMOs, alternative therapies and, <u>59</u>
Holter monitor, 23
Homeopathy, 58–60
Home remedies, 172–78
herbs to avoid in, <u>177</u>
for skin, <u>288–89</u>
Hormone(s). *See specific hormones*
Hormone-replacement therapy (HRT)
Estratab for, <u>45</u>
natural progesterone for, 43–46
SERMs as alternative to, 77
synthetic progesterone for, 42–43
Horse chestnut, health benefits of, <u>180</u>
Horseradish, for congestion, 177
Hot flashes, 68–69, <u>68</u>, <u>69</u>
Household tasks, conflict over, 235
HRT. *See* Hormone-replacement therapy
Hunger. *See* Appetite
Hydrodistention and cystoscopy, 19
HydroDiuril, interaction with herbs, 181
Hydroxycitric acid (HCA), 193
Hydroxyzine, for interstitial cystitis, 19
Hypercholesterolemia, familial, <u>108</u>
Hyperthyroidism, 20, 21–22, 117
Hypnosis, for allergies, 126
Hypothyroidism, 20–21, 22, 117–18
Hysterectomy, menopause after, <u>71</u>
Hysteroscopic resection, for fibroid removal, <u>35</u>

I

Ibuprofen, for breast pain, <u>37</u>
IC, 18, 19–20
ICA, 19, 20
IgE, interception of, to prevent allergic reactions, <u>122</u>
Impotence
heart disease related to, <u>96</u>
herbal remedies for, <u>253</u>
Viagra and (*see* Viagra)
Impulses
giving in to, 270–71
managing, 268
Indigestion, home remedy for, 174
Infections
herpes virus, lemon balm for, <u>180</u>
urinary tract, <u>250</u>
vaginal, 33–34
Infidelity, 244–48
achieving fidelity and, 247–48
emotional well-being vs. sex and, 245–46
statistics on, <u>246</u>
In-laws, agreeing on visits from, 236–37
Inositol hexaphosphate, to prevent cancer, 85–87
Insect bites and stings, home remedy for, 176
Insurance coverage, for alternative medicine, <u>59</u>
Interstitial cystitis (IC), 18, 19–20
Interstitial Cystitis Association (ICA), 19, 20
Inventions, improving women's lives, <u>264</u>
Iron, 287
Irritability, perimenopausal, 70–71

J

Jealousy, of other couples, 240–41
Jenny Craig, <u>190–91</u>

K

Kava, for menopausal symptoms, 71
Kegel exercises, 38–39, <u>242</u>
Kidney disease, assessing risk for, 30
Kidney stones, osteoporosis related to, 112–13, 119–20

L

Lactose intolerance, osteoporosis and, 120
Language, gender differences in, _233_
Lasers, 297–303
    for acne scars, 299
    for age spots, birthmarks, brown spots,
        red blood vessels, and sun spots, 301
    facials using, 303
    finding specialists for, _300_
    hair removal using, 302–3
    for spider veins, 299, 301
    for stretch marks, 301–2
    tattoo removal using, 302
    to smooth skin, 298
    to whiten teeth, 297–98
LDL level, 32, _90_, _94_
Lead, hair-color products containing, _306_
Lemon balm, health benefits of, _180_
Lemon balm tea, _175_
Lemon juice, as hair conditioner, 305
Libido, oral contraceptives and, _52_
Librium, interaction with herbs, 182
Lignans, in whole grains, 153
Linoleic acid
    for hair, 291–92
    for scaliness, 290
Lip(s), diet and, 290
Lipoic acid, to prevent heart disease, _91_
Lipoprotein (a) level, _90_
Liposuction, _280_
Liver cancer, prevention of, 85
Liver disease
    assessing risk for, 30
    oral contraceptives and, 67
Longevity, gender difference in, _64–65_
L'Oréal Futur-E, 285
Love, long-term, _241_
    passion vs., 241–42
Love letters, _237_
Low body weight, osteoporosis related to,
    114–15
Low-density lipoprotein (LDL) level, 32,
    _90_, _94_
Ludiomil, side effect of, 9
Lung cancer
    gender differences in, 17
    natural products to prevent, _84_, 85
    smoking and, 9
Lyerix vaccine, 132–33
Lyme disease, 131–33
    prevention of, 132, _132_
    risk of developing, 131
    vaccine for, 132–33

M

Ma huang, interaction with drugs, 179
Mammograms, 26–28, _27_, _28_
MAO inhibitors, interaction with herbs,
    179
Marplan, interaction with herbs, 179
Masque, homemade, _288_
Mayonnaise, as hair conditioner, 305
Medical tests
    needed by women, 24–32, _25_, _27_
    results of, _28_
Medications. _See also specific types of med-_
    ications and specific drugs
    gender difference in metabolism of, 9
    for heart disease, as contraindication to
        Viagra, 251
    interaction with herbs, 179, 181–82
    for pain management, 130
    side effects of, 9
    to lower blood pressure, 100
    to prevent cancer, 73–77, _74_, _76_, _106_, 111
    to treat breast cancer, 73–77, _74_, _76_
    for weight loss, 193
Medicine. _See_ Gynecologists; Health
    care; Physicians
Melanomas. _See_ Skin cancer
Melatonin, in herbs, _182_
Memory, perimenopausal problems of,
    71–72
Men. _See also_ Gender differences
    equation of good health with sexual
        function by, 13–14
    impotence in
        heart disease related to, _96_
        herbal remedies for, _253_
        Viagra and (_see_ Viagra)
    persuading to get checkups, _31_
Menopause
    allergies and, _125_
    heart disease related to, 93
    after hysterectomy, _71_
    physical changes with, _230_
    sexual changes with, _230–31_
    staying in shape after, 223–27, _225_, _227_
    symptoms of, 66–72
        exercise for, _70_
        flaxseed for, _70_
        home remedy for, 176
        hormone-replacement therapy for (_see_
        Hormone-replacement therapy)
        natural progesterone for, 43–46, _43_
        oral contraceptives for, 49
        relaxation for, _70_

Menstrual cycle. *See also* Periods
   allergies and, <u>125</u>
   disturbances of
      oral contraceptives for, 49
      vitex for, <u>39</u>
Mental decline, blueberries to reverse,
   <u>147</u>
Meridia, 193
Migraines, oral contraceptives for, <u>53</u>
Milk, health benefits of, 146, 148
Ministrokes, <u>100</u>
Minoxidil, 310
Mircette, 51
Misdiagnosis, 18–24
   of interstitial cystitis, 18, 19–20
   preventing, <u>21</u>
   of PSVT, 22–23
   of thyroid problems, 20–22
Moisturizers
   homemade, <u>288</u>
   with vitamin E, 285
Mold, allergic reactions to, 123–24
Moles, melanoma potential of, 80
Monascus purpureus, for heart disease, <u>94</u>
Monoamine oxidase (MAO) inhibitors,
      interaction with herbs, 179
Monounsaturated fat, 169–70
Mornings
   conflict over using bathroom in,
      234–35
   slowing pace of, 260–61
Motion sickness, home remedy for,
      176–77
Motivation, to lose weight, gender differ-
      ence in, 185
Motrin, for breast pain, <u>37</u>
Mucilage, herbs containing, drug absorp-
      tion and, 182

N

Nails
   diet and, 290
   vitamin B for, 284
Naproxen sodium, for breast pain, <u>37</u>
Nardil, interaction with herbs, 179
NasalCrom, 126
Natural progesterone, 43–46
   in pill form, 44–45
   as vaginal gel, 45–46
   wild yam cream, <u>43</u>
Naturetin, interaction with herbs, 181
Naturopathy, 60

Nausea
   home remedies for, 174
   oral contraceptives and, <u>52</u>
NEAT, <u>188</u>
Night cream, homemade, <u>288–89</u>
Night sweats, 69
   home remedy for, 176
Nitroglycerin, as contraindication to
      Viagra, 251
Nolvadex. *See* Tamoxifen
Nonexercise activity thermogenesis
      (NEAT), <u>188</u>
Nonsteroidal anti-inflammatory drugs,
      for breast pain, <u>37</u>
Norgestimate, 51
Nursing, oral contraceptives and, <u>53</u>
Nut(s), health benefits of, 148
Nutri/System, <u>191</u>
Nutrition. *See* Diet; *specific foods*

O

Oily skin, 294–95
Olive oil, 169
Omega-6 fatty acids, 170–71
Omega-3 fatty acids, 166–69
   in capsule form, <u>166</u>
   health benefits of, 167–68
   sources of, 168–69
Onions
   for allergies, 124
   health benefits of, 148
Oral contraceptives, 47–54
   benefits of, 48–49, <u>48</u>
   for breast pain, <u>37</u>
   cancer risk associated with, 54
   components of, 49, 51
   contraindications to, 52–54, 67
   correct use of, 35–36
   drug interaction of, 9, 39, 53–54
   for menopausal symptoms, 67, 68, 70
   safety of, 47–48
   "scheduling" periods using, 36, 38
   skipped doses and, <u>50</u>
   skipped periods and, <u>50</u>
   smoking and, 95
   to prevent ovarian cancer, <u>106</u>
   types of, <u>52–53</u>
Oranges, health benefits of, 148
Orgasm, after menopause, <u>230</u>
Orly Nails for Males, <u>283</u>
Osteopathy, 60
Osteopenia, 112

Prometrium, 44–45
    for menopausal symptoms, 67, 68
Propecia, 310
Prophylactic surgery, to prevent cancer,
    106, 111
Prostate cancer
    growth of, garlic suppression of, 82
    natural products to prevent, 84
Protein, for brittle nails, 290
Provera, 67
Pro-vitamin B$_5$, 284
Prozac, 193
PSVT, 22–23
Puffiness, in face, 287

Q

Qi, 55
Quadriceps, exercise for, *220*
Quercetin, for allergies, 124

R

Racewalking, 208–9
Radiologists, finding, 27
Rain, allergies and, 122–23
Raloxifene, 73, 74–75
    deciding whether to take, 76
    for menopausal symptoms, 77
    side effects of, 75
    tamoxifen compared with, 75
RazorGuard, 283
Reconciliation, 278
Rectal cancer, prevention of, 84
Red pepper, for colds, 178
Red yeast, for heart disease, 94
Regulating periods, 36, 38, 39
Relationships
    conflict management and, 232–38,
        233, 236, 237
    Viagra's effect on, 253
Relaxation, for menopausal symptoms,
        69, 70, 71–72
Renova, 282–83
Requests, refusing, 261
Resveratrol, to prevent cancer, 87–88
Retin-A, 282–83
Retinol, 283
Rewards, building willpower and, 271
Rhinitis, allergic, seasonal, 121
Riboflavin, for lips, 290

Rifampin, interaction with oral contra-
        ceptives, 53
Rock climbing, for weight loss, 192
Rogaine, 310
Rosemary tea, 175
    for headache, 174–75
RPE, 204
Rules, willpower and, 266, 267

S

Sage
    for colds, 178
    for night sweats, 176
St. John's wort
    with ephedra, 193–94
    interaction with drugs, 179
    melatonin in, 182
Saluron, interaction with herbs, 181
Sassafras, caution regarding, 177
Saturated fats, reducing, to prevent
        genetic disease, 109
Scales
    high-tech, 189
    putting aside, 226–27
Scaliness, diet and, 290
Sea buckthorn, health benefits of, 180
Seasonal allergic rhinitis, 121
Sedatives, interaction with herbs, 182
Seldane, side effect of, 9
Selective estrogen receptor modulators
        (SERMs). *See* Raloxifene; Tamox-
        ifen
Selenium, to prevent cancer, 84
Self-efficacy, weight loss and, 197–99
Sensitive skin, 295
SERMs. *See* Raloxifene; Tamoxifen
Serotonin, calming effect of, 136–37
Servings, definition of, 158–59
Sesame seeds, for toothache, 173
Sexual activity, 239–43
    couple envy and, 240–41
    "good-enough" sex and, 243
    infidelity and (*see* Infidelity)
    "normal," 239–40
    passion vs. long-term love and,
        241–42
    realism about, 242–43
    surgical tightening of vagina and, 242
    urinary tract infections due to, 250
    Viagra and (*see* Viagra)
Sexual desire, communicating about,
        237–38

Sexual function
    after 50, gender differences in, <u>230–31</u>
    men's equation of good health with,
      13–14
Sexually transmitted diseases (STDs),
    gender difference in vulnerability
    to, 8
Shampooing, 305, 307
Sibutramine, 193
Sildenafil citrate. *See* Viagra
Silent treatment, <u>276</u>
Silica, for hair, 292
Sinus pain or pressure, home remedy for,
    175–76
Skin
    antiaging balm for, <u>180</u>
    combination, 296
    dry, 293
    oily, 294–95
    protecting from exposure, <u>294</u>
    sensitive, 295
    winter care for, <u>295</u>
Skin cancer, 78–80
    checking yourself for, 79
    diagnosis of, 78–79
    finding dermatologists and, 79–80
    warning signs of, <u>79</u>
Skipping meals, appetite and, <u>187</u>
Sleep
    annoying habits of partner and, <u>236</u>
    disturbance of, perimenopausal, 69–70,
      <u>70</u>
    improving, 259–60, <u>259</u>
Smoking
    cessation of, 17
      failures at, 266
      to prevent stroke, 101–2
    gender difference in consequences of, 9
    genetic diseases and, 109
    oral contraceptives and, 52, 95
    osteoporosis and, 118–19
Snack(s), low-fat, 162–65
Snack mixes, low-fat, 163
Social breaks, at work, 262–64
Sodium, limiting intake of, 287
Sore throat, home remedies for, 178
Soy, for menopausal symptoms, 67
Spearmint tea, for sagging energy, 178
Spices, as home remedies, 172–78
Spider veins, 287
    laser treatment of, 299, 301
Spinal fractures, osteoporosis and, 115
Spinning, <u>214</u>
Spot reducers, 191–92

Spotting, oral contraceptives for, <u>52</u>
Stairclimbing, 208
Statins, to reduce blood cholesterol, <u>94</u>,
    103, <u>108</u>, 111
STDs, gender difference in vulnerability
    to, 8
Steroids
    for allergies, 126
    osteoporosis and, 116–17
Stinging nettle, for allergies, 124
Strength training
    after menopause, 226
    to lower blood pressure, <u>99</u>
    for weight loss, 192
Stress
    food cravings and, 136
    gender differences in, <u>256–57</u>
    management
      kava for, 71
      tips for, <u>257</u>
      to prevent heart disease, 96
    negative feelings and, 273
Stretch marks, laser treatment of, 301–2
Stroke, 97–104
    assessing risk for, 30
    blood pressure control and, 99–100, <u>99</u>,
      103–4
    diabetes and, 101
    gender differences in, 102
    ministrokes and, <u>100</u>
    oral contraceptives and, 67
    prevention of
      cholesterol lowering for, 103
      exercise for, <u>99</u>, 103
      weight loss for, 100–101, 102–3
    risk of, 98
    smoking cessation and, 101–2
    suicide related to, <u>104</u>
    types of, 98
    warning signs of, 97, <u>98</u>
Suicide, stroke related to, <u>104</u>
Sunlight
    vitamin C to protect against, 284
    vitamin E to protect against, 285
Sun spots, laser treatment of, 301
Support, emotional, for pain, <u>128</u>
Surgery
    cosmetic, gender differences in use of,
      <u>280–81</u>
    for fibroid removal, <u>35</u>
    heart, gender differences in effective-
      ness of, 16
    prophylactic, to prevent cancer,
      <u>106</u>, 111

T

Tamoxifen, 73, 74–75
  deciding whether to take, 76
  for menopausal symptoms, 77
  need for, determining, 74
  raloxifene compared with, 75
  side effects of, 75
  to prevent breast cancer, 106, 111
Tapes
  to improve sleep, 259
  for walking or jogging, 213
Tattoos, laser removal of, 302
TCM, 61–62
Teeth
  bleaching, 297–98
  diet and, 291
Temperature
  cold compresses for breast pain and, 37
  to improve sleep, 259
Tend Skin, 283
T4 test, 22
Theophylline, interaction with oral contraceptives, 39
Thiazide diuretics, interaction with herbs, 181
Thyme, for
  colds, 178
  cough, 178
  sinus pain or pressure, 175–76
Thyroid problems, 20–22
Thyroxine, osteoporosis and, 117–18
TIAs, 100
Tick removal, 132
Tiredness, perimenopausal, 72
Tobacco. See Smoking
Tofranil, interactions with
  herbs, 179
  oral contraceptives, 39
Tomatoes, health benefits of, 148
Toothache, home remedies for, 173
Touch sense, after menopause, 231
Trace minerals
  for graying hair, 292
  in whole grains, 154, 154
Traditional Chinese medicine (TCM), 61–62
Tranquilizers, interaction with oral contraceptives, 39
Trans fats, avoiding, 169
Transient ischemic attacks (TIAs), 100
Transition time, after work, 232–34
Tricyclic antidepressants. See Antidepressants

Triggers, willpower and, 268
Triglyceride level, 32
  lowering, 94
TSH test, 21–22
Turmeric, for heartburn, 173

U

Ultrasound, endovaginal, 25
Urinary tract infections (UTIs), in women, 250
Urinary tract problems, home remedy for, 178
Urtica dioica, for allergies, 124
UTIs, in women, 250

V

Vaccine, for Lyme disease, 132–33
Vagina
  infections of, 33–34
  surgery to tighten, 242
Valerian, for menopausal symptoms, 69
Valium, interactions with
  herbs, 182
  oral contraceptives, 39
Varicose veins, horse chestnut for, 180
Vegetables, 149–51. See also specific vegetables
  for beauty, 291
  color of, 151
  cooking, 150, 151
  health benefits of, 157–61, 159
  with most fiber, 150
  phytochemicals in, 149
  serving, 151
Very low density lipoprotein (VLDL) level, 32
Viagra, 249–53
  effect on relationships, 253
  how to use, 251
  men benefiting from, 249, 251
  side effects of, 251–52
  for women, 252–53
Vinegar, as hair conditioner, 305
Visualization, for menopausal symptoms, 67–68, 68
Vitamin A
  for eyes, 291
  for wrinkles, 282–83, 286–87
Vitamin B-complex, for hair and nails, 284

Vitamin B₂, for lips, 290
Vitamin C
    for bruising, 287
    for skin, 284–85
Vitamin D, to prevent osteoporosis, 114
Vitamin E, for
    breast pain, 37
    menopausal symptoms, 68
    skin, 285
Vitex, to regulate periods, 39
VLDL level, 32
Vomiting, home remedies for, 174

W

Walking, 201–10
    backward, 210
    get-started plan for, 201–3
    maximum calorie-burn plan for, 206–7
    plateau-busting plan for, 203–5
    posture for, 209
    tapes for, 213
    toning circuit plan for, 208–10
    for weight loss, 191–92
Walnut oil, omega-3 fatty acids in, 168
Warfarin, interaction with herbs, 181
Water, drinking
    for lips, 290
    for scaliness, 290
    to avoid spider veins, 287
    to boost mood and motivation, 262
    to prevent urinary tract infections, 250
Weekends, planning, 234
Weight gain, oral contraceptives and, 53
Weight loss, 183–227
    diet programs for, 190–91
    exercise for, 191–92
    feel-good plan for, 195–200
    gadgets for, 189–91
    gender differences in, 184–85
    herbs to avoid in, 193–94
    medications for, 193
    after menopause, 223–27, 225, 227
    methods for, 187–89, 188
    Pilates exercises for, 218, 219–22
    real-life stories about, 211–17
    Spinning for, 214
    success stories of, 197, 198, 200
    supplements to avoid in, 194
    to lower blood pressure, 100–101, 102–3
    walking for, 201–10, 203, 204, 209
Weight Watchers International, 190

Whitening teeth, 297–98
Whole grains
    color of bread and, 155
    increasing intake of, 155–56, 156
    nutrients in, 153–54, 154
Wild yam cream, 43
Willpower, 265–71
    accepting failures and, 271
    fulfillment vs. denial and, 266
    handling impulses and, 268
    keeping diaries and, 270
    positive attitude for, 268–70
    realistic goals and, 266–67
    reasonable approach to, 270–71
    rules and, 266, 267
    treats and, 271
    understanding your triggers and, 268
Women's health centers, 2–3
Work
    making meaningful, 263
    social breaks during, 262–64
    transition time after, need for, 232–34
Workaholics, 235–36
Wrinkles
    laser treatment of, 298
    masque for, 288
    vitamin A for, 282–83, 286–87
Writing
    communicate feelings by, 237
    to build willpower, 270
    to gain control of feelings, 262

X

Xanax, interaction with oral contraceptives, 9, 39

Y

Yin and yang, 61
Yohimbe
    caution regarding, 177
    for impotence, 253

Z

Zinc
    for scaliness, 290
    for thinning hair, 292